Aesthetic, Regenerative and Cosmetic Gynecology

Aesthetic, Regenerative and Cosmetic Gynecology

Editor

Preeti Jindal MD DNB MRCOG (UK) FICOG
IVF, Recurrent Miscarriage, and High Risk Pregnancy Expert
Robotic Surgeon and Cosmetic Gynecology Expert
Director–The Touch Clinic (Advanced Cosmetic, Gynae, IVF and High Risk Pregnancy Centre), Mohali
Senior Consultant Gynecologist, Fortis Hospital, Mohali, Punjab, India
Past President, Mohali Obstetrics and Gynaecology Society
General Secretary, Indian Society of Aesthetic and Reconstructive Gynecology (INSARG)

JP medical publishers
London • New Delhi

Published by Jaypee Brothers Medical Publishers,
4838/24 Ansari Road, New Delhi, India

Tel: +91 (011) 43574357 Fax: +91 (011)43574390

Email: info@jpmedpub.com, jaypee@jaypeebrothers.com
Web: www.jpmedpub.com, www.jaypeebrothers.com

JPM is the imprint of Jaypee Brothers Medical Publishers.

ISBN: 978-1-78779-184-8

British Library Cataloguing in Publication Data
A catalogue record for this book is available from the British Library

Library of Congress Cataloging in Publication Data
A catalog record for this book is available from the Library of Congress

Publishing Manager: Nikita Chauhan

Editorial Assistant: Ashwani Kumar

Cover Design: Seema Dogra

Dedicated to

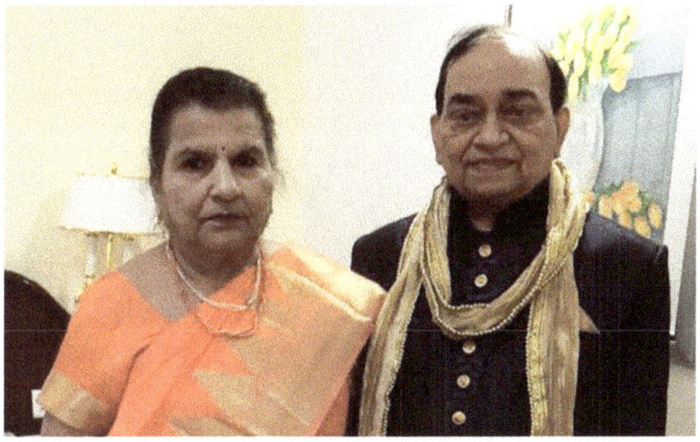

My dear parents (Dr Urmila Agarwal and Dr JP Agarwal) who inspired me always and made me capable of accomplishing the task of writing this beautiful book.

Contributors

Akashdeep Singh MBBS MD
Consultant
Department of Anesthesia and Intensive Care
Fortis Hospital
Mohali, Punjab, India

Amel Ibrahim Almaeeni
MD MSc JBOG FACS
Consultant Obstetrics and Gynecology
Fujairah Hospital
UAE

Ami Shukla
MD FRCOG Diploma in Medical Law Diploma in Medical Ultrasound
Consultant Urogynecologist
Northampton General Hospital
Northampton, UK

Anita Shyam MBBS MD (Psychiatrist)
Consultant
Psychiatrist and Sexual Medicine Expert
Private Practice
Founding Member and CMO, Qurex
New Delhi, India

AV Raveendran MBBS MD
Former Assistant Professor
Department of Medicine
Government Medical College
Kozhikode, Kerala, India

Avinash Desousa
MBBS DPM MPhil PhD (PsyD)
Consultant Psychiatrist and Founder Trustee
Desousa Foundation
Mumbai, Maharashtra, India

Ayman El Attar MD FAAFP AAACS
President, American Board of Cosmetic Gynecology
Founder and President, International Aesthetic Gynecology Congress
Dubai and Asia Pacific
President, American Aesthetic Association
New Jersey, USA

Bela Shah Jain
MBBS MS DNB FMAS ART and Reproductive Medicine (Germany)
Consultant Obstetrician and Gynecologist
Fertility Specialist and Cosmetic Gynecologist
Department of Gynecology
Asian Institute of Infertility Management
Indore, Madhya Pradesh, India

Cherry Malhi MBBS MS (Obs and Gyne)
Consultant
Department of Gynecology
The Touch Clinic
Mohali, Punjab, India

Doaa Saleh MD (Obs and Gynae)
Professor
Cosmetic Surgeon
Al-Azhar University
Cairo, Egypt

Gauri Sachdeva
BDS MDS (Oral and Maxillofacial Surgery)
Consultant
Department of Oral and Maxillofacial Surgery
Genesis Institute of Dental Sciences and Research
Ferozepur, Punjab, India

Gurkiran Kaur MBBS MD (Obs and Gyne)
Fellow
Department of Reproductive Medicine
Rainbow IVF
Agra, Uttar Pradesh, India

Indranil Banerjee
MBBS MS MRCOG Postgraduate Diploma in Leadership and Management PGCert in Medical Education
Northampton General Hospital
Northampton, UK

Jaideep Malhotra
MBBS MD FICOG FICMCH FRCOG FICS FMAS AFIAP
Managing Director
Rainbow IVF
Agra, Uttar Pradesh, India

James Dsilva MS MCh DNB
Managing Director
Dr James D'Silva Cosmetic Clinic
Mumbai, Maharashtra, India

Jasmeet Kaur MBBS MD
Consultant
Department of Anesthesia and Intensive Care
Fortis Hospital
Mohali, Punjab, India

Kanika Singh
MBBS DNB (Obs and Gyne) Fellowship Cosmetic Plastic Gynecology (USA) FICCG Laser Training, LAHA Europe
Founder Director
Woman with Vibrance
Meerut, Uttar Pradesh, India

Keshav Malhotra
MBBS MCE ESHRE Certified
Director
Embryology ART-Rainbow IVF
Agra, Uttar Pradesh, India
Chair, SIG ASPIRE

Manvi Verma
MBBS MD DNB (Obs and Gyne) MCh (Cosmetic Gynecology)
Assistant Professor
Department of Gynecology
MGM Medical College and Hospital
Navi Mumbai, Maharashtra, India

Mohan Thomas MD FACS FAACS
Managing Director
The Cosmetic Surgery Institute
Pune, Maharashtra, India

Molina Patel MD Dip RM FCG
Aesthetic Gynecologist and Fertility Expert
Akanksha Hospital and Research Institute
Anand, Gujarat, India

Muneer Ahmad Para
MBBS MS (General Surgery)
Para Consultant Vascular and Endovascular Surgery
Fortis Hospital
Mohali, Punjab, India

Muskaan Mittal MBBS MD
Consultant Gynecologist
The Touch Clinic
Mohali, Punjab, India

Narendra Malhotra
MBBS MD FICOG FICMCH FRCOG FICS FMAS AFIAP
Managing Director
Global Rainbow Healthcare
Ujala Cygnus Rainbow Hospital
Agra, Uttar Pradesh, India

Naval Milind Shah
MBBS MS ART and Reproductive Medicine (Germany)
Consultant Obstetrician and Gynecologist, Fertility Specialist and Cosmetic Gynecologist
Department of Gynecology
Naval Maternity and Nursing Home
Mumbai, Maharashtra, India

Nayana Patel MBBS, MD
Director
Akanksha Hospital and Research Institute
Anand, Gujarat, India

Neharika Malhotra
MBBS MD (Obs and Gyne) FICMCH FMAS
Infertility Consultant
Department of Gynecology
Rainbow IVF
Agra, Uttar Pradesh, India

Niket Patel MBBS MD
Director
Akanksha Hospital and Research Institute
Anand, Gujarat, India

Nutan Upadhaya
MBBS MD FICOG (Obstetrician, Gynaecologist and Infertility Specialist)
Director, Santosh Hospital
Saharanpur, Uttar Pradesh, India

Piyush Chaudhary MS (Surgery)
Consultant Vascular and Endovascular Surgery
Fortis Hospital
Mohali, Punjab, India

Poonam Mishra
MBBS DNB (Obs and Gyne) FAM FCG
Director
Manas Hospital and Manas Gynae Cosmetology and Laser Center
Lucknow, Uttar Pradesh, India

Pragati Tandon MBBS MD
Resident Doctor
The Touch Clinic
Mohali, Punjab, India

Preeti Jindal MD DNB MRCOG (UK) FICOG
IVF, Recurrent Miscarriage, and High Risk Pregnancy Expert
Robotic Surgeon and Cosmetic Gynecology Expert
Director
The Touch Clinic (Advanced Cosmetic, Gynae, IVF and High Risk Pregnancy Centre), Mohali
Senior Consultant Gynecologist, Fortis Hospital, Mohali, Punjab, India
Past President, Mohali Obstetrics and Gynaecology Society
General Secretary, Indian Society of Aesthetic and Reconstructive Gynecology (INSARG)

Prerna Keshan
MBBS DGO FICOG FICMCH FIAOG
Owner
Horizon Maternity and Fertility Clinic
Tinsukia, Assam, India

Rachana Kaveri
MBBS DNB (Obs and Gyne) MNAMS FMIS FRM
Fellowship in Cosmetic Gynaecology (UAE)
Obstetrician, Gynecologist, Laparoscopic Surgeon and Cosmetic Gynecologist
Dr Rachana Kaveri Clinic
Mumbai, Maharashtra, India

Ragini Agrawal MS FICOG FICMCH
Director
AA Dermascience Complete Clinic for WOMEN-HER Life Matters
Gurugram, Haryana, India

Ravul Jindal MBBS DNB FRCS FIVS FAMS
Director
Department of Vascular Surgery
Fortis Hospital
Mohali, Punjab, India

Renu Datta BDS MDS
Professor and Head
Department of Dental Care
Sri Sukhmani Dental College and Hospital
Derabassi, Punjab, India

Ridhi Kalra MBBS MD (Obs and Gyne)
Consultant
Department of Gynecology
The Touch Clinic
Mohali, Punjab, India

Salwa Bahkali MD (Obs and Gyne)
Accredited Faculty Member
North American Academy of Aesthetic Medicine the Institute of Laser and Aesthetic Medicine in India, and the Institute of Aesthetic Medicine
Cairo, Egypt

Shabjot Dhillon MBBS MD
Consultant Vascular and Endovascular Surgery
Fortis Hospital
Mohali, Punjab, India

Shahad Saeed Alzaabi MD ABOG
Consultant Obstetrics and Gynecology
Fujairah Hospital
UAE

Shivani Jain
BDS MDS (Oral and Maxillofacial Surgery)
Consultant
Department of Dental Care
Genesis Institute of Dental Sciences and Research
Ferozepur, Punjab, India

Shradha Goel MBBS MS DNB FICOG
Head and Director
PCOSmetic Gyne Clinic
Jaipur, Rajasthan, India

Sumitu Sahdev MBBS MD
Consultant Embryologist and IVF Specialist
Department of Gynecology
The Touch Clinic
Mohali, Punjab, India

Tanuja Uchil MBBS MD (Obs and Gyne)
Consultant
Department of Gynecology
Oma Fertility Hospital
Mumbai, Maharashtra, India

Taranvir Kaur MBBS MS (Surgery)
Consultant Vascular and Endovascular Surgery
Fortis Hospital
Mohali, Punjab, India

Tarika Datta Pursuing BDS
Internship, Bhojia Dental College and Hospital
Baddi, Himachal Pradesh, India

Vivek Malhotra MBBS MD (Dermatology)
Consultant
Department of Dermatologist
Beau Visage Skin Clinic
Chandigarh, India

Preface

The field aesthetic gynecology has emerged as a transformative and empowering branch of medicine, dedicated to enhancing the quality of life for women through a combination of medical and aesthetic interventions. This book is an endeavor to provide a comprehensive resource for practitioners, offering insights into the latest techniques, technologies, and trends that shape this evolving specialty.

Aesthetic gynecology encompasses a broad spectrum of procedures, from vaginal rejuvenation and labiaplasty to nonsurgical treatments aimed at improving both form and function. These interventions are not merely cosmetic: they address significant physical and psychological concerns, contributing to the overall well-being and confidence of women.

My goal in this book is to bridge the gap between traditional gynecology and the growing demand for aesthetic solutions. I have brought together leading experts to share their knowledge, experience, and best practices. Each chapter delves into specific procedures, patient selection criteria, surgical techniques, and post-operative care, ensuring that practitioners are well equipped to deliver safe and effective treatments.

Moreover, there is utmost importance of a holistic approach to patient care. Aesthetic gynecology requires sensitivity, empathy, and a deep understanding of the unique needs and desires of each patient. This book emphasizes the ethical considerations and patient-centered approach essential for building trust and achieving optimal outcomes.

As aesthetic gynecology continues to advance, I hope this book will serve as a valuable guide and reference for both seasoned practitioners and those new to the field. By fostering a deeper understanding and appreciation of this specialty, the aim is to contribute to the ongoing developments and enhancement of women's health and well-being.

I am sincerely grateful to the contributors who have shared their expertise and to the readers who are committed to expanding their knowledge and skills in aesthetic gynecology. Together, we can make a meaningful difference in the lives of women worldwide. Striding towards the goal of optimizing women health.

Preeti Jindal

Acknowledgments

"A reader lives a thousand lives before he dies.....The man who never reads lives only one."

–George RR Martin

Hopefully this book is good enough to ignite the desire in every doctor of adapting aesthetic and regenerative gynecology in their practice. Big thanks to all chapter contributors to take out time and share their knowledge through the chapters they have written.

I imbibed this field in my clinical practice, all thanks to my dear husband **Dr Ravul Jindal** (Director–Vascular Surgery Department, Fortis Hospital, Mohali), whose futuristic vision made me believe in importance of this field and introduced me to lasers.

I would like to thank my loving sons (Adit and Kush) for always supporting me and bearing with my long working hours.

A big appreciation to my clinic—"The Touch", staff for being with me always and helping me not only in handling patients but also in my academic pursuits. Thanks to my Senior Manager, Aanchal, without whose support and coordination compiling this book was not possible. Thanks Dr Ridhi, Dr Sumitu, Dr Pragati and my sisters Jyoti Agarwal and Arti Agarwal for being there always for me.

A big gratitude to Shri Jitendar P Vij (Group Chairman), Mr Ankit Vij (Managing Director), Ms Chetna Malhotra (Senior Director—Professional Publishing, Marketing, and Business Development), and their team Priyansh Saxena (Development Editor), Ruby Sharma (Business Manager) of M/s Jaypee Brothers Medical Publishers (P) Ltd, New Delhi, India for believing in me and giving me this opportunity.

Thanks to my mentors—Dr Shakuntala Chhabra and Dr Kala Vashishtha.

Thank to Dr Ragini Agrawal and Dr Narendra Malhotra who have always been my guiding light and supported me in all my endeavors.

Last but not the least thanks to **all my patients** from whom I learn so much every day.

Contents

CHAPTER 1

Aesthetic and Regenerative Gynecology: An Overview

Preeti Jindal

INTRODUCTION

Human being has always desired to remain young and immortal. With increase in longevity of life, the role of aesthetic and regenerative gynecology has come in limelight. It is known by various names—cosmetic gynecology, aesthetic gynecology, and regenerative gynecology. Women are becoming aware of their own body and want to achieve their dream bodies. Also because of free access to internet studies have shown that women are watching more porn-related sites than men **(Fig. 1)**.[1] It is important to know that aesthetic gynecology covers not only cosmetic aspects of women but also has antiaging regenerative role.

Who all are practicing it?

It is multidisciplinary branch practiced by gynecologists, dermatologists, urogynecologists, urologists, vascular surgeons, plastic surgeons, and few aspects are covered by dentists and cosmetologists.

HISTORY

Cosmetic is a Greek word derived from "kosmetikos" meaning to adorn. Since time immemorial world has tried to improve beauty. Sushruta, an Indian physician is considered as world's first plastic surgeon practicing labiaplasty as early as 600 BC **(Fig. 2)**.[2] In Renaissance period, Pierre Donis described labiaplasty. Jeffcote published vulval reconstructive surgeries in detail in 1957. Recently in 2008, Jamie McCartney, an artist in England made an art work depicting different vulval shapes of women reviving new interest in this field.

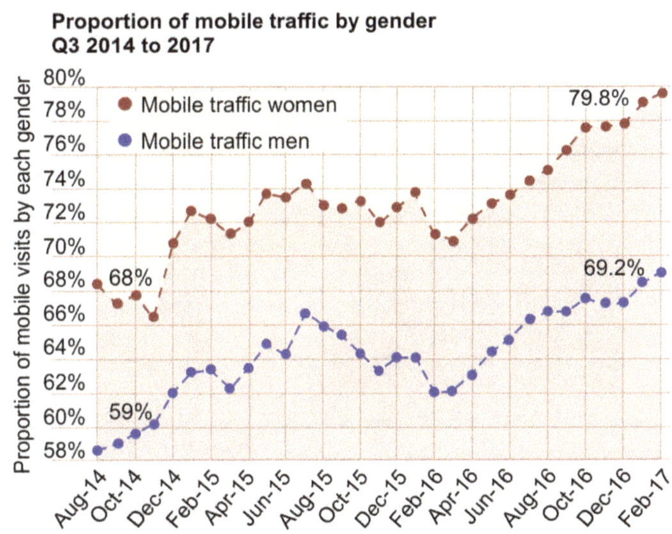

Fig. 1: Proportion of mobile visits by each gender.

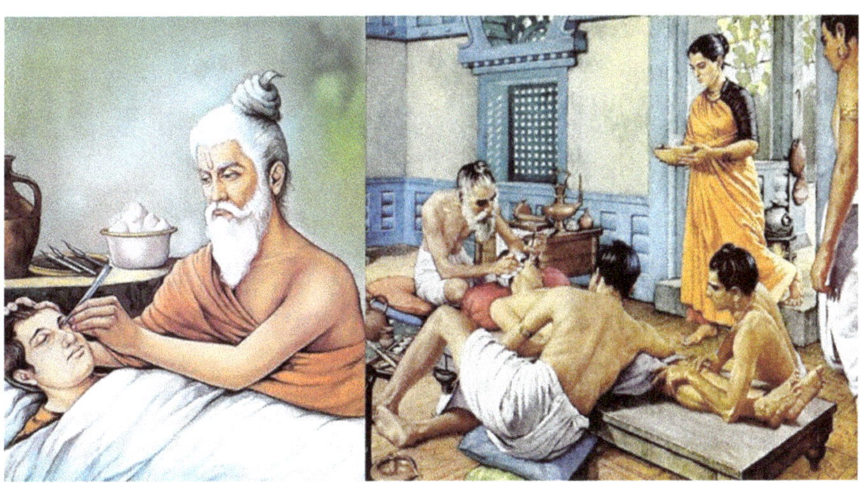

Fig. 2: Sushruta, performing plastic surgeon practicing labiaplasty.

PROCEDURES COVERED IN THIS BRANCH

There are surgical and nonsurgical procedures.

Surgical procedures mainly include mons pubis reduction or augmentation, labia majora augmentation or reduction, labiaplasty, cliteroplasty, clitoral hood reduction, hymenoplasty, colpoperineorrhaphy, posterior commissure procedures, vaginoplasty, vaginal reconstruction, vaginal septum resections, and transgender plastic procedures.

Nonsurgical procedures encompass doing all above procedures with energy-based devices, high-intensity focused ultrasound (HIFU), platelet-rich plasma, threads, fillers, botulinum, fat grafting, stem cells, mesotherapies, carboxytherapy, plasma pens, and ever evolving newer modalities **(Fig. 3)**.

Few unique cosmetic procedures are female orgasmic enhancing procedures like G shot, clitoral injections, hair removals, stretch mark treatments, breast procedures, body celluloid treatment, vulval bleaching, noninvasive treatments of genitourinary syndrome, stress urinary incontinence, vulvodynia, vaginismus, recurrent vaginal infections, and vaginal rejuvenations. **Table 1** shows cosmetic genital procedures.[3,4]

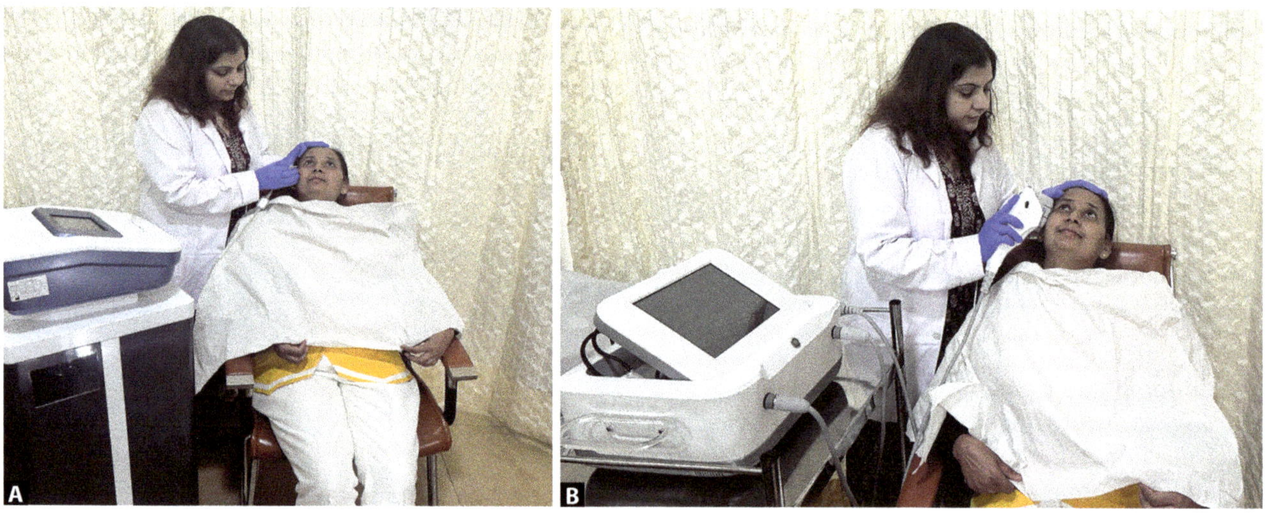

Figs. 3A and B: (A) High-intensity focused ultrasound (HIFU) for skin tightening; (B) Carboxytherapy for under eye circles.
Source: Adapted with permission from Jindal P, et al.

TABLE 1: Cosmetic genital procedures.

Type of procedure	*Purported benefit*	*Procedures used*	*Reported or potential complications*
Surgical procedures			
Clitoral hood reduction	To improve sexual function by increasing sensitivity and allowing more direct clitoral contact	Hoodectomy *Note:* Often combined with labiaplasty to create labia minora symmetry and prevent clitoral hood sagging	• Scarring • Infection • Hematoma • Hypersensitivity • Damage to the glans
Labiaplasty	To eliminate unwanted tissue of the labia minora or labia majora	• Trim or edge resection • Wedge resection using a V-shaped or Y-shaped incision • Z-plasty • De-epithelialization	• Scarring • Infection • Hypersensitivity or loss of sensation • Dyspareunia • Wound dehiscence
Labia majora augmentation	To create a full, symmetric look	• Autologous fat transplantation • Injectable fillers (hyaluronic acid)	Palpable fatty cysts

Contd...

Contd...

Type of procedure	*Purported benefit*	*Procedures used*	*Reported or potential complications*
Hymenoplasty	To recreate the virginal state of the hymen; has cultural roots in regions that place a value on an unmarried woman's virginity	Reconstruction of hymenal remnants, vaginal mucosal flaps, or both	Wound dehiscence
Vaginoplasty	To tighten vaginal contour and increase sexual satisfaction	• Anterior, posterior, or lateral colporrhaphy • Rugation restoration • Energy-based devices	• Infection • Dyspareunia • Dehiscence • Fistula
Energy-based interventions			
Energy-based vaginal procedures	To tighten vaginal contour and increase sexual sensation	Laser radiofrequency	• Burns • Scarring • Pain during sexual intercourse • Recurring or chronic pain
Injections			
G-spot amplification	To augment G-spot and heighten sexual satisfaction	• Autologous fat transfer • Hyaluronic acid	• Urinary tract infection • Infection

CONCLUSION

This is very interesting, extensive, nascent, and rising field. Everyday the demand for these procedures is increasing. It is important for clinicians to take adequate training, give realistic goals to patients, invest in good standard machines, take proper consents, and follow good ethical evidence-based practice. Also one should try to publish as much data as possible so that more evidence-based practices can be developed.[5]

REFERENCES

1. Dailymail.com. (2020). Women reveal the biggest mistakes that men make in the bedroom. [online] Available from www.dailymail.co.uk/femail/article-8947809/ Women-reveal-biggest-mistakes-men-make bedroom.htm [Last accessed May, 2024].
2. Bhagyashri S, Lalitkumar V. Concept of cosmetology in ancient India with special reference to Sushruta Samhita. Int A Med J. 2018;6(4):893-4.
3. Goodman MP, Placik OJ, Benson RH III, Miklos RJ, Moore RD, Jason RA, et al. A large multicenter outcome study of female genital plastic surgery. J Sex Med. 2010;7:1565-77.
4. Goodman MP. Female cosmetic genital surgery. Obstet Gynecol. 2009;113:154-9.
5. Jindal P, Malhotra N, Joshi S (Eds). Aesthetic and Regenerative Gynecology. Singapore: Springer Nature; 2022.

CHAPTER 2

Tracing the History of Aesthetic Gynecology

Tanuja Uchil

INTRODUCTION

The history of aesthetic gynecology is a journey through time, reflecting the evolution of societal norms, medical progress, and cultural attitudes toward women's health and beauty. From ancient civilizations to the modern era, the field has seen various stages of development.

Throughout history, societies have not only valued beauty but have also defined and classified it. These standards of beauty have been arbitrary and have varied significantly from one culture to another and over different periods.

Since the dawn of civilization, people have been concerned with their outward appearance. In ancient times, doctors made efforts to improve aesthetics by exploring new surgical techniques. Practices like piercing, scarification, and tattooing were popular, with specialized methods, such as injections, tearing, cutting, and stitching used to enhance body features. These early practices also laid the foundation for reconstructive surgeries.

In ancient civilizations, practices related to women's beauty often held cultural and religious significance. Some societies placed importance on body modifications and rituals associated with fertility and womanhood.

Additionally, women in ancient times used herbal remedies and natural substances for personal hygiene and health, although the primary focus was not necessarily on aesthetics. These practices and cultural beliefs played a crucial role in shaping the early understanding and development of aesthetic gynecology.

ANCIENT INDIA

Ancient India holds a significant place in the history of surgical techniques, with Sushruta often regarded as one of the world's earliest cosmetic surgeons. His pioneering work dates back to the 10th century BC, as documented in his book **(Fig. 1)**. Sushruta's groundbreaking contributions included the practice of skin grafting, where pieces of skin from other parts of the body were used to correct facial appearances. This technique, involving skin and vessel-rich grafts, led to revolutionary reconstructions including early forms of labiaplasty. Beyond surgical techniques, ancient Indian texts like the "Sushruta Samhita"[1] and "Ratirahasya"[2] delved extensively into female sexuality. Interestingly, the now-patented technologies of the G shot and O shot find their roots in these ancient texts, providing insights into enhancing sexual pleasure. Furthermore, the tradition of herbal vaginal smoking for tightening and rejuvenation mirrors the principles of modern laser vaginal surgeries, highlighting a remarkable continuity in the quest for female aesthetic and sexual wellness across centuries.

THE EGYPTIAN ERA

During the Egyptian era, beauty was highly esteemed, and the Egyptians left a substantial historical legacy of their endeavors to enhance appearance. Their reverence for complexion, symmetry, and youth is evident in their practices, making them among the earliest known civilizations to use makeup, dating back over 6,000 years.

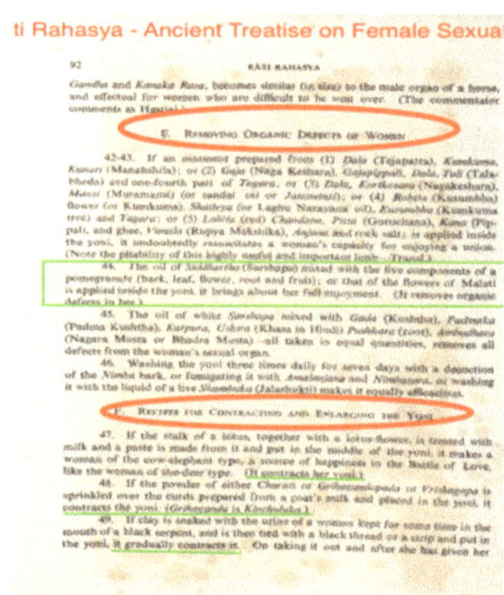

Fig. 1: Page from Sushruta Samhita book.

The exact origins of female genital mutilation (FGM) remain debated. Some scholars suggest Ancient Egypt (present-day Sudan and Egypt) as its possible origin, citing circumcised mummies from the fifth century BC. Others theorize that FGM spread through the routes of the slave trade, extending from the western shore of the Red Sea to southern and western African regions, or was transmitted from the Middle East to Africa through Arab traders.[3,4] In the third century AD, Philumenus of Alexandria described the excision of the hypertrophied clitoris because it was deemed "ugly and disgraceful." This practice was later abstracted by the Byzantine physician Aetios of Amida in the fourth century in his work "Sixteen Books on Medicine." In spite of their admiration for beauty, their treatment of the female genitalia was the precursor for FGM. It is important to note that the excision of the nonhypertrophied clitoris in Egypt was not driven by cosmetic motives but rather to prevent premarital girls from developing any desire for coitus. These historical insights shed light on the complex origins and practices surrounding female genital surgery in ancient Egypt.

THE GRECO-ROMAN ERA

The Greco-Roman era serves as a pivotal period in the early history of cosmetic gynecology, offering valuable insights into its practices. One notable figure from this time is Soranus of Ephesus, a Greek physician who practiced in Alexandria and Rome during the first and second centuries AD. Soranus recorded the earliest instances of surgical procedures on female genitalia for cosmetic purposes. His work, particularly his four-volume treatise on Gynecology, translated by Muscio in the 6th century, details the excision of a hypertrophied clitoris. This procedure was not only performed for cosmetic reasons but also to reduce excessive sexual stimulation, a technique credited to Philumenus, a respected Greek contemporary.

Further advancements in cosmetic gynecology were documented by another prominent figure in the seventh century AD Paul of Aegina (Paulus Aegineta), a Byzantine physician. In his "Medical Compendium in Seven Books," Paul outlined two distinct surgical operations. The first was his technique for excising the hypertrophied clitoris, referred to as the Nympha. Additionally, Paul described excising enlarged labia minora, known as Cauda Pudendi or pudendal tail.

Alongside these developments in surgical techniques, the concept of the *hymen* and its association with virginity emerged as a significant cultural and societal notion. The intact hymen was widely considered a symbol of a woman's virginity, leading to profound consequences for those who deviated from this expectation. The origin of this belief likely stems from a phonetic similarity between two Greek words, "Hymen" and "Hymn." "Hymen" meaning "membrane" led to the term "hymen vaginalis" for the membranous remnant of the vagina. On the other hand, "hymn" derived from "Hymenaeus," a minor god in Greek mythology linked to marriage ceremonies. Songs sung in honor of this god during weddings were called "hymn." However, this mythological association with virginity appears to be a misunderstanding. In Greek mythology, Goddess Hera represented marital relationships, while Goddess Aphrodite (Venus) was associated with extramarital affairs. The god Hymen, presiding over marriages, had no influence over sexual intercourse. This misinterpretation persisted through the ages, leading to harmful societal consequences for women who did not conform to the expectation of an intact hymen. The perpetuation of this myth, deeply rooted in ancient cultural beliefs, sheds light on the complexities and misconceptions surrounding female sexuality and cosmetic gynecology practices during the Greco-Roman era.

EARLY MEDIEVAL TIMES

Entering the Medieval era, we find significant developments in gynecological surgery, particularly in the technique of suturing vaginal lacerations during childbirth. This method laid the foundation for modern vaginoplasty techniques. In 1050 AD, a pioneering female physician named Trotula dé Ruggiero **(Fig. 2)** from La Scuola Medica Salernitana, the first medical school

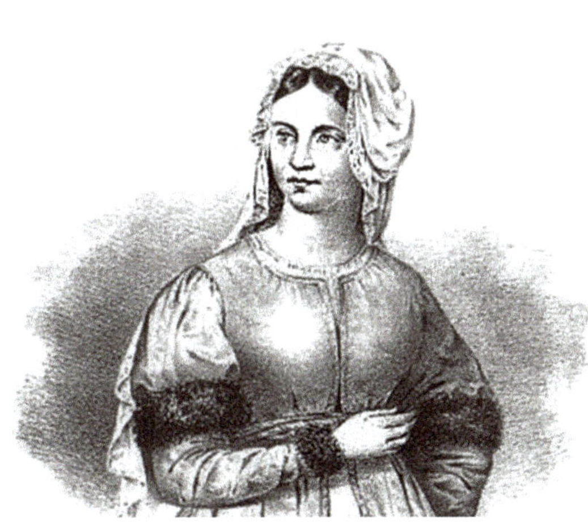

Fig. 2: Trotula dé Ruggiero (1050–1097).

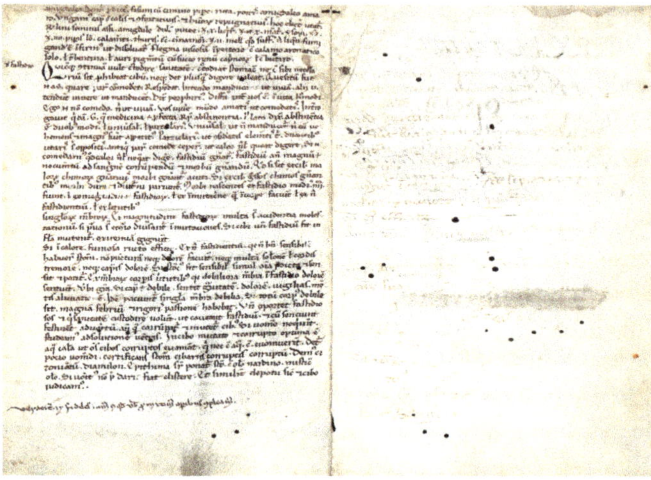

Fig. 3: Page from Trotula dé Ruggiero book.

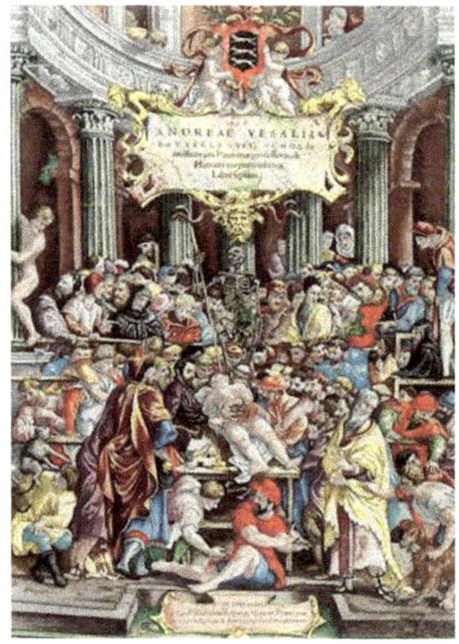

Fig. 4: Armamentarium Chirurgicum.

in Europe, described this procedure in detail. Trotula dé Ruggiero not only wrote treatments for women but also made substantial contributions to numerous other medical works **(Fig. 3)**. It was during this time, in the 11th century, that the origins of vaginoplasty can be traced back to the groundbreaking work of Trotula dé Ruggiero of Salerno. Her insights and techniques formed a crucial part of the early advancements in gynecological surgery during the medieval period.[5]

THE RENAISSANCE

During the Renaissance period, art underwent a transformation, portraying the female form with more realism and detail. This artistic shift influenced societal perceptions of beauty, with renowned artists like Leonardo da Vinci and Michelangelo contributing to a more accurate understanding of anatomy. Meanwhile, the use of cosmetics became more prevalent during this time, although the concept of aesthetic gynecology as a distinct field had not yet emerged. In the late 1600s, Parisian surgeon Pierre Dionis described the excision of the nymphae (known as labiaplasty) in his work "Cours d'opérations de chirurgie" (1707), which was based on his experiences in the court of Louis XIV. Similarly, Spaniard Roderigo de Castro (1546–1627) detailed clitoridectomy using a horsehair ligature in his work "Philosophiae Ac MedicinaeDoctoris per Europumnotissimi," first published in 1604. The German surgeon Johann Schultes (1595–1645) provided the first illustration of excision for clitoral hypertrophy in his posthumously published "Armamentarium Chirurgicum" in 1655. While the Renaissance era brought significant advances in anatomical knowledge through cadaver dissections, particularly highlighted by Vesalius (1514–1564) at the University of Padua in "De Humani Corporis Fabrica" **(Figs. 4 to 7)**, this knowledge became more widely disseminated with the invention of the printing press. However, it was not until later that surgeon like Ambroise Paré (1510–1590) and his pupil Jacques Guillemeau (1550–1612) described repairs of rectovaginal lacerations during childbirth in their respective works. In the 18th century, German military surgeon Lorenz Heister (1683–1758) provided a detailed description of labia minoraplasty in his widely popular illustrated surgical text "Institutiones Chirurgicae" (1739). Heister emphasized the practical need for such surgeries, noting that enlarged nymphae could cause discomfort and hindrance in daily activities for women.

19TH AND EARLY 20TH CENTURIES: INDUSTRIALIZATION AND MEDICAL ADVANCES

Industrialization and medical advances: The industrial revolution, with its societal transformations, also influenced attitudes toward beauty and hygiene during the 19th century. This period saw significant medical advances, enabling safer surgical procedures to be developed. While early surgical interventions for gynecological issues did take place during this time, aesthetics were not the primary concern in these procedures.

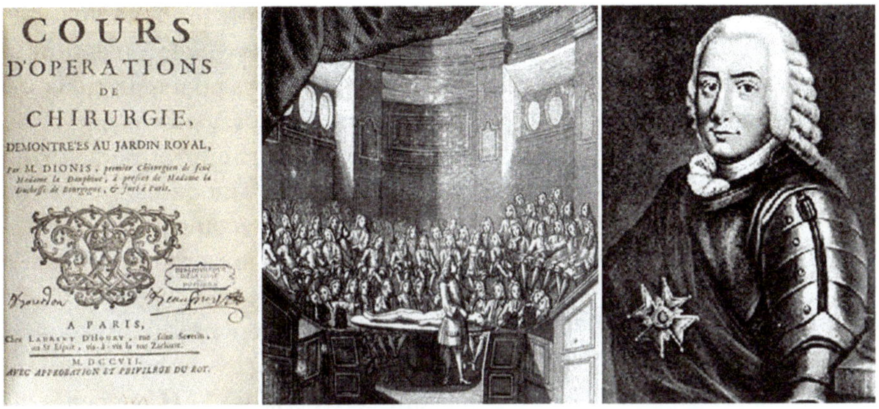

Fig. 5: Pierre Dionis in the court of Louis XIV, Paris 1690.

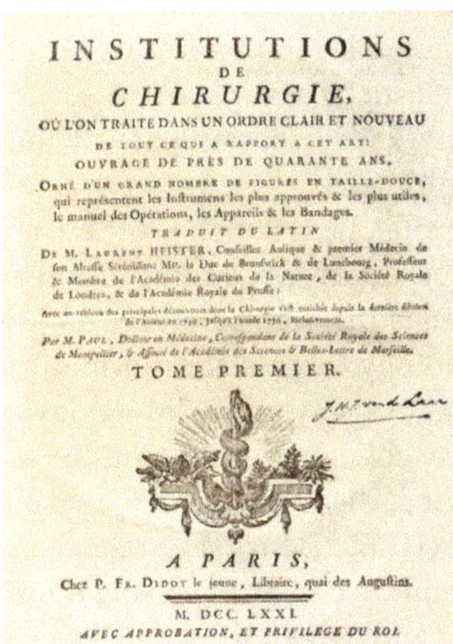

Fig. 6: Page from Armamentarium Chirurgicum book.

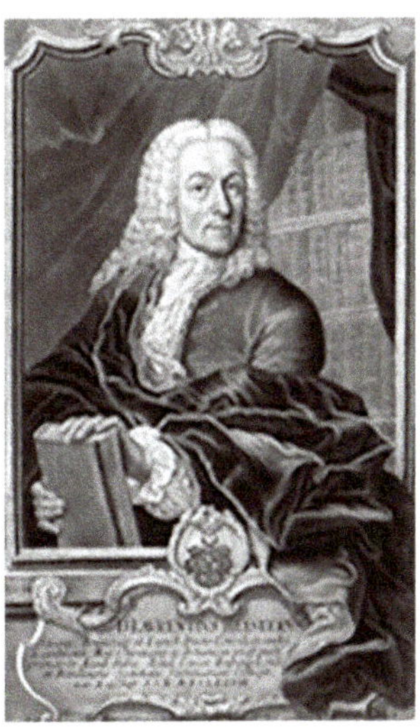

Fig. 7: Pierre Dionis.

MID-20TH CENTURY

During the mid-20th century, the women's liberation movement emerged, reshaping perspectives on women's bodies and questioning conventional beauty norms. This movement had a profound impact on societal attitudes toward female appearance. Concurrently, advancements in plastic surgery techniques during this era allowed for more precise and refined procedures. This led to a surge in interest and demand for cosmetic enhancements as women sought to redefine beauty on their own terms.

LATE 20TH CENTURY: RISE OF COSMETIC GYNECOLOGY

The first documented cosmetic labiaplasty in modern times, published in medical literature in 1976, involved a woman whose "labia minora protruding in wing-like fashion" was classified among the "abnormalities of the vulva." Surgery was performed to achieve what was considered "normal female genitalia" by Radman.[6]

The specialized field of cosmetic gynecology has evolved significantly over time, offering procedures like labiaplasty, vaginoplasty, and hymenoplasty. Here is a chronological overview of its introduction and growth:

In 1975, Dr James Burt, a surgeon from Ohio, made a groundbreaking contribution with his book titled "The Surgery of Love." This publication was the first of its kind, outlining procedures such as vaginoplasty and hoodectomy. Dr Burt's work was controversial, as he described a woman's vagina as "structurally inadequate for intercourse."

The field gained further recognition in 1978 when the European Journal of Obstetrics and Gynecology published the first paper on medical labiaplasty, titled "Benign Enlargement of the Labia Minora."

By 1984, medical literature was acknowledging cosmetic vaginal surgery, particularly in the Journal of Plastic Reconstructive Surgery.

In 1996, Dr David Matlock performed the inaugural vaginal rejuvenation procedure, later patenting and trademarking his technique, which helped solidify advancements in the field.

The late 1990s to early 2000s marked a significant turning point, with vaginoplasty and labiaplasty garnering substantial attention. These procedures became focal points of mainstream articles in popular publications, such as Cosmopolitan, Harper's Bazaar, and Marie Claire. This era saw a noticeable shift toward public awareness and discussion surrounding these cosmetic gynecological procedures.[6]

The 21st Century

In the 21st century, aesthetic gynecology underwent significant transformations with the advent of new technologies and increased global accessibility to procedures and information. Technological advancements, particularly in laser technology and noninvasive procedures, opened up fresh avenues for aesthetic gynecological treatments.

The term "cosmetic gynecology" was introduced in 2004 by Dr Pelosi II, who has since made notable contributions to various surgical cosmetic gynecology procedures. In 2005, Dr Alinsod from Long Beach brought forward the concept of the "Barbie" look, describing a smooth genital area appearance without visible labia minora.

Addressing the growing interest in procedures such as labiaplasty, the American College of Obstetricians and Gynecologists issued a statement in 2007 emphasizing the importance of informing women about the long-term benefits and potential risks. By 2011, the British Journal of Medicine revealed that 40% of surveyed women expressed a desire for vaginal rejuvenation. In 2012, the United States witnessed nearly 2,000 vaginal rejuvenation procedures alone, indicating a steady annual rise in numbers, despite the American Society for Plastic Surgery no longer tracking specific statistics on this procedure.

The 21st Century: Technological Advancements

In the 21st century, the field of cosmetic gynecology has witnessed a significant rise in technological advancements, particularly with the introduction of laser technology. While lasers have been used for skin conditions, their application in vaginal rejuvenation emerged prominently in the mid-2010s. Various types of lasers, such as fractional CO_2 lasers, erbium-doped yttrium aluminum garnet (Er:YAG) lasers, diode lasers, and radiofrequency ablation devices, have become key tools in this field.

CO_2 lasers, for example, create microscopic incisions in vaginal tissue, triggering a healing response that boosts collagen production and thickens the vaginal skin. This process enhances lubrication and elasticity. Similarly, erbium YAG lasers are utilized for nonsurgical gynecological procedures, employing thermal-only SMOOTH-mode pulses to induce vaginal collagen hyperthermia, leading to collagen remodeling and the synthesis of new collagen fibers. This results in improved tightness and elasticity of vaginal tissue.

Radiofrequency devices operate by increasing tissue molecular mobility, generating heat within the tissue. This heat activates heat shock proteins and initiates an inflammatory response, prompting fibroblasts to produce collagen and elastin. High-intensity focused ultrasound (HIFU) technology targets the dermal and superficial musculoaponeurotic system (SMAS) layers of the skin, promoting new collagen production for skin tightening, toning, and lifting. High-intensity focused electromagnetic technology (HIFEM) targets pelvic floor muscles, involuntarily contracting and relaxing them to strengthen the pelvic floor and tighten the vaginal canal.

In addition to these methods, newer techniques such as carboxytherapy, platelet-rich plasma (PRP), stem cell therapy, and exosomes are now also utilized in cosmetic gynecology. These advancements in technology have revolutionized the field, offering nonsurgical options for women seeking vaginal rejuvenation and tightening, with improved safety, effectiveness, and minimal downtime.

CURRENT TRENDS: HOLISTIC APPROACHES AND ETHICAL CONSIDERATIONS (CONCLUSION)

The evolution of aesthetic gynecology mirrors broader shifts in medicine and cultural attitudes toward women's health and beauty. One significant factor contributing to this evolution has been the changing cultural attitudes toward openness about women's health and body image. These shifting perspectives have played a crucial role in the growth of aesthetic gynecology as a specialized field.

In contemporary times, there is a notable trend toward holistic approaches in women's healthcare. This approach emphasizes not only the physical aspects but also the psychological and emotional well-being of women. Aesthetic gynecology is increasingly incorporating these holistic perspectives, recognizing that a woman's sense of beauty and confidence is interconnected with her overall health and happiness.

The field of aesthetic gynecology needs to navigate these current trends thoughtfully. While technological advancements continue to expand treatment options, ethical considerations, and a deep understanding of women's needs and desires should remain central. By embracing these holistic approaches and staying attuned to changing cultural norms, aesthetic gynecology can continue to evolve in a way that prioritizes the well-being and empowerment of women.

REFERENCES

1. Bandhopadhyay S. Surgery in Ancient India and Sushruta Samahita. In: Bhattacharya N (Ed). The History and Philosophy of Science: An Indian Perspective. Routledge: London; 2022.
2. Upadhyay SC. Rati Rahasya of Pandit Kokkoka. Bombay; DB Taraporevala; 1965.
3. Andro A, Lesclingand M, Grieve M, Reeve P. Female genital mutilation. Overview and current knowledge. Population. 2016;71(2):215-96.
4. Ross CT, Strimling P, Ericksen KP, Lindenfors P, Mulder MB. The Origins and Maintenance of Female Genital Modification Across Africa: Bayesian Phylogenetic Modeling of Cultural Evolution under the Influence of Selection. Hum Nat. 2016;27(2):173-200.
5. https://en.wikipedia.org/wiki/Trotula
6. Radman HM. Hypertrophy of the labia minora. Obstet Gynecol. 1976;48(1 Suppl):78S-79S. https://pubmed.ncbi.nlm.nih.gov/940641/

CHAPTER 3

The Mechanisms of Aging

Narendra Malhotra, Neharika Malhotra, Jaideep Malhotra, Keshav Malhotra, Gurkiran Kaur

INTRODUCTION

Aging is defined as physiological changes that are progressive in nature and lead to senescence and a general decline of biological functions of the body.[1] It involves decline of physiological functions which lead to progressive increase in risk of disease and mortality and finally with passage of time, mortality (death). It is a universal biological phenomenon, and all living organisms age. We know its inevitability is a fundamental aspect of existence, but scientists have been ceaselessly driven to solve the intricate mysteries that underlie the aging process. Since a long time, an association between aging and chronic diseases has been suggested. In addition, it is well known that the risk of various chronic diseases increases with aging, such as diabetes mellitus, Alzheimer's disease, parkinsonism, cardiovascular disorders, osteoporosis, and osteoarthritis **(Fig. 1)**.[2-6] A combined approach is required in these cases to improve the symptoms as well as the quality of life.[7] Based on this observation, it is hoped that a better understanding of the processes and mechanisms of aging will enable to identify therapeutic measures for such diseases. In this comprehensive article, we will address the multifaceted mechanisms that converge to orchestrate aging, providing an in-depth exploration of how our bodies undergo transformation as the sands of time slip through the hourglass.

MOLECULAR AND CELLULAR MECHANISMS OF AGING

Cellular damage and accumulation of the damaged cellular DNA such as DNA mutations or misfolding of proteins, leads to loss of normal cellular function. This ultimately leads to the accumulation of abnormal cells and loss of normal mechanisms of homeostasis, causing a limitation of regenerative potential, low-grade inflammation, and altered intercellular and intertissue communication. This molecular damage accumulation along with factors such as epigenetic modifications,

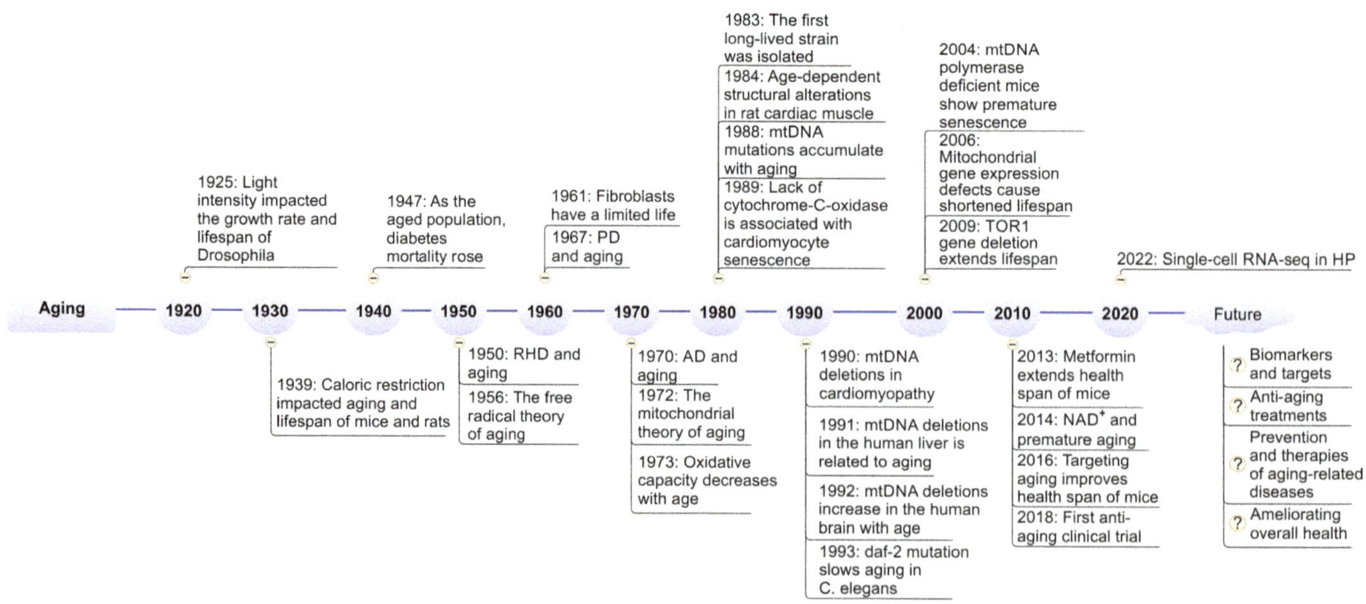

Fig. 1: Timeline of research on aging and aging-related diseases. (AD: Alzheimer's disease; HP: heterochronic parabiosis; mtDNA: mitochondrial DNA; NAD^+: nicotinamide adenine dinucleotide; PD: Parkinson's disease; RHD: rheumatic heart disease)

abnormal gene expression, and endocrine balance, is the main force behind the process of aging **(Fig. 2)**.

These mechanisms can be divided and studied at three levels: (1) the molecular level (genomic instability, telomere dysfunction, epigenetic alterations, loss of proteostasis, compromise of autophagy, mitochondrial dysfunction), (2) the cellular level (cellular senescence, stem cell exhaustion, and intercellular communication), and (3) systemic level (deregulated nutrient sensing) **(Figs. 3 and 4)**.

GENOMIC INSTABILITY

Genomic instability in an organism causes altered gene expression leading to abnormal physiological functions, hampered cell growth, and eventually cell death.[8]

NUCLEAR DNA DAMAGE ACCUMULATION

Genomic instability is mostly caused by double-stranded DNA breaks.[9] DNA damage occurs due to any cause, mostly due to endogenous and exogenous genotoxins. DNA can be damaged in many ways, making it a major cause of aging, such as spontaneous deamination, base modifications, strand breaks and crosslinks, and the most important being increased mutations.[10] Strand breaks when left unrepaired leads to impaired replication and transcription. Even if repaired inaccurately, it may lead to accumulation and propagation of abnormal nuclear material and mutations leading to aberrant chromosomal expression and hence senescence.[11]

The DNA damage response (DDR) of a cell is composed to regulatory and repair processes that help to identify DNA damage, arrest the cell cycle, and hence repair the damage. This is the stage at which the fate of the cell is decided, whether it will survive or undergo senescence. If the breaks are repaired adequately, the DDR signaling stop and the predamage state is returned. But if the repair is not successful, the DDR signaling will continue, leading to eventually cell senescence and death.[12]

MITOCHONDRIAL DNA

Mitochondrial DNA (mtDNA) differs from nuclear DNA in that it is composed of only exons. It lacks the histone packaging that may function as protection, and a system for gene repair. Therefore, the mtDNA may be more prone to damage and mutations than nuclear DNA.[13] mtDNA structure as well as copy numbers may be affected.[14] It has been recently found that a decrease in the levels of melatonin due to aging leads to impaired mitochondrial homeostasis, leading to stimulation of the cGAS/STING/IRF3 pathway, and hence increased production of cytokines and other inflammatory markers.[15]

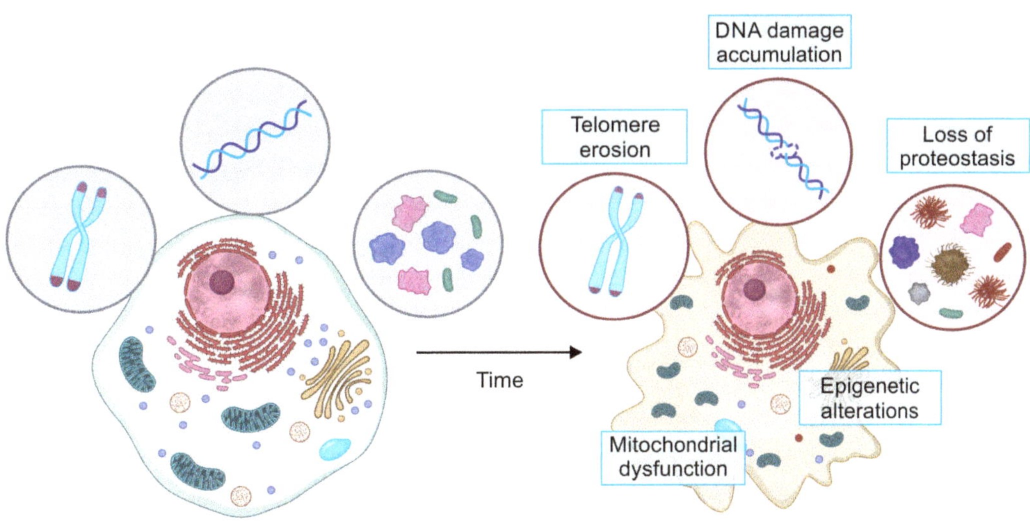

Fig. 2: The molecular wear-and-tear of aging. Time-dependent accumulation of cellular damage, namely lesions and mutations in the deoxyribonucleic acid (DNA) and misfolded proteins, can induce mitochondrial dysfunction and impair cellular function. Additionally, with each *somatic cell* division, *telomeres* shorten. Persistent DNA lesions and critically short telomeres are known to trigger a persistent *DDR* that can lead the cell into a senescent state. Gradual alterations in a cell's *epigenetic* landscape capable of altering a cell's fate or identity also accumulate over time. (DDR: DNA damage response)

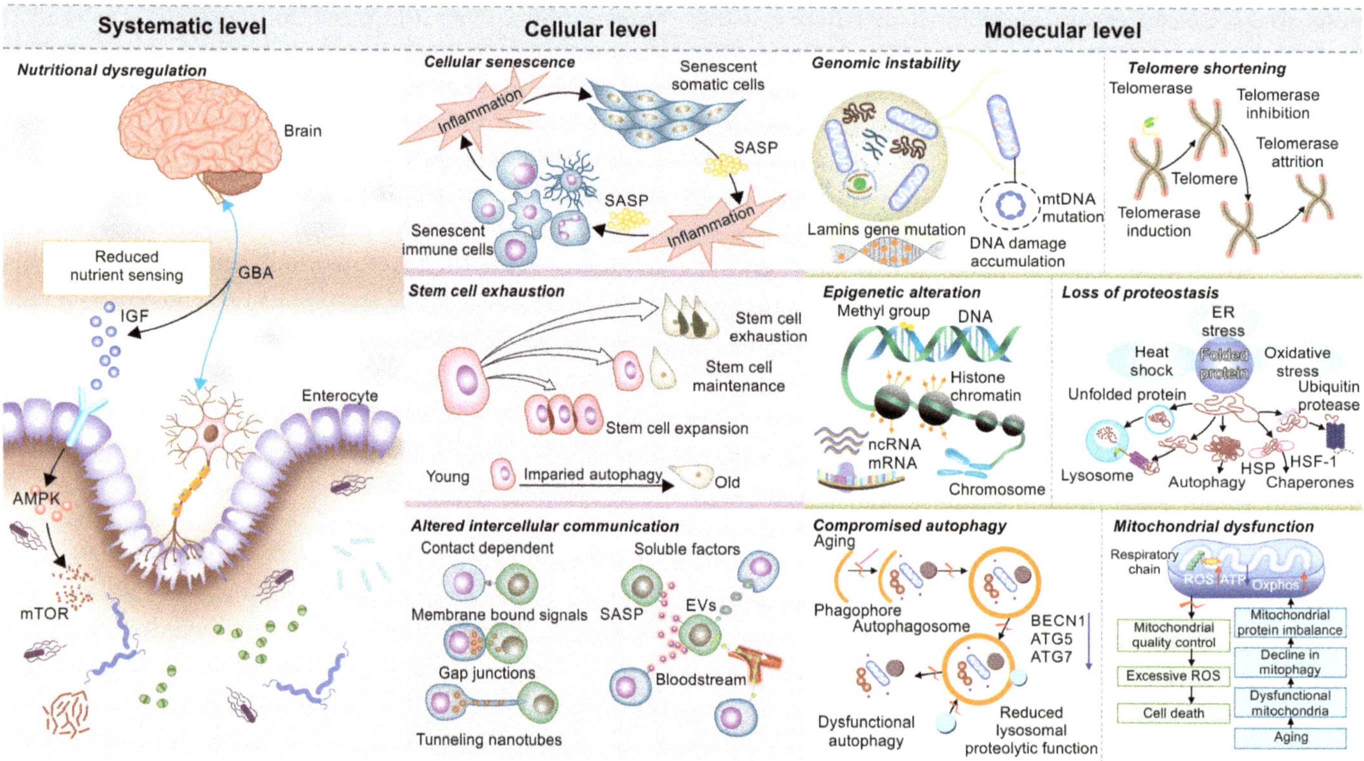

Fig. 3: The 10 hallmarks of aging are subdivided into three categories: molecular hallmarks (genomic instability, telomere dysfunction, epigenetic alterations, loss of proteostasis, compromise of autophagy, and mitochondrial dysfunction), cellular hallmarks (cellular senescence, stem cell exhaustion, and altered intercellular communication), and systemic alterations (deregulated nutrient sensing). (AMPK: protein kinase AMP-activated catalytic subunit α1; ATG5: autophagy-related 5; ATG7: autophagy-related 7; ATP: adenosine triphosphate; BECN1: Beclin 1; ER: endoplasmic reticulum stress; EVs: extracellular vesicles; GBA: gut–brain axis; HSF-1: heat shock factor-1; HSP: heat shock protein; IGF: insulin-like growth factor-1; mtDNA: mitochondrial DNA; mRNA: messenger RNA; mTOR: mechanistic target of rapamycin kinase; ncRNA: noncoding RNA; OXPHOS: oxidative phosphorylation; Rb: retinoblastoma; ROS: reactive oxygen species; SASP: senescence-associated secretory phenotype)

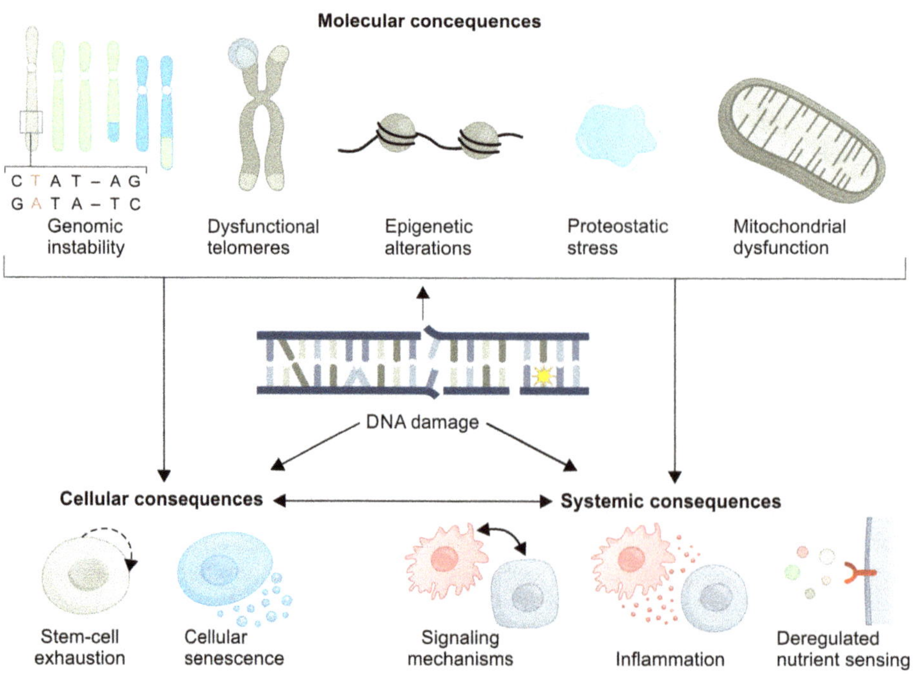

Fig. 4: Deoxyribonucleic acid (DNA) damage as a mechanism of aging.

NUCLEAR ARCHITECTURE

Lamin A and C are produced by the *LMNA* gene and are responsible for the maintenance of nuclear architecture.[16] *LMNA* gene mutations may be found in many neurodegenerative disorders, such as neuropathies, muscular dystrophy, and Hutchinson–Gilford syndrome.[16] Lamin B1 levels are directly related to aging, with a decrease in the levels associated with cellular senescence.[17]

JUNK DNA

Junk DNA is composed of repetitive DNA sequences that do not code for proteins.[18] It is believed that VNTR2-1, a junk DNA sequence actually functions to improve the activity of telomerase. Therefore, the telomerase gene activity may be found increased in people who have longer VNTR2-1 sequence.[19] Hence, junk DNA may also have a role in the mechanisms of aging.

TELOMERES DYSFUNCTION

Deoxyribonucleic acid damage and shortening at the level of telomere up to a critical level induces a DDR. This leads to arrest of the cell cycle and release of proinflammatory factors which ultimately cause aging.[20] Telomerase controls the length of the telomere; therefore, an increase in the activity of telomerase may prolong the lifespan of an organism **(Fig. 5)**.

TELOMERES

Telomeres are composed of tandem hexameric DNA sequence repeats (TTAGGG).[20] They are located at the terminal end of the chromosome arm. They help to maintain stability of the genome.[21] Telomere length is a major factor that determines its functional capacity, and telomere length has an inverse relationship with age, therefore may be used to predict the lifespan of a species.[22] Telomere shortening occurs until a threshold level, after which it stimulates the DDR, which further leads to cell dysfunction and senescence.[22]

TELOMERASE

Cells of the human embryo show a high telomerase activity, which then goes on decreasing with age.[23] The process of aging is hence a gradual process, in which telomerase activity may be reactivated at some critical points to allow the process to go on smoothly. When the critical telomere length is attained, telomerase expression occurs. It has been shown that failure of expression of telomerase in human skin cells leads to a critical length of the telomere

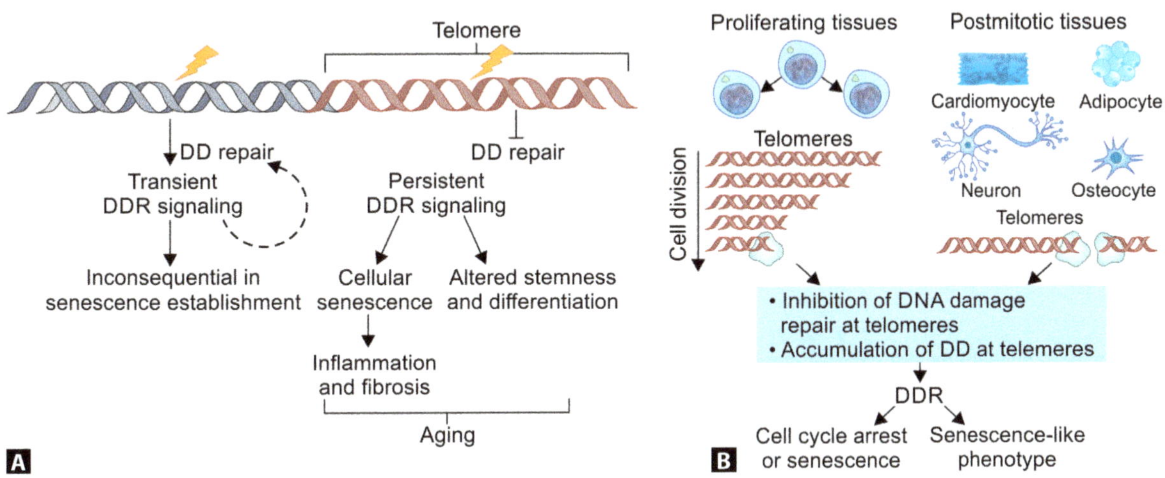

Figs. 5A and B: Telomere shortening and damage and their consequences. (A) Genomic DNA damage (DD) triggers a transient DNA damage response (DDR) that may not be sufficient for senescence establishment. Alternatively, an irreparable, therefore persistent, DNA damage at telomeres causes a protracted DDR and cellular senescence that are associated with senescence-associated secretory phenotype (SASP)-mediated inflammation and consequent fibrosis. These events in a stem-cell context impair stem-cell properties and alter differentiation. Overall, this contributes to organismal aging.[17] (B) In proliferating tissues, telomeres are shortened with cell cycle divisions and, when critically short, they trigger a DDR. In nonproliferating, postmitotic tissues, telomere dysfunction can be driven by irreparable DNA damage within telomeres. In both cases, the persistent DDR activation sustains a senescent phenotype that is characterized by arrested proliferation and SASP activation.

and DNA damage in less time as compared to cells that attain telomerase expression.[24]

EPIGENETIC ALTERATIONS

Epigenetic alterations may be caused by any changes in phenotype or gene expression due to mechanisms other than changes in DNA sequences.[25] These alterations may affect tissue function and survival by affecting the cell's response to damage.[26] These mechanisms include DNA methylation, histone modifications, chromatin remodeling, and transcriptional alteration by noncoding RNAs (ncRNAs) **(Fig. 6)**.

DNA METHYLATION

Deoxyribonucleic acid methylation accumulates gradually in the cell and is a marker of aging.[27] It may lead to changes in transcription and translation, thereby affecting gene expression, leading to eventually, cell senescence.[28]

HISTONE MODIFICATION

These include acetylation, methylation, phosphorylation, ubiquitination, glycosylation, adenosine diphosphate (ADP)-ribosylation, deamination, and proline isomerization.[29] Out of these, acetylation and methylation are the major modifications involved in aging and senescence.[29]

CHROMATIN REMODELING

Chromatin undergoes changes at local and global level with age.[30] Heterochromatin loss is associated with aging, as evidenced by markers HP1 and H3K9me3.[31]

TRANSCRIPTIONAL ALTERATIONS

It is now known that an unstable genome gives rise damage to double-stranded RNA (dsRNA) that lead to aging.[32] Recently, expression of circular RNA (circRNAs) present throughout the genome has been found to be increased in aging, with a strong correlation in this aspect. This increase in levels of circRNAs globally may be due to the highly stable nature of circRNAs.[33]

LOSS OF PROTEOSTASIS

Proteostasis refers to the state of protein homeostasis, in which the proteins stay in a precise folded three-dimensional structure. This requires a highly coordinated process consisting of chaperones and protein-degradation machineries **(Figs. 7A and B)**.[34] These mechanisms are responsible for the folded orientation of proteins since

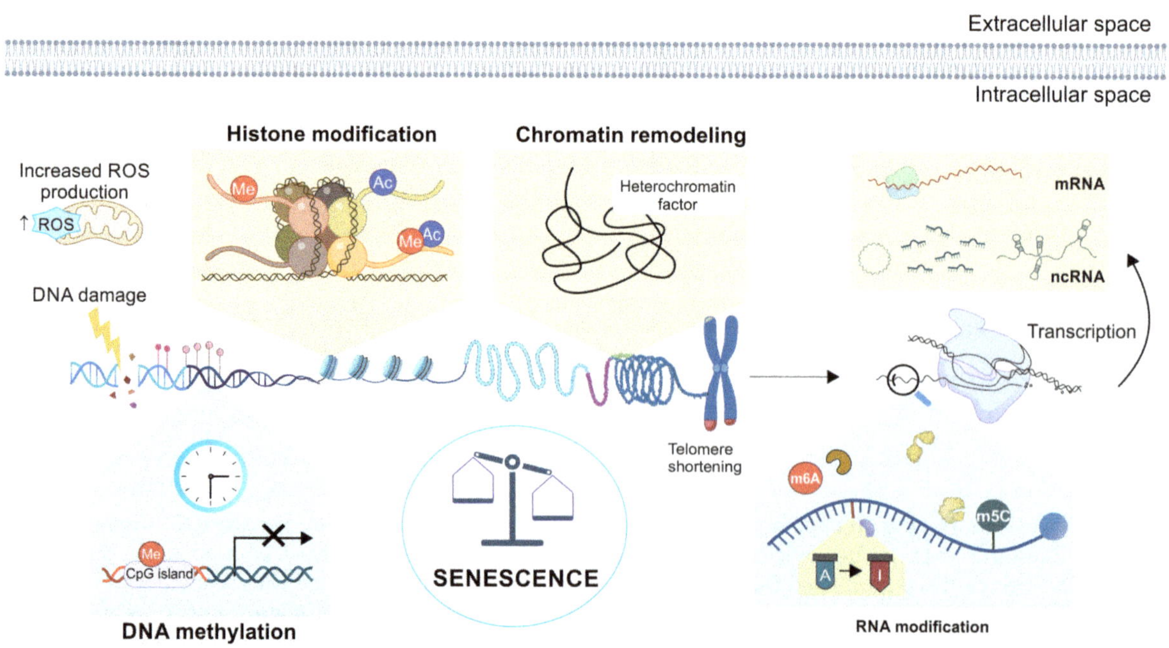

Fig. 6: An overview of the aging epigenome. During aging and the emergence of cellular senescence, a series of epigenetic changes occur in cells including alterations in DNA methylation, chromatin remodeling, histone modification, RNA modification, and ncRNA regulation. (DNA: deoxyribonucleic acid; mRNA: messenger RNA; ncRNA: noncoding RNA; ROS: reactive oxygen species)

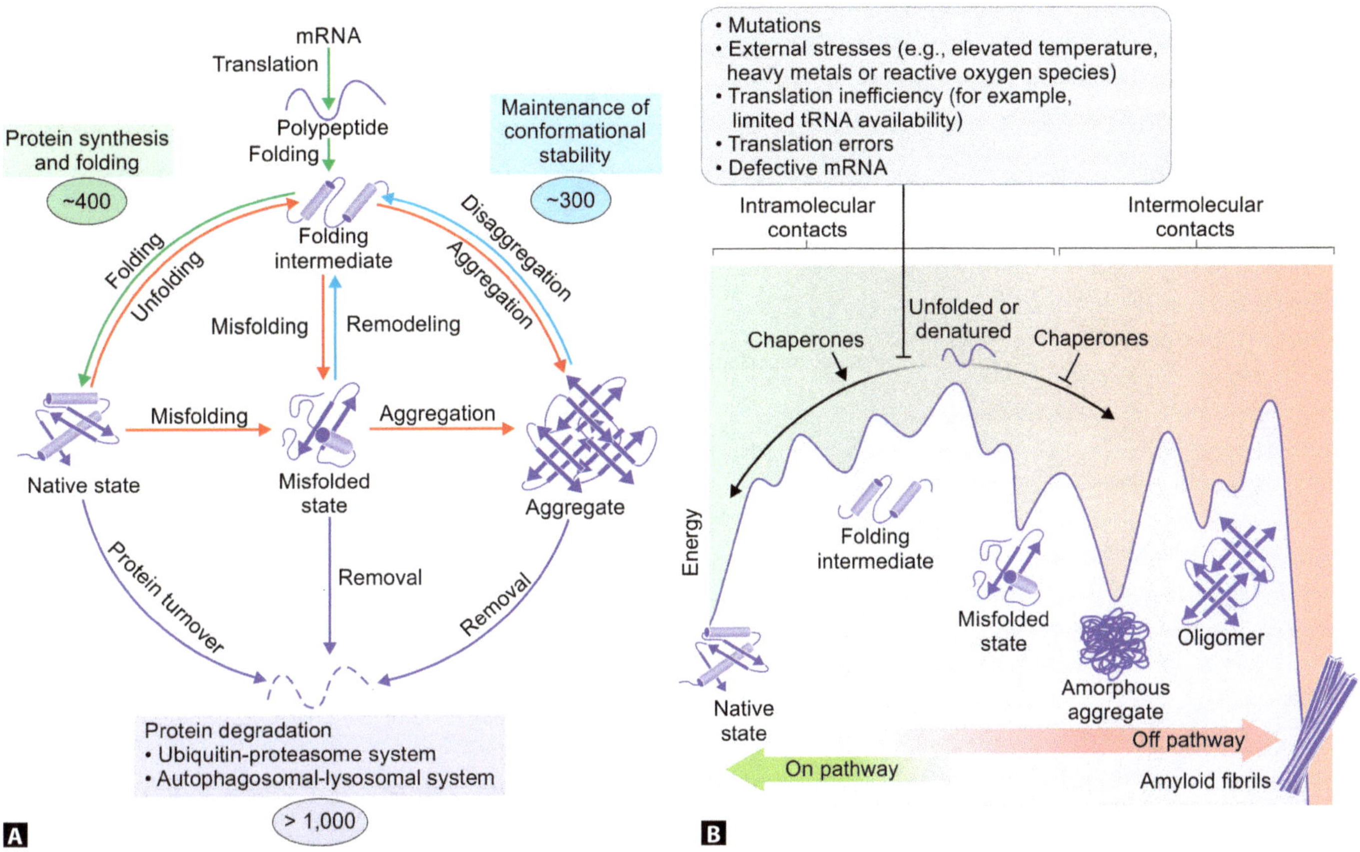

Figs. 7A and B: The proteostasis network and its decline in aging. (mRNA: mRNA: messenger RNA; tRNA: transfer RNA)

their production, and failure to adopt and maintain this state during and after synthesis leads to degradation.[34] This process may be affected if DNA mutations occur in the component of proteostasis, leading to improper folding and hence degradation and aging. Proteostasis may be altered, leading to age-related degenerative disorders like Alzheimer disease, Parkinson disease, and Huntington disease.[34,35]

COMPROMISE OF AUTOPHAGY

Autophagy is the process of degradation of cellular components like organelles with defective structure or misfolded protein structures in lysosomes.[36] Activity of autophage is seen to decline with age, leading to increased cellular damage and age-related disorders.[37]

Recently, levels of transition metals such as iron and copper have been found to be increased in senescent cells than in nonsenescent cells **(Fig 8)**.[38] It is believed that accumulation of iron occurs due to a defect in autophagy and degradation of ferritin in lysosomes.[38] Also, defective mitochondria undergoes accumulation of ferritin on its outer membranes. This leads to mitophagy, which is a form of autophagy that controls the production of damaged mitochondria via specific molecules and receptors.[39]

MITOCHONDRIAL DYSFUNCTION

Mitochondria are highly prone to damage with aging, resulting in loss of function of the organism due to oxidative damage, and hence aging **(Fig. 9)**.[40]

Mitochondrial dysfunction due to aging may occur due to accumulation of mtDNA mutations, mitochondrial proteins damage and dysfunction, and defective clearance of damaged mitochondria by mitophagy. Mitochondrial dysfunction is believed to occur due to nuclear DNA repair deficiencies.[41]

As an effect of this dysfunction, the respiratory chain is disrupted, leading to increased electron leakage, reduced adenosine triphosphate (ATP) production, and increased ROS.[41] This leads to cell senescence and death.[42] Therefore, cell function and lifespan may be improved by improving mitochondrial function via NAD^+ repletion.[43]

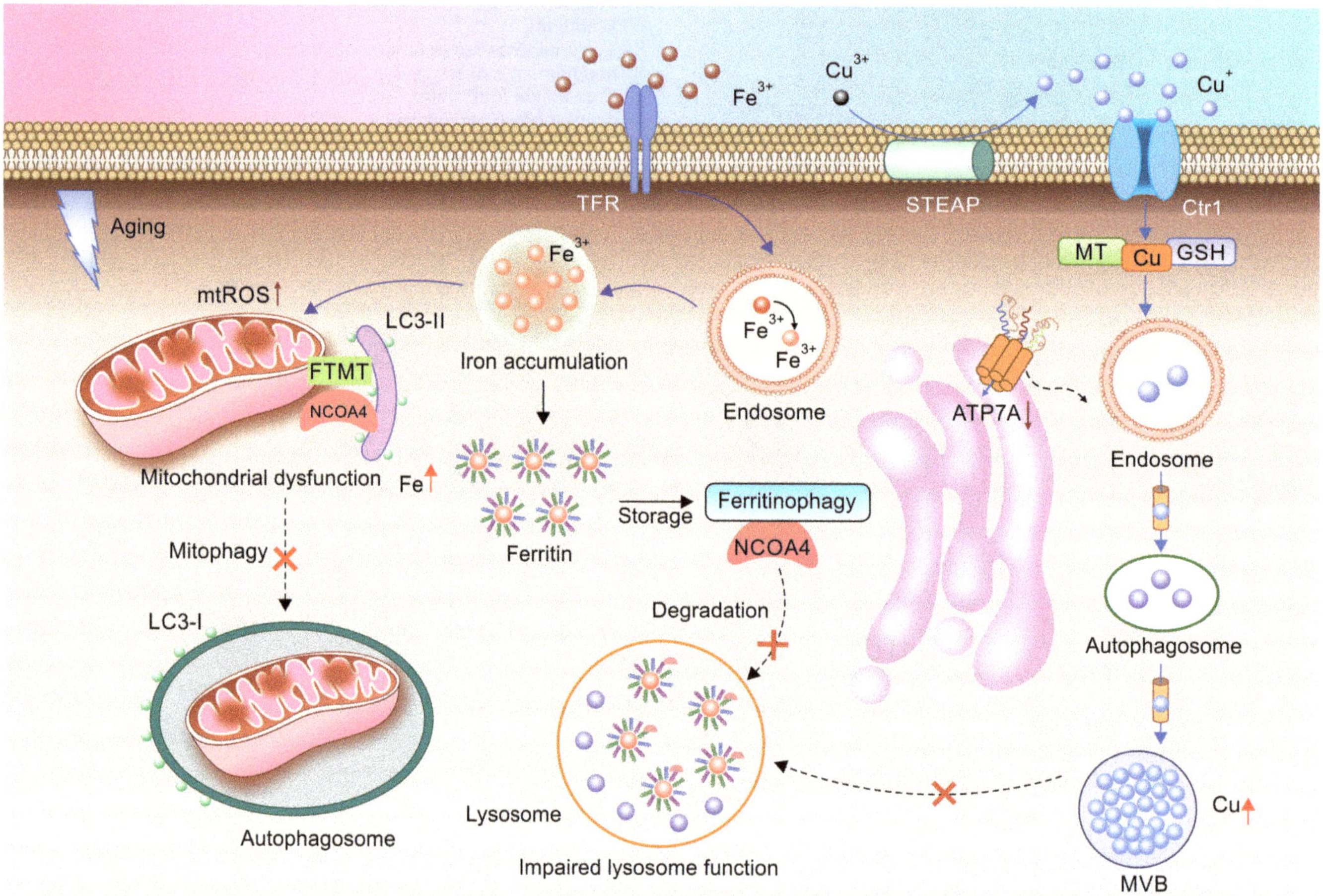

Fig. 8: Iron and copper accumulate in senescent cells. In senescent cells, iron accumulation is due to defective autophagic degradation of ferritin by lysosomes. In addition, in aging cells, FTMT accumulates on the outer membranes of defective mitochondria and promotes mitophagy by specifically interacting with the autophagic cargo receptor NCOA4 coupled to the LC3-II double-membrane phagophore. Furthermore, in senescent cells, reductions in the levels of ATP7A (a copper exporter) block autophagic—lysosomal degradation of copper. (ATP7A: copper-transporting ATPase 1, Ctr1: copper transporter 1; FTMT: mitochondrial ferritin; LC3-I: cytosolic form of LC3; LC3-II: LC3-phosphatidylethanolamine conjugate; mtROS mitochondrial ROS; MVB: multivesicular body; NCOA4: nuclear receptor coactivator 4; TFR: transferrin receptor)

SENESCENCE AND INFLAMMATION

Cellular senescence can be divided into two categories: (1) Replicative senescence and (2) Stress-induced premature senescence. Replicative senescence is a form of premature senescence that occurs after a limited number of divisions and shortening of telomeres. This leads to cessation of cell proliferation and differentiation.[12,44] Stress-induced premature senescence is a form of premature senescence that occurs due to some damaging factors, such as DNA damage and oxidative stress.[45]

The process of aging causes an increase in the immune cells that help in the clearance of aging cells. These immune cells then further have an inflammatory action due to production of cytokines.[46] In contrast, premature T-cell failure is found to cause aging. T-cell failure may be evidenced by thymic degeneration, mitochondrial dysfunction, genetic and epigenetic alterations, and loss of protein homeostasis.[46] This process of immune dysfunction and slow clearance may explain the accumulation of abnormal and senescent cells and increased low-grade systemic inflammation (inflammaging) **(Fig. 10)**.

STEM CELL DEPLETION

Stem cell depletion has been associated with tissue dysfunction and decreased potential of regeneration

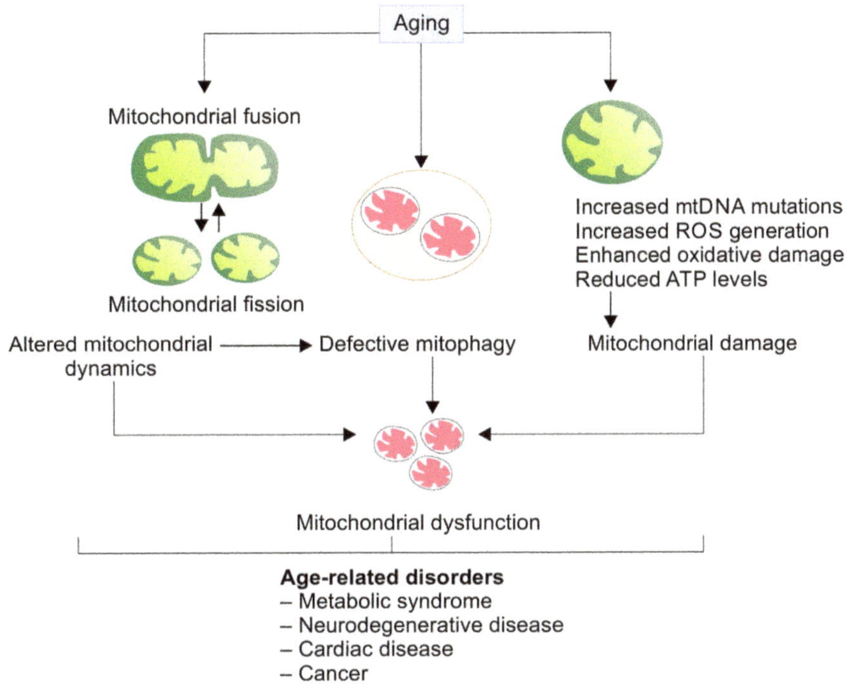

Fig. 9: Mitochondrial dysfunction during aging and age-related disorders. Aging is associated with progressive mitochondrial dysfunction that occurs due to accumulation of mitochondrial DNA (mtDNA) mutations and increased reactive oxygen species (ROS) production that causes oxidative damage to cellular macromolecules, thereby leading to reduced respiratory chain activity and adenosine triphosphate (ATP) generation. Mitochondrial fission and fusion play a vital role in the regulation of mitochondrial function, metabolism, and quality control. Altered mitochondrial dynamics with chronological age can inhibit mitophagy leading to accumulation of damaged or dysfunctional mitochondria in cells.

of cells.[47] Many mechanisms like DNA damage and accumulation, telomere shortening, loss of proteostasis, epigenetic modifications, and mitochondrial dysfunction have been found to reduce stem cell populations. Processes such as autophagy and diet modifications may help to preserve stem cells **(Fig. 11)**.[48]

ALTERATIONS IN CELL FUNCTION AND FATE

Deoxyribonucleic acid damages and epigenetic modifications may cause altered gene expression, cellular dysfunction leading to aging.[49] These set of changes cause accumulation of somatic mutations that may be seen in blood cells and body tissues such as skin and esophageal epithelium **(Fig. 12)**.[50,51] Skin cell mutations may have a specific pattern that resembles UV exposure and is found in skin malignancies.[5352] Mutation rates may be lower in the esophagus than in skin.[51] This accumulation of mutations over time leads to increase in senescent cells and loss of stem cell populations.

CONCLUSION

A lot of insight has been gained in the past decade into the mechanisms of aging, the damage at cellular and molecular levels and their impact on age-related chronic diseases. Recently, DNA damage and its accumulation has been studied in the assessment of biological age and the morbidities associated with aging. The process of aging and factors that affect aging is a complex mechanism, with each step being a scope in itself for therapeutic options in the age-related disorders. Therefore, it is an area with so many mysteries and possibilities, making the scientists even more intrigued and curious each day.

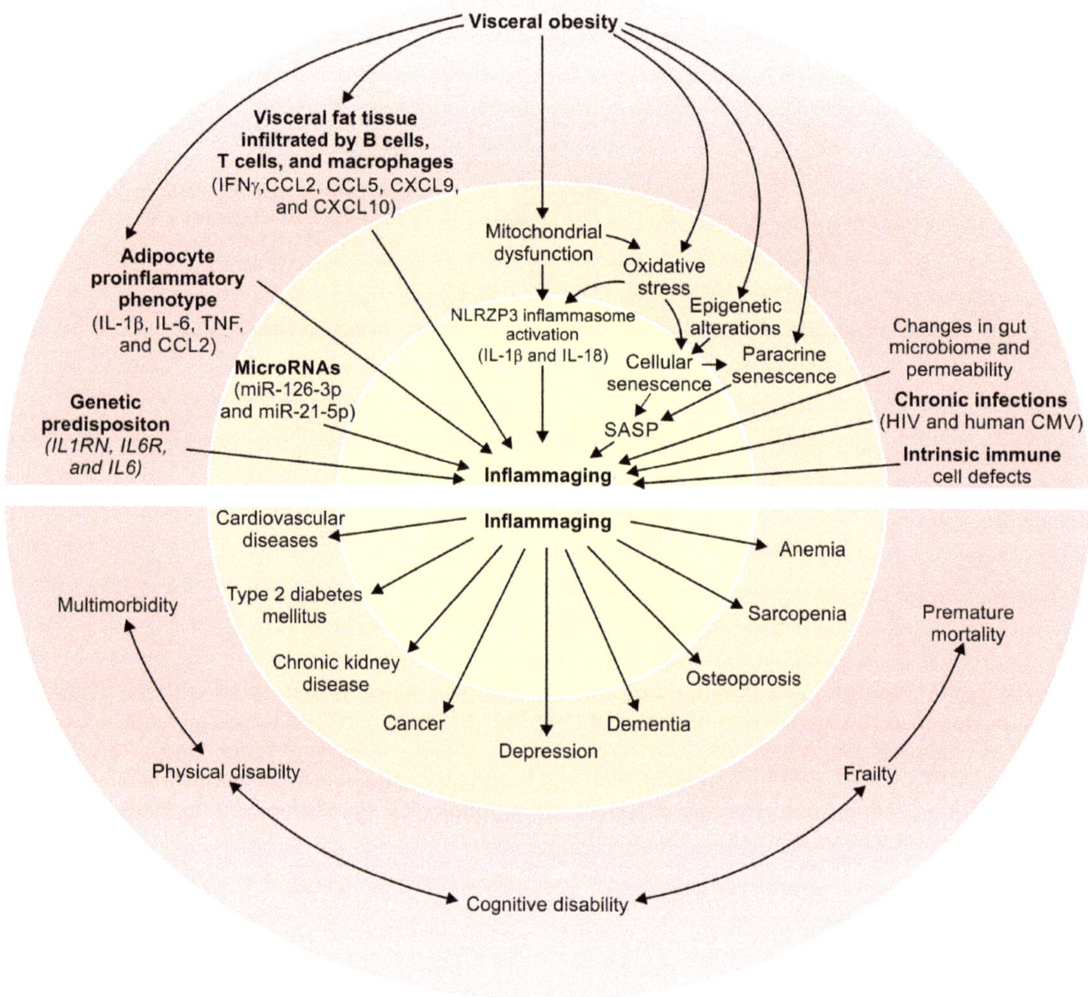

Fig. 10: Inflammaging: Chronic inflammation in aging. (CMV: cytomegalovirus; SASP: senescence-associated secretory phenotype; HIV: human immunodeficiency virus)

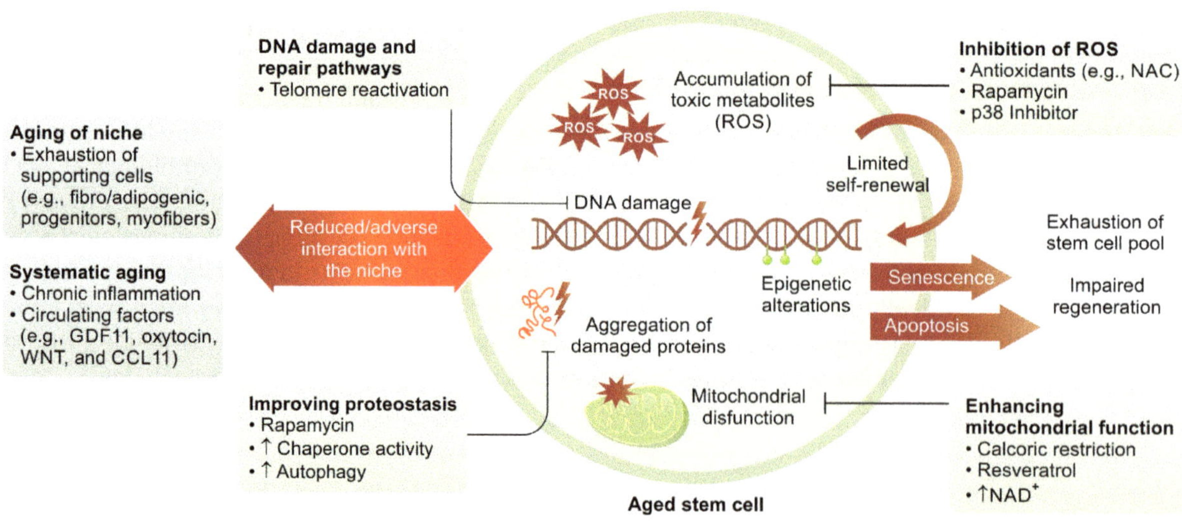

Fig. 11: Stem cell exhaustion in aging. (DNA: deoxyribonucleic acid; NAC: N-acetyl cysteine; NAD^+: nicotinamide adenine dinucleotide; ROS: reactive oxygen species)

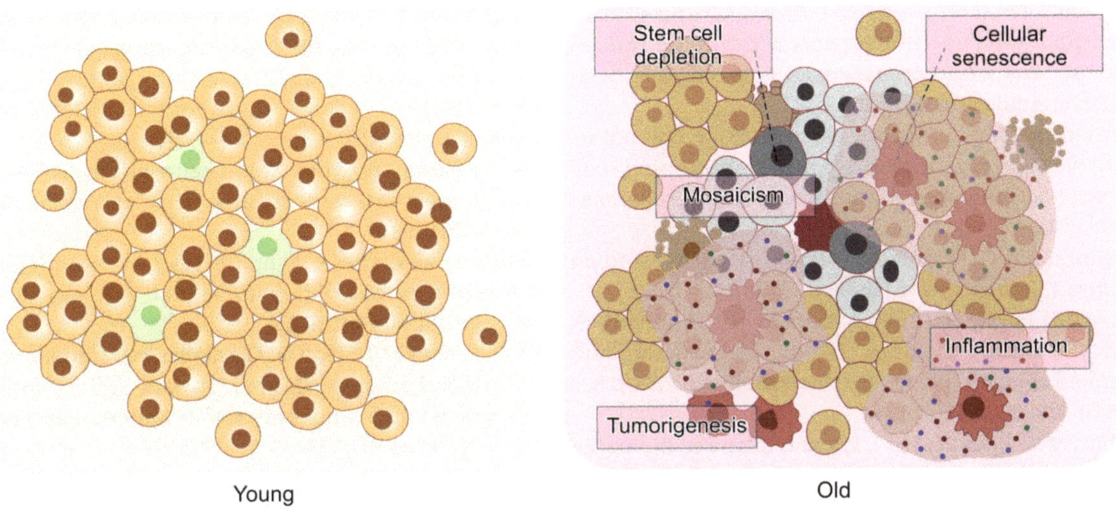

Fig. 12: Alterations in cell function and fate drive tissue dysfunction. Accumulation of molecular damage drives an age-dependent increase in cell-to-cell variability and introduces cellular heterogeneity within tissues. Over time, the pools of stem cells within tissues (left panel, green) become depleted and numbers of senescent cells increase (right panel, red). Senescent cells, via the SASP (right panel, small dots), establish a proinflammatory microenvironment (right panel, red areas) affecting neighboring cells. Accumulation of genomic mutations can cause cells to become tumorigenic (right panel, dark red cells) and explains the age-dependent increase in clonal mosaicism of somatic cells within tissues (right panel, gray). (SASP: senescence-associated secretory phenotype)

REFERENCES

1. Guarente LP, Rogers K, Petra S. "aging". Encyc Britannica. 2023.
2. Niccoli T, Partridge L. Ageing as a risk factor for disease. Curr Biol. 2012;22(17):R741-52.
3. Cortes-Canteli M, Iadecola C. Alzheimer's Disease and Vascular Aging: JACC Focus Seminar. J Am Coll Cardiol. 2020;75(8):942-51.
4. Yan M, Sun S, Xu K, Huang X, Dou L, Pang J, et al. Cardiac aging: from basic research to therapeutics. Oxid Med Cell Longev. 2021;2021:9570325.
5. Hernández Cordero AI, Yang CX, Yang J, Horvath S, Shaipanich T, MacIsaac J, et al. Airway aging and methylation disruptions in HIV-associated chronic obstructive pulmonary disease. Am J Respir Crit Care Med. 2022;206(2):150-60.
6. Chen X, Gong W, Shao X, Shi T, Zhang L, Dong J, et al. METTL3-mediated m6A modification of ATG7 regulates autophagy-GATA4 axis to promote cellular senescence and osteoarthritis progression. Ann Rheum Dis. 2022;81(1): 87-99.
7. Zhao Y, Seluanov A, Gorbunova V. Revelations about aging and disease from unconventional vertebrate model organisms. Annu Rev Genet. 2021;55:135-59.
8. Aguilera A, García-Muse T. Causes of genome instability. Annu Rev Genet. 2013;47:1-32.
9. Siametis A, Niotis G, Garinis GA. DNA Damage and the aging epigenome. J Invest Dermatol. 2021;141(4S):961-7.
10. da Silva PFL, Schumacher B. DNA damage responses in ageing. Open Biol. 2019;9(11):190168.
11. Osorio FG, Rosendahl Huber A, Oka R, Verheul M, Patel SH, Hasaart K, et al. Somatic mutations reveal lineage relationships and age-related mutagenesis in human hematopoiesis. Cell Rep. 2018;25(9):2308-2316.e4.
12. Fitsiou E, Pulido T, Campisi J, Alimirah F, Demaria M. Cellular senescence and the senescence-associated secretory phenotype as drivers of skin photoaging. J Invest Dermatol. 2021;141(4S):1119-26.
13. Kauppila TES, Kauppila JHK, Larsson NG. Mammalian mitochondria and aging: an update. Cell Metab. 2017;25(1):57-71.
14. Chiang JL, Shukla P, Pagidas K, Ahmed NS, Karri S, Gunn DD, et al. Mitochondria in ovarian aging and reproductive longevity. Ageing Res Rev. 2020;63:101168.
15. Jauhari A, Baranov SV, Suofu Y, Kim J, Singh T, Yablonska S, et al. Melatonin inhibits cytosolic mitochondrial DNA-induced neuroinflammatory signaling in accelerated aging and neurodegeneration. J Clin Invest. 2020;130(6):3124-36.
16. Gonzalo S, Kreienkamp R, Askjaer P. Hutchinson-Gilford progeria syndrome: a premature aging disease caused by LMNA gene mutations. Ageing Res Rev. 2017;33:18-29.
17. Bin Imtiaz MK, Jaeger BN, Bottes S, Machado RAC, Vidmar M, Moore DL, et al. Declining lamin B1 expression mediates age-dependent decreases of hippocampal stem cell activity. Cell Stem Cell. 2021;28(5):967-977.e8.
18. Fagundes NJR, Bisso-Machado R, Figueiredo PICC, Varal M, Zani ALS. What We Talk About When We Talk About "Junk DNA". Genome Biol Evol. 2022;14(5):evac055.

19. Xu T, Cheng D, Zhao Y, Zhang J, Zhu X, Zhang F, et al. Polymorphic tandem DNA repeats activate the human telomerase reverse transcriptase gene. Proc Natl Acad Sci U S A. 2021;118(26):e2019043118.
20. Zhu Y, Liu X, Ding X, Wang F, Geng X. Telomere and its role in the aging pathways: telomere shortening, cell senescence and mitochondria dysfunction. Biogerontology. 2019;20(1):1-16.
21. Laberthonnière C, Magdinier F, Robin JD. Bring It to an End: Does Telomeres Size Matter? Cells. 2019;8(1):30.
22. Howard JT, Janak JC, Santos-Lozada AR, McEvilla S, Ansley SD, Walker LE, et al. Telomere shortening and accelerated aging in US military veterans. Int J Environ Res Public Health. 2021;18(4):1743.
23. Blackburn EH, Epel ES, Lin J. Human telomere biology: a contributory and interactive factor in aging, disease risks, and protection. Science. 2015;350(6265):1193-8.
24. Sun L, Chiang JY, Choi JY, Xiong ZM, Mao X, Collins FS, et al. Transient induction of telomerase expression mediates senescence and reduces tumorigenesis in primary fibroblasts. Proc Natl Acad Sci U S A. 2019;116(38):18983-93.
25. Sen P, Shah PP, Nativio R, Berger SL. Epigenetic mechanisms of longevity and aging. Cell. 2016;166(4):822-39.
26. da Silva PFL, Schumacher B. Principles of the molecular and cellular mechanisms of aging. J Invest Dermatol. 2021;141(4S):951-960.
27. Horvath S, Raj K. DNA methylation-based biomarkers and the epigenetic clock theory of ageing. Nat Rev Genet. 2018;19(6):371-84.
28. Michalak EM, Burr ML, Bannister AJ, Dawson MA. The roles of DNA, RNA and histone methylation in ageing and cancer. Nat Rev Mol Cell Biol. 2019;20(10):573-89.
29. Paluvai H, Di Giorgio E, Brancolini C. The histone code of senescence. Cells. 2020;9(2):466.
30. Kane AE, Sinclair DA. Epigenetic changes during aging and their reprogramming potential. Crit Rev Biochem Mol Biol. 2019;54(1):61-83.
31. Wood JG, Hillenmeyer S, Lawrence C, Chang C, Hosier S, Lightfoot W, et al. Chromatin remodeling in the aging genome of Drosophila. Aging Cell. 2010;9(6):971-8.
32. Tarallo V, Hirano Y, Gelfand BD, Dridi S, Kerur N, Kim Y, et al. DICER1 loss and Alu RNA induce age-related macular degeneration via the NLRP3 inflammasome and MyD88. Cell. 2012;149(4):847-59.
33. Knupp D, Miura P. CircRNA accumulation: a new hallmark of aging? Mech Ageing Dev. 2018;173:71-9.
34. Hipp MS, Kasturi P, Hartl FU. The proteostasis network and its decline in ageing. Nat Rev Mol Cell Biol. 2019;20(7):421-35.
35. Santra M, Dill KA, de Graff AMR. Proteostasis collapse is a driver of cell aging and death. Proc Natl Acad Sci U S A. 2019;116(44):22173-78.
36. Aman Y, Schmauck-Medina T, Hansen M, Morimoto RI, Simon AK, Bjedov I, et al. Autophagy in healthy aging and disease. Nat Aging. 2021;1(8):634-50.
37. Kitada M, Koya D. Autophagy in metabolic disease and ageing. Nat Rev Endocrinol. 2021;17(11):647-61.
38. Zeidan RS, Han SM, Leeuwenburgh C, Xiao R. Iron homeostasis and organismal aging. Ageing Res Rev. 2021; 72:101510.
39. Aman Y, Cao S, Fang EF. Iron out, mitophagy in! A way to slow down hepatocellular carcinoma. EMBO Rep. 2020;21(11):e51652.
40. Fakouri NB, Hou Y, Demarest TG, Christiansen LS, Okur MN, Mohanty JG, et al. Toward understanding genomic instability, mitochondrial dysfunction and aging. FEBS J. 2019;286(6):1058-73.
41. López-Otín C, Blasco MA, Partridge L, Serrano M, Kroemer G. The hallmarks of aging. Cell. 2013;153(6): 1194-217.
42. Korolchuk VI, Miwa S, Carroll B, von Zglinicki T. Mitochondria in Cell Senescence: Is Mitophagy the Weakest Link? EBioMedicine. 2017;21:7-13.
43. Zhang H, Ryu D, Wu Y, Gariani K, Wang X, Luan P, et al. NAD^+ repletion improves mitochondrial and stem cell function and enhances life span in mice. Science. 2016;352(6292):1436-43.
44. Rhinn M, Ritschka B, Keyes WM. Cellular senescence in development, regeneration and disease. Development. 2019;146(20):dev151837.
45. Cai Y, Song W, Li J, Jing Y, Liang C, Zhang L, et al. The landscape of aging. Sci China Life Sci. 2022;65(12):2354-454.
46. Mittelbrunn M, Kroemer G. Hallmarks of T cell aging. Nat Immunol. 2021;22(6):687-98.
47. Ermolaeva M, Neri F, Ori A, Rudolph KL. Cellular and epigenetic drivers of stem cell ageing. Nat Rev Mol Cell Biol. 2018;19(9):594-610.
48. García-Prat L, Martínez-Vicente M, Perdiguero E, Ortet L, Rodríguez-Ubreva J, Rebollo E, et al. Autophagy maintains stemness by preventing senescence. Nature. 2016;529(7584):37-42.
49. Nikopoulou C, Parekh S, Tessarz P. Ageing and sources of transcriptional heterogeneity. Biol Chem. 2019;400(7): 867-78.
50. Machiela MJ, Chanock SJ. The ageing genome, clonal mosaicism and chronic disease. Curr Opin Genet Dev. 2017;42:8-13.
51. Martincorena I, Fowler JC, Wabik A, Lawson ARJ, Abascal F, Hall MWJ, et al. Somatic mutant clones colonize the human esophagus with age. Science. 2018;362(6417):911-7.
52. Martincorena I, Roshan A, Gerstung M, Ellis P, Van Loo P, McLaren S, et al. Tumor evolution. High burden and pervasive positive selection of somatic mutations in normal human skin. Science. 2015;348(6237):880-6.

CHAPTER 4

Anatomy and Physiology: In Relation to Aesthetic and Regenerative Gynecology

Prerna Keshan

INTRODUCTION

A thorough knowledge of the anatomy and physiology of the vulvovaginal complex is a must to understand the physiology of aging and the anatomical changes associated with the same. Aesthetic, functional, and regenerative gynecology call for an in-depth dive into the very basics of the anatomical and physiological preview of the female genitalia. The motive of this chapter is to enhance the basics of functional anatomy for all clinicians delving into this field of aesthetics.

VULVOVAGINAL COMPLEX

The vulvovaginal complex **(Fig. 1)** classically comprises in a sequential manner of the following structures:

- The upper most part is called the mons pubis which is also known as the "Venus Mount".
- Thereafter, it is the clitoral hood underneath which lies the most sensitive organ of sexual arousal—the clitoris.
- Bilaterally, there are two pads of fat tissue known as the "labium majus".

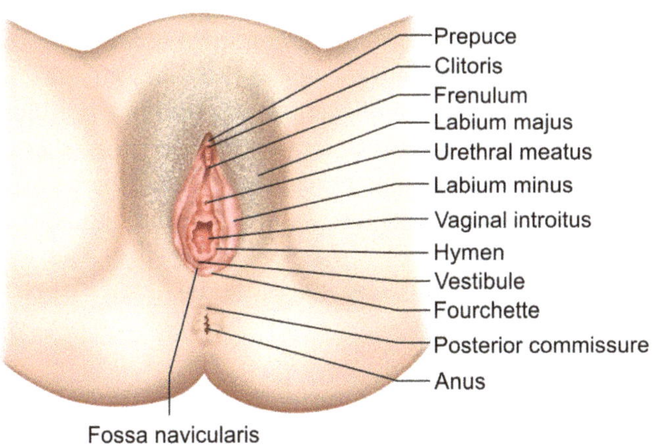

Fig. 1: Vulvovaginal complex.

- Besides the labium majus, bilaterally there lies the two thin leaf-like structures called the "labia minora".
  1. Hymen
  2. Vestibule
- At the central alignment below the clitoral body, there lies the urethral meatus.
- Bilaterally, there are the two Bartholin's glands, they are also known as the "greater vestibular glands".
- Beside the Bartholin's glands, there lie the minor vestibular glands which are of not much functional significance.
- The glands lying alongside the urethra are known as the "paraurethral glands".
- Vagina

Mons Pubis

Gross anatomy—under the bony prominence of the symphysis pubis lies this dense pad of fat which serves as a protective cushion. This mound is a triangle in shape and comprises adipose connective tissue in the subcutaneous strata.

Changes

- The mons pubis is subjective to alter during various phases of aging. It becomes considerably less elevated with the onset of menopause. On the contrary, it becomes more elevated during the onset of puberty. This mound also alters with weight gain and significant weight loss wherein the elevation can increase or decrease respectively.
- Coarse and thick hair cover the pubic mound which is also called the "escutcheon". This escutcheon has the tendency to decrease as age advances more so during the postmenopausal phase of life.
- It is of utmost importance to understand that the deviance of the degree of angulation of the pubic rami also determines the elevation of the mons pubis. This is in addition to the amount of adipose connective tissue in the mons pubis.

Labium Majus

- Starting from the pubic mound anteriorly and extending uptill the perineal body, the two labium majus runs bilaterally as pad of dense skin folds. Posteriorly, there lies the commissure which is of great functional and applied anatomical significance.
- The exterior part of the outer lips (labia majora) bilaterally is covered with hair and the interior portion comprises abundant apocrine and eccrine sweat glands lacking hair.
- It is covered by squamous epithelium.
- Both the outer lips comprise dense subcutaneous tissue and fibrofatty tissue. The labia majora are highly vascular with intricate supply of veins.
- Labia majora do not consist any macular tissue.

Changes

The variations in the labia majora extend in the following manner—they can be full/tight/lax/baggy. The documentation per se can be labeled to be empty or redundant labia.

Labia Minora

- These are the two leaf-like thin structures running alongside the labium majus medially and bilaterally.
- At the upper end of the labia minora there is a division into two lamellae, the frenulum of the clitoris is formed by the inferior portion whereas the superior portion runs into the prepuce.
- In the most inferior part, it is the fourchette which is formed by the fusion at the central alignment.

Structurally

- The labia minora are composed of connective tissue with many vessels, elastin fibers, and some smooth muscle fibers.
- There are numerous sweat glands in labia minora, but they are devoid of any hair cuticles.
- The labia minora bilaterally have loose connective tissue thereby imparting free cutaneous movement during the act of coitus.

Hart Line of the Labia Minora (Fig. 2)

- This is a linear demarcation of the outer aspect of the interior portion of the labia minora in which the epithelium is stratified squamous.

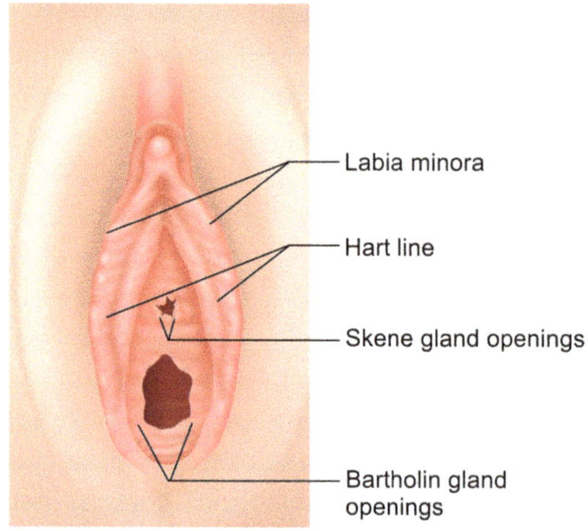

Fig. 2: Hart line of the labia minora.

- On the medial aspect of the Hart line, each labium has nonkeratinized squamous epithelium.

Variations

- A well-defined deep sulcus separates the labia majora from the labia minora. However in few subjects, it is seen that occasionally the sulcus has tendinous segmental insertions and sometimes it is even not seen. This leads to an ill-defined separation between the outer and the inner lips.
- Appearance and shape of the labia minora has many anatomic variations, asymmetrics being the most common.
- The skin quality may vary from tight to loose and rugose.

Clitoris (Fig. 3)

- It is the principal female erogenous organ. At the upper end, the clitoris is situated beneath the hood of the clitoris. This arrangement can however vary widely. This particular knowledge of the wide variation in the shape and size of the clitoral hood has significant applied anatomical value in the practice of aesthetics.
- The entire clitoris is not what it looks like from the exterior. The internal structure is homologous to the male penis and comprises the following—the glans clitoris, the body of the clitoris, and bilaterally the crura.

Glans Clitoris

- The glans clitoris comprises a magnanimous nerve supply which is the basis of its being the most sensitive structure for human sexual arousal reflex.

- Usually the hood of the clitoris merges with the upper part of the labia minora.

Variations

- Clitoral hood may be small. In this, the frenulum continues with the labia minora.

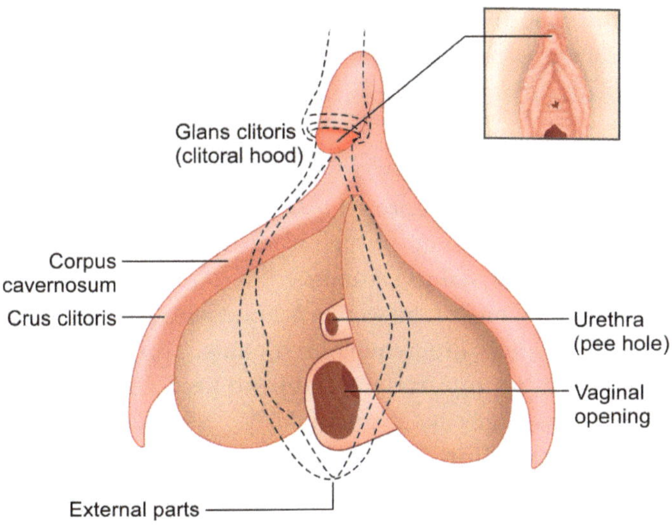

Fig. 3: The clitoris: Inside the body.

- Clitoral hood may be heavy.
- At times the clitoris is laterally divided and that looks like a double-folded clitoris at the lateral end.
- There may also be the presence of many folds in the clitoris laterally rather than only two.
- An important structural change of applied aesthetic significance is that the body of the clitoris which is bigger in size has a much heavier covering hood. Clitoral hood reduction surgery is a very commonly done surgery in this field of aesthetic and functional gynecology.

Body of the Clitoris

- From the hood of the clitoris bilaterally radiates the corpora cavernosa.
- The divergence bilaterally from the clitoral body creates a narrow area called crura.

VASCULAR ANATOMY (FIG. 4)

- Beneath the perineal membrane there lies the internal pudendal artery. The parent arterial supply is from this internal pudendal artery. The outer and the inner

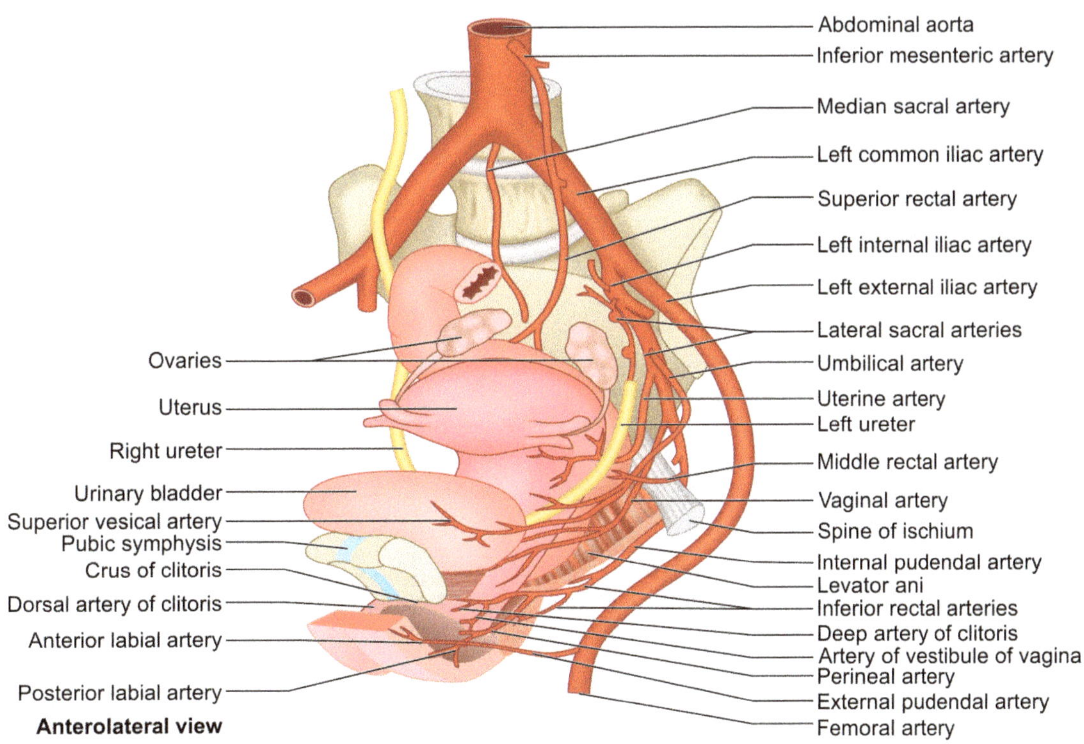

Fig. 4: Vascular anatomy.

lips have the vascular supply from the posterior labial artery and the perineal artery respectively.

- The clitoris and its entire length is supplied by the dorsal artery of clitoris.
- Georgiou et al. have reported the following in the vascular supply of the vulvovaginal complex. There is one artery that is dominant and is identified at the center, two arteries coming from the posterior end and one small artery at the anterior end.

Nerve Supply (Fig. 5)

- The primary nerve supply of the vulvovaginal complex is via the pudendal nerve.
- The branches of the pudendal nerve namely the superficial and the deep perineal nerves supply the entire extent starting at the juncture of the superficial perineal muscle.
- Later in its course, the posterior labial nerve arises from the superficial branch and the dorsal nerve to the clitoris arises from the deep branch of the perineal nerves.

Vestibule (Fig. 6)

- The boundaries of the vestibule comprises the following structures—on the lateral aspect is the Hart line, on the medial aspect is the outer surface of the hymen, on the anterior aspect is the frenulum of the clitoris, and on the posterior aspect is the juncture of the fourchette. This gives an almond shape to the vestibular area.
- There are six openings which perforate the vestibule namely the urethral meatus, the vagina, bilaterally the vestibular gland ducts, and the glands of Skene.
- The area between the fourchette and the vagina is termed as the fossa navicularis which lies at the most posterior aspect of the vestibule.

Vaginal Opening and the Hymen

- The most important organ of the external genitalia is the vaginal opening which is located at the posterior most aspect of the vestibule.
- The distal end of the vagina is lined with the hymen or at times only the hymenal remnants. This knowledge has a huge implication in applied aesthetic anatomy for procedures like hymenoplasty.
- Vagina comprises both collagenous and elastic connective tissues. This knowledge is of importance in aesthetic procedures as maximum vaginal rejuvenative procedures are based on collagen remodeling and neovascularization. The epithelial lining is of stratified squamous type in both the inner and outer aspects of the vaginal wall.

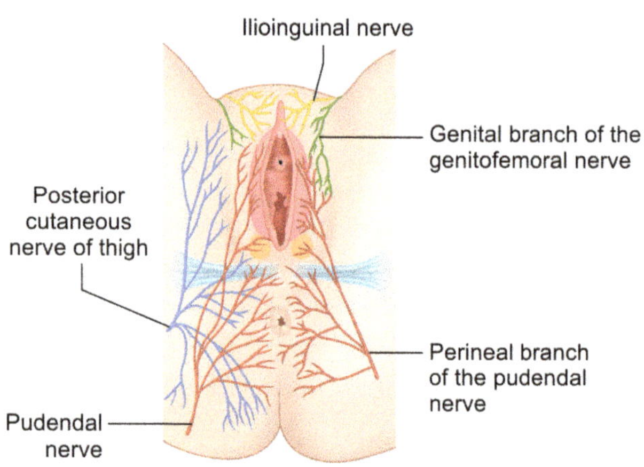

Fig. 5: Nerve supply.

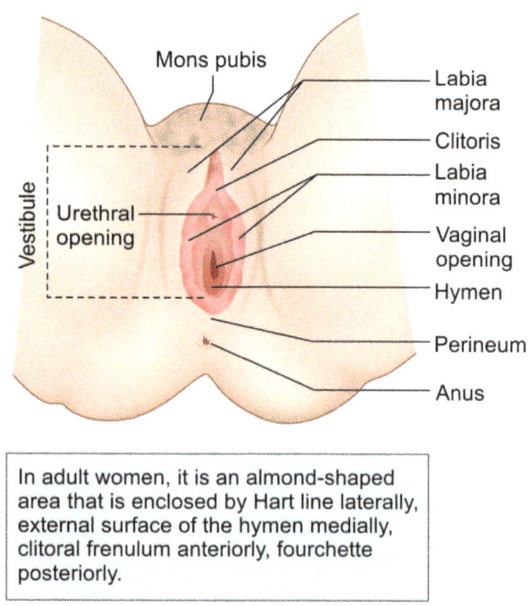

Fig. 6: Vestibule.

Various Types of Hymen (Fig. 7)

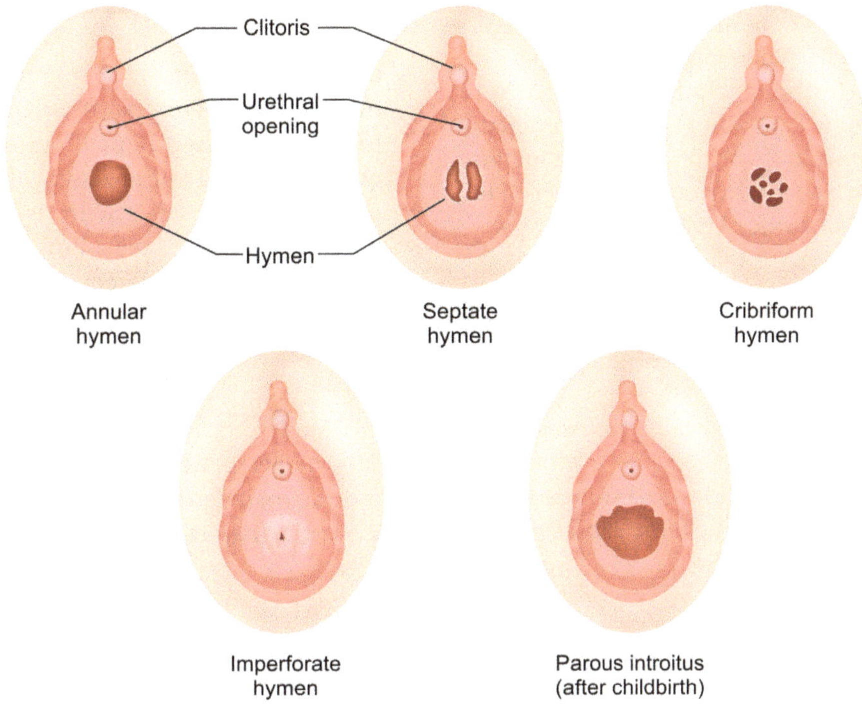

Fig. 7: Various types of hymens.

Vagina

- The lining of the vagina has a weak inner coat of circular fibers and a stronger outer longitudinal fiber coat.
- Vaginal pH is strongly acidic; pH is 4–5, due to Döderlein's bacillus.

Changes

- The characteristics of the vagina change during intercourse, throughout menstrual cycle, pregnancy, and with age.
- With increasing age the walls become lax and dry due to estrogen deficiency.

CLASSIFICATION OF FEMALE GENITAL ANATOMY FOR AID IN AESTHETIC AND REGENERATIVE PROCEDURES

For better understanding of the variation in the labial anatomy and correction of the same in required population, Motakef classified the degree of labial (labia minora) protrusion.[1] This classification is based on the length of the labia minora that extends beyond the anterior aspect of the labia majora. Based on this, the following are the degrees of labial (labia minora) protrusions. This knowledge is of utmost importance for all practicing aesthetic gynecologists because labioplasty is one of the most commonly done procedures in this field and it requires an apt knowledge of the degree of protrusion because undercorrection is always better than overcorrection in cases of hanging labia or labial hypertrophies. Labial hypertrophies may act as hindrance in pleasurable coitus as well as other cosmetic and functional issues revolving around the vagina.[2]

- *Class I:* 0–2 cm
- *Class II:* 2–4 cm
- *Class III:* More than 4 cm

Later, FRANCO AND FRANCO 8 in 1993, also classified labia minora hypertrophy into various types:

- Less than 2 cm enlargement is termed as type I hypertrophy.
- 2–4 cm enlargement is termed as type II hypertrophy.
- 4–6 cm enlargement is termed as type III hypertrophy.
- More than 6 cm enlargement is termed as type IV hypertrophy.

Later based on the position of enlargement of the labia minora in its length depending on whether there upper, middle or lower third enlargement, Banwell classified labia minora hypertrophy as the following:

- Enlargement of the upper one-third of the labia minora is termed as type I hypertrophy.

- Enlargement of the middle one-third of the labia minora is termed as the type II hypertrophy.
- Enlargement of the lower one-third of the labia minora is termed as the type III hypertrophy.

This classification further includes symmetrical or asymmetrical hypertrophy depending on the symmetry of enlargement of the labia minora beyond the labia majora.

The takeoff between the labia minora and the perineum is also known as the labial perineal takeoff.

This emphasizes upon the distance between the posterior attachment of the labia minora and the perineum. This measurement can vary through a wide range and its proximity to the perineum can be classified as the following:

- If the posterior attachment of the labia is closest to the perineum, it is called *low* "labial perineal takeoff".
- If the posterior attachment of the labia is little farther from the perineum, it is called *medium* "labial perineal takeoff".
- If the posterior attachment of the labia is very far from the perineum, it is called *high* "labial perineal takeoff".

The aesthetic and functional implication of the low perineal takeoff is that it might be connected to the posterior fourchette, the knowledge of which is important for labioplasty procedures.

In addition to this, there may also be asymmetrical perineal takeoff.

Clitoral Labial Complex

- The clitoral labial complex is subjected to a wide variety of anatomic differences.
- Traditionally, the body of the clitoris and the clitoral hood should be small.
- The body of the clitoris and the hood might be hyperplastic and even disproportionate to the labia minora.
- There can be a vestigial clitoral hood, the significance of which is very pertinent in aesthetic procedure commonly done that is clitoral hood reduction.

Sexual Response Cycle

Understanding of the sexual response cycle is of importance to understand the changes associated with it to further treat functional and anatomic aberrancies of the same. It is divided into four phases:

1. Excitement or the arousal phase
2. Plateau phase
3. Orgasm
4. Resolution phase

Aesthetic Ideals

- Ideally there is no standard anatomic appearance or standard aesthetic appearance of the female genitalia or the intimate organs.
- An individual's body has its own standard based on her functional and aesthetic requirements. The desirable appearance and improvement of functionality in terms of comfort and self-esteem is to be regarded as the basis of aesthetic ideal. Proportionate rectifications more preferably undercorrection than overcorrection is the mainstay of vulvovaginal aesthetic, functional, and regenerative gynecology.

Applied Anatomy

- Prior to aesthetic treatment of the female genitalia, a thorough anatomical knowledge of the standards and the wide anatomic variations of the vulval complex is a must.
- Careful documentation of the anatomy prior to aesthetic treatment is mandatory.

CONCLUSION

It is of paramount importance that a thorough anatomical and physiological knowledge should be considered the basis of any aesthetic management. With the wide range of normal anatomic variations it is the responsibility of the care provider to reassure a client about her physiological variations and the need of correction only when functional or aesthetic concern arises. Undercorrection is always better than overcorrection and that is possible only with the perfect eye to the vulvovaginal anatomy. The procedural learning curve associated with this stream of aesthetic, functional and regenerative gynecology may be short but in depth anatomical knowledge of the female genitalia is the very basic of a successful outcome of any treatment revolving around the very sensitive vulvovaginal and urogenital complex.

REFERENCES

1. Motakef S, Rodriguez-Feliz J, Chung MT, Ingargiola MJ, Wong VW, Patel A. Vaginal labiaplasty: current practices and a simplified classification system for labial protrusion. Plast Reconstr Surg. 2015;135(3):774-88.
2. Banwell PE. Anatomy and classification of the female genitalia: implications for surgical management. In: Hamori CA, Banwell PE, Alinsod R (Eds). Female Cosmetic Genital Surgery: Concepts, Classification, and Techniques. New York: Thieme Publishers; 2017. pp. 14-7.

CHAPTER 5

Counseling and Consenting in Cosmetic Gynecology

Bela Shah Jain, Naval Milind Shah

INTRODUCTION

Cosmetic gynecology, also known as, aesthetic and regenerative gynecology is a new and emerging branch of medicine. It includes surgical and nonsurgical procedures to enhance not just the appearance of the female genital area but also improve the sexual function in females and thereby improvement in overall quality of life.[1]

The field of cosmetic gynecology has undergone significant growth in recent years, spurred by advancements in medical technology, increased public awareness, financial independence in women, and shifting societal norms regarding body aesthetics. The growing demand for these procedures underscores the importance of establishing robust counseling protocols and ensuring informed consent to address patients' needs, concerns, and expectations effectively. This chapter explores the nuanced aspects of counseling and consent in cosmetic gynecology, aiming to provide a comprehensive understanding of how healthcare providers can navigate these processes ethically and effectively.

UNDERSTANDING PATIENT MOTIVATIONS

Patient motivations for seeking cosmetic gynecological procedures are multifaceted and deeply personal. While dissatisfaction with genital appearance is a common driver, other factors such as functional discomfort, sexual dysfunction, and psychological distress also play significant roles.[2] Cultural and societal influences, including social media and societal norms, further shape patients' perceptions of genital aesthetics and contribute to their motivations for seeking intervention. Understanding these diverse motivations requires healthcare providers to adopt a holistic approach, acknowledging the complex interplay of psychological, social, and cultural factors that influence patients' attitudes toward their bodies.

It enables healthcare providers to tailor counseling and treatment plans to meet the unique needs of each patient.

INDIAN SCENARIO

In the Indian context, cosmetic gynecology has emerged as a rapidly growing field, reflecting the evolving attitudes toward female genital aesthetics and women's health. Traditionally, discussions about female genitalia were considered taboo in Indian society. However, with increasing globalization and exposure to Western influences, there has been a gradual shift toward greater acceptance and openness regarding discussions about intimate health and appearance.[3]

Cultural influences play a significant role in shaping patient motivations and treatment preferences in India. Traditional beliefs surrounding femininity, modesty, and marital expectations contribute to the demand for certain cosmetic gynecological procedures. For example, hymenoplasty, a procedure aimed at reconstructing the hymen, is often sought by women as they prepare for marriage to adhere to societal expectations of virginity.[4] Additionally, procedures such as labiaplasty and vaginal tightening may be motivated by cultural ideals of beauty and modesty, as well as concerns about sexual satisfaction and marital harmony.[5]

However, alongside cultural influences, there is a growing emphasis on individual autonomy and empowerment in India, particularly among urban, educated women. Women are increasingly seeking cosmetic gynecological procedures to address personal concerns, improve self-confidence, and enhance their quality of life.[3] Factors such as childbirth-related changes, aging, and changes in body image contribute to the demand for procedures aimed at restoring genital aesthetics and function.[6]

Healthcare providers in India face unique challenges in providing cosmetic gynecology services while navigating cultural sensitivities and upholding ethical standards. It is essential for providers to offer culturally sensitive counseling and informed consent processes that respect patients' values and preferences.[7] By fostering open communication and understanding, providers can empower women to make informed decisions about their bodies and achieve optimal outcomes in cosmetic gynecological care.

INFORMED CONSENT PROCESS

Informed consent serves as the cornerstone of ethical practice in cosmetic gynecology, ensuring that patients are fully informed about the nature, risks, and benefits of the procedures they are considering. It holds extreme importance particularly in the context of cosmetic gynecology, where patients' expectations and perceptions of outcomes can vary widely. The informed consent process involves more than just obtaining a signature on a form; it requires active engagement with patients, providing them with comprehensive information in a manner that is accessible and understandable. This includes discussing the goals and expected outcomes of the procedure, potential risks and complications, alternative treatment options, and postoperative care requirements.[8]

Healthcare providers must ensure that patients fully understand the nature of the procedure including its anatomical implications and potential impact on sexual function and satisfaction. Patients' emotional state and cognitive capacity should be taken into consideration during this process and the communication strategies should be tailored accordingly. Moreover, the consent process should be documented thoroughly to serve as a legal and ethical safeguard for both patients and providers.

PHOTO DOCUMENTATION

Photo documentation has become extremely pertinent in cosmetic procedures, which not only acts as a valid legal document, but also helps patients assess the outcome of surgery. Photographs help to increase patient satisfaction, since they allow patients to appreciate the change they have undergone and to ascertain whether they have received the treatment they had assented to. They also safeguard doctors if certain aberrations or scars which were present prior to the surgery are attributed to the procedure undergone by the patient.

A valid written consent should be taken from all patients for photography or videography prior to any procedure.

The use of these photos or videos for publications, research, or educational purposes should be with prior consent of the patient and the identity of the patient should be concealed.

ETHICAL CONSIDERATIONS

Ethical considerations permeate every aspect of cosmetic gynecology practice, from patient selection to postoperative care. Healthcare providers must adhere to ethical principles, such as beneficence, nonmaleficence, and respect for patient autonomy throughout the treatment process.[9] This includes prioritizing patient safety, ensuring transparency in communication, and respecting patients' right to make informed decisions about their bodies. Additionally, providers must be vigilant against potential conflicts of interest and avoid performing unnecessary procedures for financial gain.

COUNSELING STRATEGIES

Effective counseling is essential for preparing patients for cosmetic gynecological procedures and managing their expectations. Counseling sessions should be tailored to the individual needs and preferences of each patient, providing a safe and supportive environment for open dialogue.[10] Preprocedural counseling sessions offer an opportunity for healthcare providers to educate patients about genital anatomy, variations, and normalcy, dispelling myths and misconceptions that may contribute to body image issues or unrealistic expectations.[2] Moreover, counseling sessions provide a platform for discussing alternative treatment options, including nonsurgical approaches and psychological support, for patients with underlying psychological issues or unrealistic expectations.[10] Providers must employ active listening skills, empathy, and cultural sensitivity to establish rapport with patients and address their concerns effectively. In addition to individual counseling sessions, group counseling or educational seminars may also be beneficial allowing patients to share their experiences and support one another during the treatment process. Collaborating with mental health professionals can further enhance the efficacy of counseling interventions and support patients' overall well-being.

MANAGING UNREALISTIC EXPECTATIONS

Despite thorough counseling and informed consent processes, some patients may harbor unrealistic expectations regarding the outcomes of cosmetic gynecological procedures. Providers must approach these situations with empathy and sensitivity, acknowledging patients' desires while also tempering unrealistic aspirations.[2] This may involve honest and transparent discussions about the limitations of medical interventions, the potential for unexpected outcomes, and the importance of self-acceptance and body positivity. Providers should strive to empower patients to make informed decisions that align with their values and goals, while also providing ongoing support and guidance throughout the treatment process.

The SOGC published a guideline[8] intended to provide evidence-based direction for Canadian gynecologists, primary healthcare providers, and surgeons offering cosmetic vaginal and vulvar procedures that fall outside the traditional realm of medically indicated reconstructions. The guideline laid out recommendations as shown in **Box 1**.

BOX 1: The SOGC published a guideline laid out recommendations.[8]

- Health providers should play an important role in educating women about their anatomy and helping them appreciate individual variations including transitions through the reproductive life cycle (strong, low)
- For women who present with requests for vaginal cosmetic procedures, a complete medical, sexual, and gynecological history must be obtained, and the absence of any major sexual or psychological dysfunction, including body dysmorphic disorder, should be ascertained. Any possibility of coercion or exploitation must also be ruled out (strong, high)
- There is insufficient evidence to support any female genital cosmetic surgery or procedure to improve sexual satisfaction and/or self-image. Physicians choosing to proceed with these cosmetic procedures should not promote these surgeries for the enhancement of sexual function or self-image (strong, low)
- Hymenoplasty is a surgical procedure that is not medically indicated. Counseling of the woman is paramount to provide both reassurance and accurate information that the procedure does not reliably result in the desired outcome of bleeding at first marital intercourse (strong, moderate)
- Laser is not recommended for genitourinary syndrome of menopause or cosmetic genital indications without further rigorous short- and long-term clinical research (strong, low)
- Counseling should be a priority for women requesting female genital cosmetic surgery and procedures that are not medically indicated. Topics should include normal variation and physiological changes over the lifespan, as well as the possibility of unintended consequences of cosmetic surgery to the genital area. The lack of both high-quality evidence and data regarding outcomes should also be discussed and considered as part of the informed decision-making process (strong, high)
- Caution should be used in advertising female genital cosmetic surgeries, to ensure such advertising is factual and not misleading (strong, high)
- Physicians who see adolescents requesting female genital cosmetic surgery require additional expertise in counseling adolescents (strong, low)
- Female genital cosmetic surgery must not be performed until genital maturity (strong, low)
- Surgery is not considered cosmetic if there is documented functional impairment, which may include structural, psychological, and/or anatomical concerns (strong, moderate)

(SOGC: Society of Obstetricians and Gynaecologists of Canada)

CONCLUSION

Counseling and consent are fundamental components of ethical practice in cosmetic gynecology, ensuring that patients are empowered to make informed decisions about their bodies. By understanding patient motivations, prioritizing patient autonomy, and fostering open communication, healthcare providers can navigate the complexities of this field with integrity and compassion. As the field of cosmetic gynecology continues to evolve, it is essential for providers to remain vigilant in upholding ethical standards and delivering patient-centered care that promotes both physical and psychological well-being.

REFERENCES

1. Joshi S. Counselling Before Cosmetic Gynecology. In: Jindal P, Malhotra N, Joshi S (Eds). Aesthetic and Regenerative Gynecology. Singapore: Springer Nature Singapore; 2022. pp. 23-7.
2. Goodman MP, Placik OJ, Benson III RH, Miklos JR, Moore RD, Jason RA, et al. A large multicenter outcome study of female genital plastic surgery. J Sex Med. 2010; 7(4 Pt 1):1565-77.
3. Desai SA, Dixit VV. Audit of female genital aesthetic surgery: changing trends in India. J Obstet Gynaecol India. 2018;68(3):214-20.
4. Dhaketa M, Acharya S, Taksande AB, Prasad R, Munjewar PK, Wanjari MB, et al. Hymenoplasty in India: A

Comprehensive Review of Contemporary Trends and Impact on Young Adults. Cureus. 2023;15(7):e41852.
5. Eftekhar T, Hajibabaei M, Veisi F, Ghanbari Z, Montazeri A. Body image, sexual function, and sexual satisfaction among couples before and after gynecologic cosmetic surgery. J Family Reprod Health. 2021;15(4):252-7.
6. Jindal P, Kundal I. Introduction to the Rising field of Aesthetic and Regenerative Gynecology. In: Jindal P, Malhotra N, Joshi S (Eds). Aesthetic and Regenerative Gynecology. Singapore: Springer Nature Singapore; 2022. pp. 1-6.
7. Crow K, Matheson L, Steed A. Informed consent and truth-telling: cultural directions for healthcare providers. JONA: J Nurs Adm. 2000;30(3):148-52.
8. Shaw D, Allen L, Chan C, Kives S, Popadiuk C, Robertson D, et al. Guideline No. 423: Female genital cosmetic surgery and procedures. J Obstet Gynaecol Can. 2022;44(2):204-14.e1.
9. Varkey B. Principles of clinical ethics and their application to practice. Med Princ Pract. 2021;30(1):17-28.
10. Ilardo ML, Speciale A. The community pharmacist: perceived barriers and patient-centered care communication. Int J Environ Res Public Health. 2020;17(2):536.

CHAPTER 6

Laser and Its Role in Aesthetic and Regenerative Gynecology

Preeti Jindal, Vivek Malhotra, Cherry Malhi

INTRODUCTION

The use of laser technology in gynecology has become widespread since the CO_2 laser was initially used by Kaplan and colleagues in 1973 for treatment of cervical erosions.[1] Laser consists of three main components, i.e., a lasing medium (solid, liquid, or gas) according to which laser is named, an energy source and an optical resonator. Many advancements in laser technology have been made and several types of lasers are now available like the CO_2, neodymium-doped:yttrium aluminum garnet (Nd:YAG), potassium titanyl phosphate (KTP), argon, diode, etc. Laser beam can be focused on target tissue with minimal impact on the surrounding area. Laser and other energy-based devices raise the temperature of target tissue to certain level and hence achieve the desired effects like rejuvenation, cutting, coagulation, or ablation.

HISTORY

Laser is an acronym that stands for *light amplification by the stimulated emission of radiation*, a concept that was developed by Einstein and popularized by Maser in 1917.[2] The first working laser developed by Theodore Maiman in 1960 used ruby as the active medium, and in 1961 the CO_2 laser was introduced.[3,4] The CO_2 laser was used in gynecology in 1973 for treatment of cervical erosions, later by Bellina for treatment of cervical intraepithelial neoplasia (CIN), as well as for microsurgery of the fallopian tube;[5,6] since then it has evolved tremendously.

LASER PHYSICS

The basic mechanism of laser beam generation involves three key processes: stimulated emission, population inversion, and feedback mechanism which results in the amplification and coherent emission of light, forming the laser beam **(Fig. 1)**. Firstly, stimulated emission—electrons in the gain medium (atoms or molecules) are excited to higher energy levels. When these electrons return to lower energy levels, they release photons. Stimulated photons trigger the release of additional photons with the same energy, phase, and direction. Secondly, population

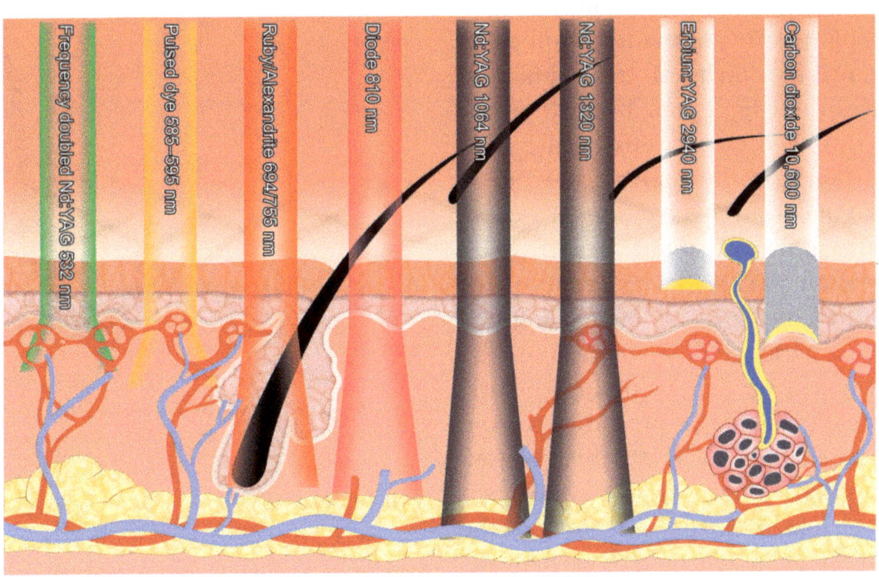

Fig. 1: Energy penetration and clinical effect of commonly used cutaneous lasers.

inversion—achieving the population inversion is crucial. More electrons are in higher energy state than in lower energy states. This is achieved through external energy input known as pumping, which can be optical, electrical, or chemical. Thirdly, feedback mechanism is obtained by placing the gain medium between two mirrors, forming an optical cavity. One mirror is highly reflective, and the other is partially transparent, allowing portion of the emitted photons to exit as laser beam. The photons reflecting between mirrors undergo stimulated emission reinforcing each other and creating a coherent intense laser beam.

Hence, a laser beam is coherent (light traveling in one phase in respect to time and space), monochromatic (single wavelength), and collimated (narrow beam of light in parallel unidirectional fashion). Lasers are classified by various criteria like gain medium, pumping mechanism, and application. Common classifications are:

- Based on gain medium—solid state lasers (Nd:YAG, Ruby, and Ti:sapphire), gas lasers (Helium-Neon, CO_2, excimer), liquid or dye lasers (Rhodamine 6G dye laser), and semiconductor lasers (diode).
- Based on pumping mechanism—optical pumping (Nd:YAG), electrical discharge pumping (Excimer), and chemical pumping (COIL) laser.
- Based on applications—industrial lasers, medical, military, and scientific lasers
- Based on output characteristics—continuous wave (CW) lasers and pulsed lasers

LASER–TISSUE INTERACTION

Laser in body works by selective photothermolysis. The absorption of light (photo) in pigmented molecules (chromophores—hemoglobin, melanin, tattoo ink, and water) transforms absorbed light into heat (thermo) causing destruction (lysis) of target cells by the high temperature. Fractional photothermolysis is when a portion or "fraction" of the skin is heated in microscopic columns creating *microthermal zones (MTZs)*. The untreated tissue between MTZs acts as reservoir of regenerative cells helping in tissue repair and healing.

There are three basic parameters that determine the amount of energy being delivered to the tissue. The first is the *wattage*. For most gynecologic procedures using the CO_2 laser, one rarely exceeds 20–30 W, which is used primarily for excision purposes. The second parameter is *time*. The longer the laser remains focused on one spot, the more energy is applied to that area. To limit tissue damage, especially in critical areas, one can simply move the beam back-and-forth, or select an intermittent, timed pulse mode, usually in fractions of a second. The third parameter that can be controlled is the *spot size* of the beam. As one gets closer to the target area, the spot size is made smaller, producing a more intense effect.

The combination of watts (power) and spot size determines the rate of tissue interaction. The higher the power density, the greater the laser's ability to vaporize and cut. This concept is expressed in watts/cm^2 (unit/area) and referred to as intensity or power density. Power density is, therefore, inversely proportional to the area of the spot size and to the beam diameter. Doubling the beam diameter reduces the power density to one-fourth. Conversely, by decreasing the diameter of the spot size, the power density is increased by four times.

Three types of tissue injury may be identified following a laser wound. The zone of vaporization is characterized by an absence of tissue and a V-shaped defect, because energy is greater in the center of the beam than on the perimeter. Immediately below the zone of vaporization is a fixed zone of stromal necrosis measuring approximately 50–100 μm in depth (in CO_2 laser), regardless of the crater's extent. Within this zone, small vessels (<1 mm) are sealed. The third zone is one of reversible injury or potential repair. Laser wounds are clean, produce minimal tissue damage, and cannot be compared with cautery wounds, in which substantial devitalized debris remains behind. Therefore, laser and scalpel wounds are similar **(Fig. 2)**.

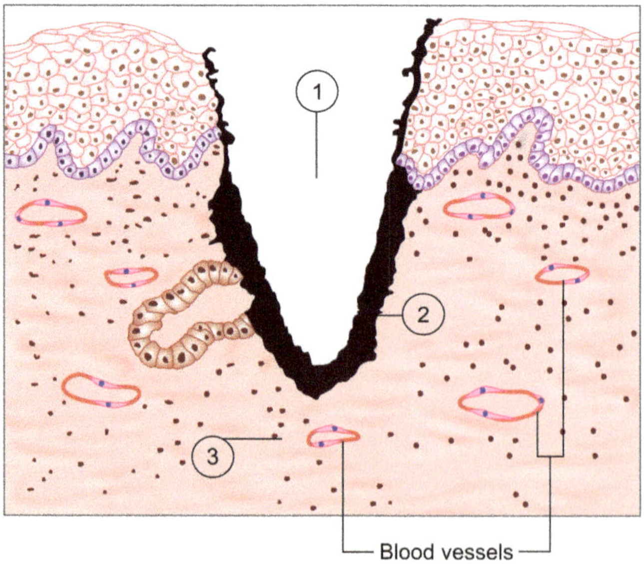

Fig. 2: A CO_2 laser beam produces a spot or crater in which three zones of tissue injury may be identified. (1) Vaporization, (2) Necrosis, and (3) Reversible injury.

CO_2 LASER

Of the various lasers available, the CO_2 laser is the most versatile and is extremely safe because of its limited depth of penetration (0.1–0.5 mm) and lateral thermal damage (0.5 mm). This allows use of the CO_2 laser in delicate areas where cautery would be unsafe, such as the bladder, lateral side wall near the ureter, and bowel serosa. Besides vaporization, the CO_2 laser can be used for excision or incision by increasing the power density. The possibilities are almost unlimited, thanks to its great vaporization, ablation, cutting, and coagulation capacity.

The CO_2 laser may serve three principal functions: as a cutting or excisional instrument, as a vaporizing or ablating instrument, and as a defocused cauterizing instrument. Though this is one of most versatile, effective, and useful laser in gynecology, there are few disadvantages of it too.

Disadvantages of the CO_2 laser are wavelength limitation as it works at 10.6 μm only. As it emits invisible infrared radiation it is not visible to eye, the helium–neon beam is added to it to give it red color. Focusing of the helium–neon beam and evacuation of smoke referred to as "plume," is needed to allow adequate visualization of the target. Machines are large, bulky, and costly. Also it is very powerful ablative instrument, so safe controlled use is required for prevention of harm to patient, operator, and staff.

LASER TREATMENT IN AESTHETIC GYNECOLOGY

"Light Amplification by Stimulated Emission of Radiation" (LASER) has been worldwide applied in medical science in past decades. It is basically harnessed energy that can be channelized for cutting, coagulating, warming, heating, and vaporizing.[7] Laser in cosmetic gynecology is used to treat the conditions, such as stress urinary incontinence, genitourinary syndrome of menopause, mild pelvic organ prolapse, recurrent vaginal infections, vulvodynia, dyspareunia, vulval rejuvenation, hair removal, and vaginal rejuvenation.

Noncosmetic benefits of laser are in surgeries as scalpel and energy source, lichen sclerosis, wart removals, Bartholin abscess drainage, etc.

ADVANTAGES OF LASER PROCEDURES

These procedures are noninvasive, painless, stitchless, coffee break procedures, and less expensive than surgeries.

CONCLUSION

Laser use has revolutionized the aesthetic gynecology. If used properly it can be a very useful tool in the armamentarium of every gynecologist.

REFERENCES

1. Kaplan I, Goldman J, Ger R. The treatment of erosions of the uterine cervix by means of the CO_2 laser. Obstet Gynecol. 1973;41(5):795-6.
2. Einstein A. Zur Quantentheorie der Strahlung. Physikalische Zeitschrift. 1917;18:121-8.
3. Maiman TH. Stimulated optical radiation in ruby. Nature. 1960;187:493-4.
4. Patel CKN. Continuous wavelength action on vibrational rotational transitions of CO_2. Phys Rev. 1964;136: A1187-A1193.
5. Bellina JH. Gynecology and the laser. Contemp Obstet Gynecol. 1974;4:24-4.
6. Bellina JH. Microsurgery of the fallopian tube with the carbon dioxide laser: Analysis of 230 cases with a two year follow-up. Lasers Surg Med. 1983;3:255-60.
7. Jindal P, Malhotra N, Joshi S (Eds). Aesthetic and Regenerative Gynecology. Singapore: Springer Nature Singapore; 2022.

CHAPTER 7

Diode Laser in Cosmetic Gynecology

Molina Patel, Nayana Patel, Niket Patel

INTRODUCTION

Developments in both technology and fashion have induced seasonal changes in the notion of beauty in the face of her unspoken issues. A silent but strong revolution to battle the age-related genital subfunctioning has started in the common woman, which aims and wants genital aesthetics and best sexual functioning at all times in her life. This has paved way to the increasing popularity and demand of the super specialized field of "aesthetic and regenerative gynecology."

Fluctuations and decline in sex hormones (mainly estrogen), trauma from childbirth, ignorance toward macro and micronutrient supplementation, lack of adequate rest, physically and mentally strenuous lifestyle, genetics are a few factors which make women vulnerable to alterations in genital anatomy and functionality with age.[1]

While conventional surgical options such as vaginoplasty, transobturator tapes (TOT), transvaginal tapes (TVT), sling surgeries and medical management options vaginal estrogen creams, hyaluronic acid and isoflavone lubricants, vaginal gels, pelvic physiotherapy, acupuncture etc., are available, women now opt for quicker, more convincing and newer options such as energy-based systems for their intimate issues. They are wary of surgery due to the risk, expense, and downtime involved.

These devices have opened up a new market for nonsurgical vulvovaginal correction procedures. Moreover, energy delivery followed by medical therapy (as maintenance) in the vaginal canal provides long-term relief and better outcome in combination.

Let us understand the various energy-based devices that are available in the field of aesthetic gynecology **(Table 1)**.

TABLE 1: Various energy-based devices available in the field of aesthetic gynecology.

(A) LASERS (light amplification by the stimulated emission of radiation) Diode LASER Er:YAG LASER Carbon dioxide (CO_2)		*Working principle:* • Angiogenesis • Microvascularization • Tissue oxygenation • Tissue lubrication • Tissue sensitivity
(B) Radiofrequency-based devices		
Monopolar	Bipolar	Multipolar
(C) HIFU (high intensity focused ultrasound)		
Guided waves		*Shear waves*

LASER

LASER "light amplification by stimulated emission of radiation" has been used in gynecology for >40 years. It is well established for the treatment of human papillomavirus (HPV)-related cervical lesions/erosions, genital wart removal etc. More recently, their use has been extrapolated for genitourinary syndrome of menopause (GSM), vaginal laxity syndrome, lichen sclerosus, vulvodynia, overactive bladder, mild-to-moderate stress urinary incontinence (SUI), pelvic organ prolapse etc.

Several ex vivo studies have suggested that LASER has the potential to modify vaginal tissue characteristics. In this regard, LASERS have been utilized and marketed as a treatment or therapy for vaginal rejuvenation and "designer LASER vaginoplasty" by the aesthetics industry.

A diode laser is a semiconductor device that emits coherent and monochromatic light in different arrangements. Depending on the wavelength, range, versatility, beam quality, size, cost and application, output energy requirement, there are >15 types of diode lasers.[2]

The diode used for laser hair removal uses 755 nm and 810 nm. However, the photonics 15 W/1470 nm diode laser has been explored for vaginal cosmetology as a quick, safe, minimally invasive, and highly effective energy delivery system.[3]

WORKING PRINCIPLE

- Intralesional fiber system that causes localized heating within a narrow range.

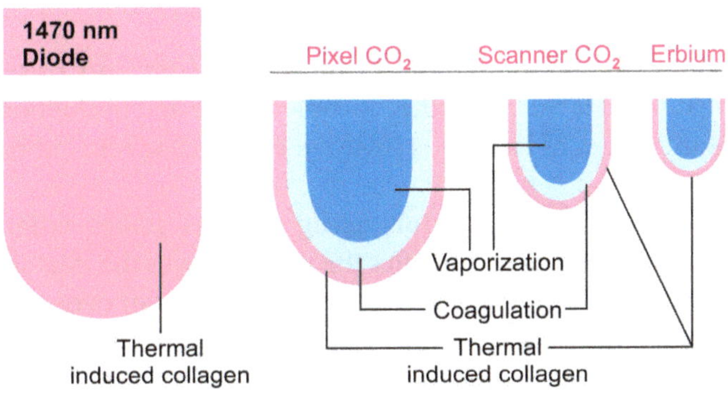

Fig. 1: Mechanism of treatment.

- Photothermal laser mucosa tissue interaction
- Water, hemoglobin particularly deoxyhemoglobin are chromophores for diode laser.
- Depth of penetration is up to 3 mm.
- Mode—continuous with 360° emission of radial light
- Local tissue moisture is vaporized + controlled thermal effect → bio modulating effect that stimulates neocollagenesis + regenerates connective tissue and epithelium → tissue remodeling.
- Outer sheath of the probe is single/multiple use (after proper sterilization)
  - Diagram from slide: **Figure 1**
  - *Description:* Mechanism of action of diode laser in comparison to CO_2 fractional laser and Erbium YAG laser

QUALIFICATION PARAMETERS

- Counseling
- Detailed history
- General health consultation
- Pregnancy test
- Evaluating for inclusion and exclusion criteria

Counseling

This is the most crucial part of any therapeutic intervention in the field of aesthetic gynecology. The following heads must be covered in detail in your counseling session with the patient before, during, and after each session:

- Benefits of undergoing laser therapy
- Understanding the patients' expectations from the laser therapy
- Pre/post precautions that the patient has to take.
- *Written and informed consent*
- Safety—patient must be ensured that energy-based devices such as diode laser are safe and noninvasive.
- Questionnaires—patient must be informed that questionnaires will be given to the patients to document their subjective response before and after the laser therapy.
- Patient must be explained that adjunct therapy such as pelvic physiotherapy/+ TENS (transcutaneous electrical nerve stimulation) therapy/+ platelet rich plasma (PRP) may be considered along with laser therapy to yield maximum results.

Detailed History

Patient must be asked about:

- History of taking any treatments including hormonal treatments
- Family history of cervical malignancy
- Recurrent urine/cervical/vaginal infections
- The last PAP (Papanicolaou test) smear report must be checked, if not, then fresh PAP test must be taken.

Examination

- A per speculum and per vaginum examination should always be done prior to starting laser therapy.
- Prolapse, if any, must be analyzed by pelvic organ prolapse quantification (POP Q) classification.
- Anatomical abnormalities of the cervix/vagina must be noted.
- Presence of intrauterine device should be noted.
- *Pregnancy test must be done when necessary.*

Inclusion Criteria

Motivated patients with genuine indication who consent to and also understand the nuances of these new energy-based devices.

Exclusion Criteria

- Active HPV/HSV (herpes simplex virus)
- Vulvar intraepithelial neoplasia (VIN) findings
- Acute vaginitis
- Genital malignancy
- Uncontrolled vaginal bleeding
- Pregnancy
- Recent vaginal injury/bleeding
- Patients on menstrual periods
- *Patients with body dysmorphic syndrome*
- *Patients with unrealistic expectations*

INDICATIONS OF DIODE LASER

- *Genitourinary syndrome of menopause*[4]
  - *Protocol*
    - 3–4 sittings, each a month apart
    - *Each sitting:* 3–5 passes of the laser probe (depending on the severity of atrophy)
    - *Power output:* 3–4 W
    - *Mode:* Pulse/repeat/continuous
    - On time = 2 seconds; Off time = 1 second
- *Stress urinary incontinence*
  - *Protocol*
    - *3–4 sittings @ 4–5 passes per sitting; 4 weeks apart*
    - *Site of application is slightly specific for SUI*
      - *Three positions:* 11–12–01 O'clock
        - 1 cm beyond mid-urethra
        - Directly under mid-urethra
        - 1 cm before mid-urethra
      - *Power output:* 3–4 W
      - *Mode:* Pulse/repeat/continuous
      - On time = 2 seconds; Off time = 1 second
- *Inflamed episiotomy/cesarean section scars/keloids*
  - Tissue ablation followed by coagulation of local blood vessels causes reduction of inflammation and causes gradual shrinkage and improves texture of the scar/keloids.
  - Local anesthetic agent is applied for 15 minutes (for example Prilox cream - 25 mg of Lignocaine + 25 mg of Prilocaine).
  - Power output is adjusted according to the scar/keloid hardness, generally starting from 3 W and increasing up to 12 W. The laser is targeted at multiple entry points along the scar at a distance of 4–6 mm.
  - Monthly sittings are continued until a satisfactory effect is achieved.
- Labial wrinkles
- Recurrent vaginal infections
- Vaginal laxity syndrome
- Dyspareunia
- Lichen sclerosus of the vagina
- Surgical indications:
  - Labiaplasty/clitoral hood reduction
  - Wart/skin tag removal

Note: The treatment protocol must be customized according to the case at the discretion and judgement of the treating aesthetic gynecologist.

SCALES FOR EVALUATION

While histopathological tissue biopsy (pre and post-treatment) is the most idea documentation and evaluation of the effect of laser, it is invasive and can be refused by patients.

Subjective evaluation using various scales when documented before and after the therapy, gives the treating aesthetic gynecologist as well as the patient, an overview of the effect, and guide any scope of improvement in a particular area if needed.

Every subjective scale is specific for its indication. They must be chosen accordingly, and few are as follows:

- VAS (visual analogue scale)
- International Consultation on Incontinence Questionnaire-Urinary Incontinence Short Form (ICIQ-UI SF) (*Gold Standard*)
- The urogenital distress inventory (UDI-6)
- Vaginal health index (VHI)
- Dermatology life quality index
- Female sexual function index (FSFI)

PRETREATMENT EVALUATION

Counseling same as above.

Post-treatment Instructions

- No sexual activity for at least 2–3 days
- Intravaginal hyaluronic acid/estrogen cream/isoflavone gel may be offered.
- Adequate hydration
- Take oral vitamin C supplements for the next 4–6 months
- Maintain good general health.
- Kegel exercises/TENS therapy started in conjunction in case of SUI.
- There might be slight blood-stained discharge in about few patients of severe atrophy in the early 3–5 days → reassurance.

ADVANTAGES OF DIODE LASER

- Compact and potable size
- Rhobust—a semi-conductor has no loose parts. So, the care needed in maintenance is much lesser than a resonator or gas/dye laser.
- Comparatively inexpensive—laser diodes are manufactured in billions and are cheaper than other types of laser.

- Available in different wavelengths—laser diodes can be manufactured in any wavelength based on its applicability.

SCIENTIFIC EVIDENCE

Research has demonstrated the tissue remodeling properties of fractional lasers in aesthetic medicine with the effect of stimulating the production of new elastin and collagen fibers.[5] However, publications and research evaluating the diode laser, specifically for vaginal cosmetology, are comparatively fewer.

A study by Sharma and Srivastav showed improvement in the vulvovaginal symptoms after analyzing the inflammatory and histopathological changes after superficial stress vascular laser diode laser. They concluded that after four diode laser treatment sessions, histopathological changes were significant and deep. Glycogenization of the vaginal epithelium, increase in the angioblastic fibroblastic activity, and reduction of inflammation of menopause are some of the demonstrable changes after diode laser therapy.

- *Therapeutic goal:*
  - Relief of symptoms
  - Restoration of the vaginal environment to a healthy state
  - Restoration of vaginal function—lubrication, tightening, and sexual function

CONCLUSION

Diode laser is a promising energy-based device in the field of aesthetic gynecology. It is safe, effective, and an advanced new age non-surgical tool to offer to women with various intimate concerns. Adequate training, appropriate counseling, ideal patient selection, and cost effectiveness of treatment are important determinants of treatment outcomes.

REFERENCES

1. Kingsberg SA, Krychman M, Graham S, Bernick B, Mirkin S. The Women's EMPOWER Survey: Identifying Women's Perceptions on Vulvar and Vaginal Atrophy and Its Treatment. J Sex Med. 2017;14(3):413-24.
2. Ruffolo AF, Braga A, Torella M, Frigerio M, Cimmino C, De Rosa A, et al. Vaginal laser therapy for female stress urinary incontinence: new solutions for a well-known issue-a concise review. Medicina (Kaunas). 2022;58(4):512.
3. Guerette NL. Safety and efficacy of hybrid fractional laser (1470 nm and 2940 nm) for symptoms of genitourinary syndrome of menopause: 12 month prospective multi-center study. J Minim Invasive Gynecol. 2019;26:S70.
4. Garzon S, Apostolopoulos V, Stojanovska L, Ferrari F, Mathyk BA, Laganà AS. Non-oestrogenic modalities to reverse urogenital aging. Menopausal Rev. 2021;20: 140-7.
5. Bojanini B, Juan F, Mejía C, Alexandra M. Laser treatment of vaginal atrophy in post-menopause and post-gynecological cancer patients. Laser Health Acad. 2014;1:65-71.

CHAPTER 8

Radio Frequency in Cosmetic Gynecology

Shradha Goel

INTRODUCTION

Radio frequency (RF) is a form of energy-based device using electromagnetic form of current that can be delivered through various tissue types to generate thermal energy.[1] RF has been used in medicine in 1920s for electrocautery.[2] It has been used in nearly all medical specialties, including cardiology, urology, dermatology, plastic surgery, and oncology.[1] It is used in collagen remodeling in shoulder ligaments instability in orthopedics.[3] Over the last 20 years, its use in aesthetic surgery has increased.

Nonsurgical modes in cosmetic gynecology are gaining popularity by eliminating downtimes, high surgery costs, incision, and anesthesia related risks. Specifically, the remarkable evolution of aesthetic gynecology has advanced the high-intensity focused ultrasound (HIFU), RF, and laser therapies to provide female patients with safe and minimally invasive treatment options capable of addressing dyspareunia, postcoital bleeding, reduced lubrication, and urinary incontinence, among other genitourinary syndrome (GUS) of menopause symptoms. While laser, HIFU, and RF technologies proved to be useful for those who need traditional surgical cosmetic gynecology methods but do not desire them in favor of daycare procedures. RF emerges as a superior treatment technology, given its ability to deliver controlled thermal energy for tissue remodeling.

Nonsurgical modes to treat skin laxity were ablative and nonablative lasers, by injuring the epidermis and dermis which causes dermal collagen remodeling and secondary skin tightening. In properly selected patients, lasers can provide excellent skin resurfacing and dermal remodeling.[4] However, the energy and subsequent heat required to generate significant skin tightening at the dermal level cannot be accomplished without injury to the epidermis—leading to complications, such as burns and irreversible pigmentation changes.[5] For this reason, lasers are limited to lighter Fitzpatrick skin types, excluding darker skinned patients.

Radio frequency devices are designed to offer precise tissue remodeling, making it most suitable for cosmetic gynecology patients; whose demand is precision.[6] RF is nonablative, making it suitable for varying skin tones and avoiding hypopigmentation and hyperpigmentation.[7] Its effects are independent of skin color and type; therefore, they have a broader spectrum of patients compared to other noninvasive and minimally invasive devices. Vaginal laxity is best treated with RF therapy since it generates heat beneath the skin at varying degrees and at varying intensities.

In 2002, the Food and Drug Administration (FDA) approved the first monopolar RF device for facial wrinkle reduction using 6 MHz device (ThermaCool; Thermage, Inc., Hayward, California).[8] Since 2002, more sophisticated RF devices have been created with additional safety measures to deliver RF radiation in bipolar, multipolar, and fractional forms.

Thus, RF proves to be the novel solution to noninvasive cosmetic gynecology; particularly regarding the genitourinary syndrome of menopause, vulval tightening, vaginal laxity, stress urinary incontinence, and even for cancer patients. Being minimally invasive, independent of skin color and type, and with varying depth of heat generation; RF application has emerged as an ideal treatment option in aesthetic gynecology.

RADIO FREQUENCY: MECHANISM OF ACTION

Since RF uses an electric current instead of a light source, it is different from lasers. In dermatology, it is often used to treat cellulite,[9] rhytides, acne vulgaris, and skin laxity.

Radio frequency technology includes any electromagnetic wave frequencies within the range of 3–300 GHz.[10] An RF field is composed of both electrical and magnetic components. The frequency range of RF devices used in skin rejuvenation ranges from approximately 0.5–40 MHz. An RF device's frequency is crucial, and it has an inverse relationship with penetration depth. It is known that the lower frequencies have higher penetration rates. So, the penetration depth of 60 MHz frequency will remain superficial compared to that of a frequency of 6 MHz.

Radio frequency does not use selective photothermolysis[11] to target particular chromophores like lasers do. Due to varying tissue resistance or impedance to the electromagnetic current, RF produces heat. This means that heat is produced when the tissues' inherent resistance converts the electrical current to thermal energy as dictated by the following formula:

$$\textit{(Ohm's law): Energy (J)} = \textit{Current}^2 \times \textit{Resistance} \times \textit{Time}$$ [12]

Adipose tissue, for instance, has a higher tissue impedance than muscle, and for a given quantity of energy, it will produce more heat than muscle which has lower impedance for a given amount of time.[11] In fact, when RF energy is directed to subdermal adipose tissue, it has been shown to generate temperatures 7-fold higher than those generated by the dermis, leading to fat necrosis with epidermal preservation.[13]

There are two mechanisms which allow RF energy to cause contraction in soft tissue and skin:

1. Instantaneous hydrogen bond cleavage in the triple helix of collagen, resulting in the collagen fibrils becoming thicker and shorter
2. Initiation of a wound healing cascade to enhance blood flow, collagen remodeling, and elastin reorganization over the next 3–4 months.

Electron microscopy evaluation of RF-heated collagen further demonstrates breakage of intramolecular bonds in the collagen fibrils, leading to increased diameter and shortening.[14] Also, messenger ribonucleic acid studies show up regulation of expression of the collagen gene following RF irradiation of the skin.[15]

At 43°C for 10 minutes, there is delayed adipocyte cellular death, while at 45°C for 3 minutes, 60% of adipocytes lose viability. This procedure allows the RF device to move clockwise and counterclockwise, covering the middle and distal areas and inducing heating that enhances microcirculation, promotes uniformity in subdermal fat distribution, and resultantly prompts vaginal and vulval skin tensioning and tightening.

Clinical studies and animal studies demonstrate that subdermal temperatures from 65°C to 68°C and skin surface temperatures ranging from 38°C to 42°C are required to obtain optimal contraction. Further, it is postulated that heated fibroblasts may be stimulated to produce collagen.[16] Importantly, if temperatures exceed a critical heat threshold, there is the potential for collagen ablation and full-thickness injury.[17] There is no single shrinkage temperature of collagen contraction.[17] Rather, the delivery of RF energy is a function of time and temperature to allow for maximal epidermal protection while optimally heating the dermal collagen. For every 5°C decrease in temperature, a 10× increase in time is required to achieve a comparable collagen contraction.[17] RF volumetric dermal heating is favorable because it avoids targeting specific dermal targets and instead leverages various tissue impedances to generate desired heat and contraction.[18] This nonspecificity means that RF is safe to use in all Fitzpatrick skin types.

COMPARISON OF DEPTH PENETRATION OF VARIOUS LASERS IN COSMETIC GYNECOLOGY

There are various lasers used in the treatment of vaginal laxity and genitourinary syndrome of menopause **(Fig. 1)**. RF proves to be the safest and ideal amongst all types of lasers as it has following unique features:

- Maximum and safe penetration as beam can reach maximum depth till dermis, subcutaneous fat with no risk of burning superficial musculoaponeurotic system (SMAS)[19]
- Epidermal protection with no risk of burns of skin unlike HIFU.

High-intensity focused ultrasound has varying degree of penetration till SMAS, with no controlled cooling at epidermis and may cause deep burns at epidermis and SMAS.

TYPES OF RADIO FREQUENCY

Radio frequency can be monopolar delivery, bipolar delivery, combination, or Fractional RF delivery.

Present-day RF devices come with two main electrode configurations—monopolar and bipolar.

Monopolar Radio Frequency Devices

One active electrode in a monopolar device transmits the electromagnetic current in the direction of a grounding

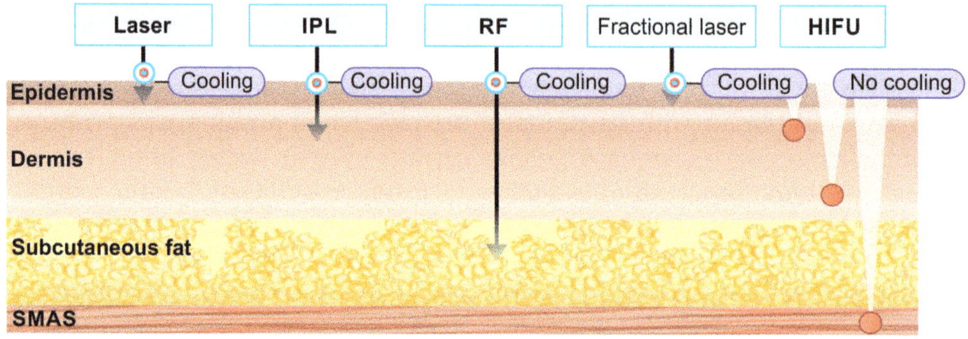

Fig. 1: Depth of penetration of various lasers used in functional gynecology. (HIFU: high-intensity focused ultrasound; IPL: intense pulsed light; RF: radio frequency; SMAS: superficial musculoaponeurotic system)
Source: Elfaki SH. Radiofrequency in cosmetic gynecology, literature review 2018-23. Gynecol Obstet Open Acc. 2024;8:182.

pad. To shield the epidermis from the volumetric dermal heating, a cooling spray may be applied in certain situations. Both capacitive and conductive couplings can be used to deliver the energy. Conductive coupling is based on energy concentrated at the distal portion of the electrode being delivered to the target tissue. This causes the skin surface in touch with the electrode to heat up, which may cause damage to the epidermis. By distributing energy over a surface, capacitive coupling produces a consistent heat zone.

Skin tightening of the face, periorbital area, belly, and extremities can be achieved noninvasively with the help of monopolar RF energy. The first monopolar RF device was the FD Thermacool device (Thermage, Inc.), which was introduced in 2001 and approved by FDA for the noninvasive treatment of periorbital rhytids and wrinkles in 2002, for full face treatment in 2004, and for body contouring in 2006.[20]

Bipolar Radio Frequency Devices

They allow current to flow between two strategically placed electrodes, bipolar devices are different from monopolar ones. The tissue to be heated and tightened is between these two electrodes, and the depth of penetration is approximately half the distance between the electrodes.[21] Thus, bipolar RF devices provide a reduced penetration depth in comparison to monopolar. Less discomfort[22] and a more controlled or localized energy distribution are offered by this arrangement, nevertheless. With these systems, the grounding pad is not required because there is no current flow through the rest of the body. Although this heat is targeted between the two electrodes, monopolar devices are believed to lead to a more uniform volumetric heating.

Hybrid and Combination Devices

Hybrid RF systems use monopolar and bipolar mechanisms (Accent RF; Alma Lasers, Ltd., Caesarea, Israel). The monopolar handpiece uses an alternating electromagnetic field to heat the skin deeply and volumetrically. Based on tissue impedance,[23] the bipolar handpiece is utilized for more superficial localized (nonvolumetric) heating. Thus, hybrid RF is useful to treat GUS of menopausal women presenting with vaginal laxity and urinary incontinence, simultaneously.

Fractional Radio Frequency Devices

Fractional RF creates microthermal zones with the energy dispensed at the measured portion.[24] It is a non-ablative approach which uses either needles (Morpheus8; InMode, Lake Forest, California) or electrodes to deliver thermal injury to the subdermis while leaving islands to tissue intact in between untreated.[24] As in fractional laser resurfacing, the unaffected areas serve to expedite recovery time. Some of the devices used in this technology include Thermage, Pelleve, Endymed microneedle, VR52, Exilis, and INFINITIM RF machines.[24] Thermage uses a monopolar head, Exilis combines RF thermal energy with ultrasound technology, while INFITINIM combines RF energy with microneedling targeting the dermis.

APPLICATIONS OF TRANSVAGINAL RADIO FREQUENCY IN FUNCTIONAL GYNECOLOGY

Genitourinary Syndrome of Menopause

Genitourinary syndrome presents with a myriad of symptoms in menopausal women, including genital, sexual and urinary tract, viz., vaginal dryness, decreased lubrication, dyspareunia, itching, burning, stress urinary incontinence, loose pelvic muscles. RF being the safest and with maximum depth and degree of penetration of skin is the novel solution to treat GUS **(Fig. 2)**. It effectively treats all abovementioned symptoms and is preferred by patients over other invasive or minimally invasive procedures. Based on numerous prospective cohort studies, RF, precisely the bipolar type has demonstrated effectiveness in treating GUS.[25,26]

Vaginal Laxity and Vulval Tightening

Multiple childbirth, aging leads to vaginal and vulval laxity which affects one's intimate relationships.

In the treatment of vaginal laxity, RF delivers controlled thermal energy to target tissues to stimulate collagen production, synthesis, and tissue remodeling. As established in a study, RF is one of the most commonly utilized energy-based devices, authorized by the FDA agency for various gynecological applications, including the treatment of loose pelvic muscles, vaginal laxity, and genital warts.[25,26] The efficacy of this technology underlies multiple prospective cohort studies which have demonstrated that RF therapy is a promising and effective treatment for vaginal laxity.[25] In another study on an animal model of multiparous swine, administering RF treatment once per week for 3 weeks showed an increased density of elastin and collagen fibers in vulvovaginal tissue[25] This study indicates that RF treatment may enhance the structural integrity and elasticity of the vulvovaginal tissue.

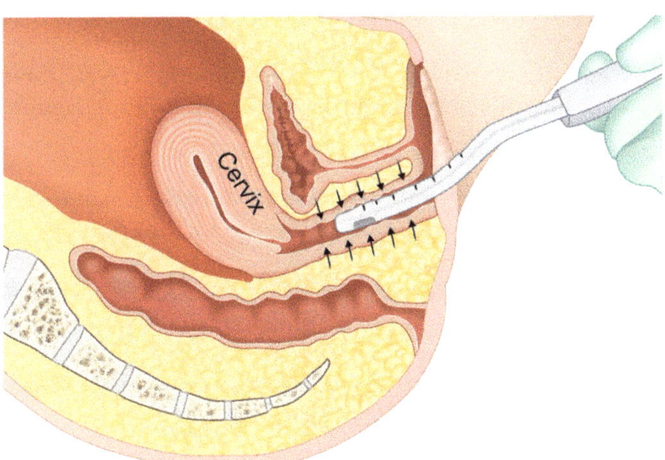

Fig. 2: Application of radio frequency (RF) probe in vagina to treat genitourinary syndrome (GUS).

Stress Urinary Incontinence

In treating stress urinary incontinence (SUI), RF technology delivers controlled thermal energy to the suburethral area to induce tissue contraction and tissue remodeling; critical in regulating urine flow.[27] According to a review of energy-based treatments for GUS of menopause RF resulted in 30% shrinking in the suburethral area of the vagina, with a significant improvement reported in stress urinary incontinence symptoms[28] This study reflects the action of RF through which the stimulation of new collagen, elastin, and blood vessels strengthens and rejuvenates loose tissues.[28,29] Therefore, despite being introduced recently, RF is an effective treatment technology for urinary symptoms of GUS of menopause and even in SUI in postpartum women.

Role in Cancer Patients

Based on the quality of RF not altering hormonal balance, makes it the best possible noninvasive therapy to treat cancer patients postradiotherapy and chemotherapy. This is an ideal treatment to treat vaginal dryness and dyspareunia in the cancer patients in whom hormone therapies are contraindicated.[30] With the approval of FDA, RF is used in the treatment of precancerous lesions. It is proved to be very effective in treating sexual dysfunction in female cancer survivors.[30]

Thus, RF provides the most feasible management option to address the GUS of menopause during and after cancer treatment.

CONCLUSION

Radio frequency is a promising innovative technique in subspecialty of noninvasive cosmetic and functional gynecology. Compared to HIFU, and other laser therapies, safety of the skin and precision of depth makes it the most breakthrough treatment approach for GUS of menopause, stress incontinence, and vaginal laxity. Besides these qualities, FDA approval and devoid of any effect on hormonal balance makes it a novel solution for treating sexual dysfunction in menopausal women and female cancer survivors. Improved techniques for measuring clinical outcomes as well as research into the ideal energy levels and treatment duration are among the fundamental questions surrounding RF that require clarification and future research.

REFERENCES

1. Greene RM, Green JB. Skin tightening technologies. Facial Plast Surg. 2014;30:62-7.
2. Fisher GH, Jacobson LG, Bernstein LJ, Kim KH, Geronemus RG. Nonablative radiofrequency treatment of facial laxity. Dermatol Surg. 2005;31:(9 pt 2)1237-41; discussion 1241.
3. Miniaci A, Codsi MJ. Thermal capsulorrhaphy for the treatment of shoulder instability. Am J Sports Med. 2006;34:1356-63.
4. Hruza GJ, Dover JS. Laser skin resurfacing. Arch Dermatol. 1996;132:451-5.
5. Atiyeh BS, Dibo SA. Nonsurgical nonablative treatment of aging skin: radiofrequency technologies between aggressive marketing and evidence-based efficacy. Aesthetic Plast Surg. 2009;33:283-94.
6. Kolczewski P, Parafiniuk M, Zawodny P, Haddad R, Nalewczyńska A, Kolasa AK, et al. Hyaluronic acid and radiofrequency in patients with urogenital atrophy and vaginal laxity. Pharmaceuticals. 2022;15:1571.
7. Mohammad S, Joshi KS, Mohammad S, Acharya N. Aesthetic Gynaecology: What Women Want? Cureus. 2023;15(8):e44251.
8. Alexiades-Armenakas M, Dover JS, Arndt KA. Unipolar versus bipolar radiofrequency treatment of rhytides and laxity using a mobile painless delivery method. Lasers Surg Med. 2008;40:446-53.
9. Lolis MS, Goldberg DJ. Radiofrequency in cosmetic dermatology: a review. Dermatol Surg. 2012;38(11):1765-76.
10. Elsaie ML. Cutaneous remodeling and Photorejuvenation using radiofrequency devices. Indian J Dermatol. 2009;54(3):201-5.
11. Greene RM, Green JB. Skin tightening technologies. Facial Plast Surg. 2014;30:62-7.
12. Alster TS, Lupton JR. Nonablative cutaneous remodeling using radiofrequency devices. Clin Dermatol. 2007;25: 487-91.
13. Youn A. Nonsurgical face lift. Plast Reconstr Surg. 2007; 119(6):1951.
14. Zelickson BD, Kist D, Bernstein E, Brown DB, Ksenzenko S, Burns J, et al. Histological and ultrastructural evaluation of the effects of a radiofrequency-based nonablative dermal remodeling device: a pilot study. Arch Dermatol. 2004;140(2):204-09.
15. Dierickx CC. The role of deep heating for noninvasive skin rejuvenation. Lasers Surg Med. 2006;38:799-807.
16. Ruiz-Esparza J, Gomez JB. The medical face lift: a noninvasive, nonsurgical approach to tissue tightening in facial skin using nonablative radiofrequency. Dermatol Surg. 2003;29:325-32; discussion 332.
17. Ruiz-Esparza J. Near [corrected] painless, nonablative, immediate skin contraction induced by low-fluence irradiation with new infrared device: a report of 25 patients. Dermatol Surg. 2006;32:601-10.
18. Ee HL, Barlow RJ. Lasers, lights and related technologies: a review of recent journal highlights. Clin Exp Dermatol. 2007;32:135-7.
19. Elfaki SH. Radiofrequency in cosmetic gynecology, literature review 2018-23. Gynecol Obstet Open Acc. 2024;8:182.
20. Narins DJ, Narins RS. Non-surgical radiofrequency facelift. J Drugs Dermatol. 2003;2:495-500.
21. Elsaie ML. Cutaneous remodeling and photorejuvenation using radiofrequency devices. Indian J Dermatol. 2009;54:201.
22. Montesi G, Calvieri S, Balzani A, Gold MH. Bipolar radiofrequency in the treatment of dermatologic imperfections: clinicopathological and immuno-histochemical aspects. J Drugs Dermatol. 2007;6: 890-6.
23. Friedman DJ, Gilead LT. The use of hybrid radiofrequency device for the treatment of rhytides and lax skin. Dermatol Surg. 2007;33:543-51.
24. Görgü M, Gökkaya A, Kizilkan J, Karanfil E, Dogan A. Radiofrequency: review of literature. Turk J Plast Surg. 2019;27:62.
25. Bujnak A, Crowder CA, Krychman ML. Energy-based devices for functional vaginal problems: issues and answers. Curr Sex Health Rep. 2021;13:1-13.
26. Palacios S, Combalia J, Emsellem C, Gaslain Y, Khorsandi D. Therapies for the management of genitourinary syndrome of menopause. Post Reprod Health. 2019;26:32-42.
27. Sarmento ACA, Lírio JF, Medeiros KS, Marconi C, Costa APF, Crispim JC, et al. physical methods for the treatment of genitourinary syndrome of menopause: a systematic review. Int J Gynaecol Obstet. 2021;153(2):200-19.
28. Kamilos MF, Costa APF, Sarmento ACA, Eleutério J Jr, Gonçalves AK. Microablative fractional radiofrequency as a therapeutical option for genitourinary syndrome of menopause: perspectives. Front Reprod Health. 2021;3:779421.
29. Soares-Júnior JM, Alves T, Aguiar Energy-based devices in gynecology: the new frontier for the treatment of genitourinary syndrome of postmenopause? Clinics (Sao Paulo). 2021;76:e3066.
30. Arab M, Vasef M, Talayeh M, Hosseini MS, Farzaneh F, Ashrafganjoei T. The effect of radiofrequency therapy on sexual function in female cancer survivors (gynecologic and breast) and non-cancer menopausal women: a single-arm trial. J Lasers Med Sci. 2023;14:e32.

CHAPTER 9

High Intensity Focused Ultrasound

Rachana Kaveri

INTRODUCTION

Quality of life (QoL) is the standard of health, comfort, and happiness experienced by an individual or group. There is now a paradigm shift in mainstream medicine, wherein, the focus has changed from treating diseases to ensuring overall well-being of an individual and QoL is an important parameter to assess this. The ultimate goal is longevity with well-being.

Cosmetic gynecology has evolved as one such subspeciality of medicine which caters to the well-being of women in a holistic, innovative, and empathetic manner.

High intensity focused ultrasound (HIFU) is a technology introduced in the field of gynecology for its ablative potential to treat fibroids, adenomyosis, placenta accreta, and cervical lesions; however, due to the versatility of this technology, it was incorporated to regenerate genital tissue at depths that cannot be reached with the photonic technology that has been used for over a decade.

White et al. reported the first dermatological aesthetic use of HIFU in 2008[1] and the Food and Drug Administration (FDA) approved HIFU for brow-lifting in 2009. Currently it is being used for facial rejuvenation, body contouring, and vaginal tightening which are all "off-label" uses.[2,3]

TAKING BACK CONTROL

Throughout all stages of life, a woman goes through various physiological and hormonal changes. Childbirth, menopause, and aging have a profound impact on a woman's body as a whole and the genitourinary system in specific. These changes affect women typically after childbirth and in the perimenopausal and menopausal stage. Genitourinary syndrome of menopause (GSM) is a chronic complex condition of multiple atrophic and dystrophic changes in estrogen-dependent tissues and structures of the lower genitourinary tract (vulva, vagina, bladder, urethra, pelvic ligaments, and pelvic floor muscles). The prevalence of vulvovaginal atrophy associated with hypoestrogenism ranged from 65 to 84% within the first 6 years of menopause.[4] Female sexual dysfunction (FSD) is another major concern for women. As high as 40% women experience FSD in some form, at some stage of their life.[5] As gynecologists, our armamentarium should have various safe and comfortable solutions for these concerns, which will enable our patients to live a fulfilling life.

THE ANATOMY OF VAGINA AND THE PELVIC FLOOR[6]

The vagina is a hollow fibromuscular tube extending from the vulvar vestibule to the uterus. The vagina is attached to the lateral pelvic wall with endopelvic fascial connections to the arcus tendineus (white line), which extends from the pubic bone to the ischial spine. This connection converts the vaginal lumen into a transverse slit with the anterior and posterior walls in apposition.

Layer of the Vagina

- *Mucosa*—nonkeratinized stratified squamous epithelium. It consists of the epithelium and the lamina propria. The mucosa has a characteristic pattern of transverse ridges and furrows known as rugae. It is hormonal sensitive and responds to stimulation by estrogen with proliferation and maturation. The mucosa is colonized by mixed bacterial flora especially with lactobacillus, which helps maintain a pH of 3.5–4.5.
- *Muscularis*—connective tissue and smooth muscle, loosely arranged in inner circular, and outer longitudinal layers.
- *Adventitia*—endopelvic fascia, adherent to the underlying muscularis.

The vagina is closely applied anteriorly to the urethra, bladder neck, and the trigonal region; posteriorly, the vagina lies in association with the perineal body, anal canal, lower rectum, and posterior cul-de-sac. It is separated from the urinary and gastrointestinal tracts by their investing layers of fibromuscular tissue known as the endopelvic fascia.

The lower urinary and genital tracts are intimately connected anatomically and functionally. The ventral urogenital diaphragm forms an interconnected complex with the compressor urethrae, vestibular bulb, and levator ani. The dorsal part connects the levator ani and vaginal sidewall via a distinct band to the ischiopubic ramus. The urogenital diaphragm includes the sphincter urethrae and the deep transverse perineal muscle. For its support, the pelvic floor relies on the complementary role of the pelvic diaphragm and its fascia resting on the perineal fibromuscular complex. It is composed of the perineal membrane (urogenital diaphragm) anteriorly and the perineal body joined to the anococcygeal raphe by the external anal sphincter posteriorly.

PRINCIPLES AND PHYSICS OF HIGH INTENSITY FOCUSED ULTRASOUND

High intensity focused ultrasound is *a noninvasive, nonionizing* procedure with bioeffects created by focusing high-intensity ultrasound in the tissue and inducing controlled heating.[7] The ultrasonic wave propagates through the mucosa to the submucosa causing heating of the deeper layers without surface overheating **(Fig. 1)**. The vaginal transducer has a diameter of 20 mm and is cylindrical shaped, which can rotate 360° to enable treatment of the whole length and circumference of vagina either by a manual or automatic mode which can be preset. There is a *concave* emission plate of 25 mm length and 10 mm width, which directs *convergent ultrasonic waves* to a specific focal depth. These convergent mechanical waves produce the molecular vibration of the water in the vaginal tissue and in turn raise the temperature of the tissue. The device is characterized by parameters such as power (0.4–1.2 J/mm^2), frequency (4–10 MHz) and the focal depth of the transducer (1.5–4.5 mm).[8]

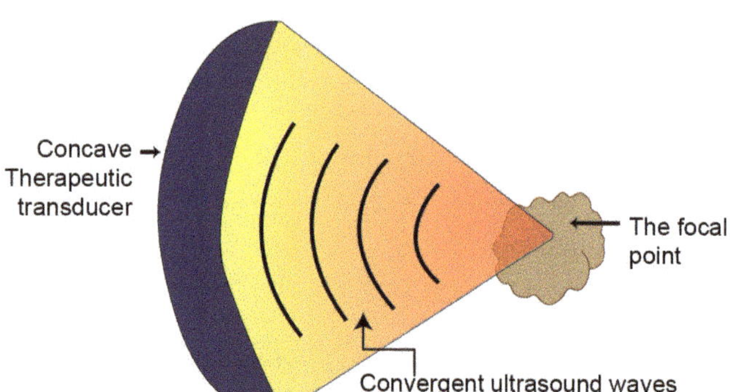

Fig. 1: Principles of high intensity focused ultrasound (HIFU) technology.

The basic mechanism of action of the HIFU device is to produce *targeted thermal coagulation points* (TCPs), with an area of <1 mm^3 and at a depth of up to 4.5 mm (in the middle and deep reticular layers of the dermis), without destroying the superficial layers.[9,10] This increases the temperature of the tissue to about 65°C leading to instant contraction and shortening of collagen. Also, the healthy tissue in between the TCPs promotes fibroblast proliferation, neovascularization, neocollagenesis, and elastogenesis. This neovascularization and collagen remodeling that occurs eventually is responsible for the rejuvenation and tightening effects of HIFU.

POSITIVE EFFECTS OF HIGH INTENSITY FOCUSED ULTRASOUND

The thermal inflammation initiates healing cascade in all the layers of the vagina. In the mucosa, there is stratification and increased glycogen in the superficial keratinocytes, which explains the reduced pH. The vaginal microbial flora also improves to a great extent. There is thickening of the epithelium and the lamina propria along with increased vascularity. Neoangiogenesis leads to an increase in the vaginal lubrication and reduces the atrophic changes hence greatly benefits women with GSM. The contraction and remodeling of collagen cause noticeable tightening effect. Also, studies demonstrate an evident rise in collagen type I compared to collagen type III after HIFU treatment.[11] There is also an increase in the elastin in the tissue.

PROCEDURE

A detailed history is inherent to find out eligibility and for proper patient selection. A gynecological examination along with a Pap smear report should be performed before the procedure. Detailed discussion about the procedure, the specific concerns of the patient, and an informed consent are important.

Customizing the parameters based on patients' concerns and examination will help to optimize the results.

Both the HIFU vaginal transducers with focal depth 3 mm (frequency 7 MHz) and focal depth 4.5 mm (frequency 4 MHz) are used during the session to deliver ultrasound pulses along a linear path. All the parameters

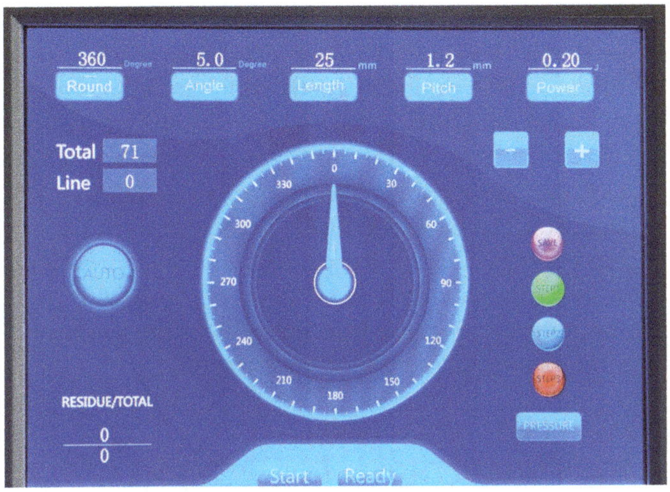

Fig. 2: High intensity focused ultrasound (HIFU) device screen to select parameters.

can be modified on the software. The parameters include intravaginal rotation of the probe: 0–360°; the angle of rotation: 3–20°; focal treatment line length: 5–25 mm; pitch (distance between each exposure zones): 1–5 mm and the power: 0.20–2.0 J **(Fig. 2)**.

The transducer is inserted into the vaginal and two rounds are performed one at 7.5 cm and the other at 5 cm inside the introitus according to the vaginal probe marking. The round is started at 12 o'clock position and the maximum angle is kept at 350°, never firing at the suburethral area twice. The angle the probe moves between each shot can be adjusted, while keeping in mind that healthy intervening tissue is essential to promote appropriate healing. The power is usually adjusted to 1.2–1.5 Joules per shot and increased to 2 Joules per shot in the second session based on the pain tolerance. The 3-mm transducer is to be used in the entire vaginal canal in all patients undergoing treatment.

- *Vaginal rejuvenation:* As we are dealing with atrophy and lack of lubrication, thermal inflammation produced on the superficial tissue is beneficial. Hence, for vaginal rejuvenation especially in GSM, the 1.5-mm and the 3-mm transducer should be used in the entire circumference of the vagina.
- *Treatment for stress urinary incontinence (SUI):* For this, additional pulses with the 4.5-mm transducer are delivered between 10 o'clock to 2 o'clock excluding the suburethral 12 o'clock position directly.
- *Vaginal tightening:* Women with laxity of vagina and introital widening received treatment with the 4.5-mm transducer throughout the vaginal cavity along with the 3-mm transducer.
- *Vulval rejuvenation protocol:* The recommended protocol is to use the 3-mm and 1.5-mm transducers, though there are studies in which the 4.5-mm transducer has been used.[12] The total number of TCP lines for the external intimate area on each side is around 20–30 lines.[13] The ideal distance between each TCP line, for both the transducers, is 1.2 mm; however, the distance can be modified based on the comfort of the woman.[14]

FOLLOW-UP

The initial two sessions are scheduled 6–8 weeks apart. Yearly maintenance sessions are advisable based on the response to treatment. Follow-up should be done at 1 month and 3 months after the second session.

OUTCOME MEASURES

- *VHI (Vaginal Health Index):* Vaginal Health Index helps us understand the degree of vaginal atrophy in patients with GSM. VHI has five parameters and each is graded from 1 to 5. The five parameters are vaginal moisture, vaginal fluid volume, vaginal elasticity, pH, and vaginal epithelial integrity. Lower the vaginal health score, higher is the degree of atrophy in the patient. A score <15 is a sign of atrophic vagina.[15,16]
- *FSFI (Female Sexual Function Index):* The FSFI is a 19-item questionnaire divided into six domains—desire, arousal, lubrication, orgasm, satisfaction, and pain, to evaluate a woman's sexual function in the past 4 weeks. All the domain scores combine to create a total score ranging from 2 to 36. A total FSFI score of 26 is recognized as female sexual dysfunction (FSD). A study done by Kolczewski P et al, not only demonstrated a significant, but also a sustained improvement in the FSFI score in the subsequent follow-up visits.[17]
- *VLQ (Vaginal Laxity Questionnaire):* Vaginal laxity can be assessed subjectively with the help of the vulvovaginal laxity questionnaire (VLQ). The patients who self-reported laxity are eligible to fill this questionnaire. Vaginal laxity can be graded as "very loose," "moderately loose," or "slightly loose," on a point Likert scale.[18,19] The questionnaire is to be filled before the first treatment and during the follow-up visits. Studies reported an average improvement in the VLQ over time.[17]

- *ICIQ-SF (International Consultation on Incontinence Questionnaire-Short Form):* The ICIQ-UI Short Form is a questionnaire for evaluating the frequency, severity, and impact on QoL of urinary incontinence in men and women. It covers urinary incontinence under four questions: How often is the leak? How much is the leak? When does urine leak? and the impact of leak on daily routine? The scoring scale is from 0 to 21 and a higher score means greater urinary leak. Treatment with HIFU has shown to improve urinary leak and reduction in the ISIQ-SF score of the patient.

APPLICATIONS OF HIGH INTENSITY FOCUSED ULTRASOUND

- *Vaginal rejuvenation:* HIFU is an excellent choice for women who are perimenopausal and menopausal and are experiencing GSM. HIFU helps improve vaginal atrophy, increases lubrication, causes collagen remodeling, and also increases estrogen receptivity. All these changes help reduce the impact of GSM and improve intimate well-being.
- *Vaginal tightening:* Vaginal laxity is a concern most commonly seen in postpartum or menopausal woman. Patients present with loss of vaginal tightness, which reduces friction during intercourse, resulting in decreased sexual satisfaction, both in the women and her partner. HIFU is beneficial in such cases as it causes collagen remodeling and neocollagenesis. This has a tightening effect on the entire length of vagina.
- *Stress urinary incontinence:* The deeper depth of action of HIFU technology can have a great advantage in the management of urinary incontinence. HIFU can help focus thermal energy to the supporting elements of the pelvic floor. Thus, providing a noninvasive option for the treatment of SUI.
- *Vulval rejuvenation:* Appearance of the external intimate area may sometimes trigger a negative psychological response. Thus, it can have an impact on a woman's self-esteem and sexual function. HIFU can be used in the vulval region for rejuvenation. It can help reduce the wrinkling and has a lifting effect in the intimate area.
- *Sexual dysfunction:* Neocollagenesis and neo-angiogenesis are seen after HIFU treatment. This causes a generalized anatomical restoration. There is improvement in the elasticity of the vagina owing to the elastin production which helps women with dyspareunia. Improved vascularity also improves sensation, leading to a better sexual gratification.
- *Prolapse:* The pubococcygeus and puborectalis group of muscle can be reached with the 4.5 mm transducer. This can cause retraction and regeneration which explains the improvement in prolapse. Though it is important to note that HIFU cannot replace surgery for treating prolapse; it provides some relief in patients who cannot or do not wish to be operated. Also, theoretically, regenerative changes owing to thermal stimulation can improve surgical results.

MERITS OF HIGH INTENSITY FOCUSED ULTRASOUND

Treatment with HIFU is quick, noninvasive, and cost effective. The various plus points of treatment with HIFU are enlisted in **Box 1**.

CONTRAINDICATIONS

A detailed medical and menstrual history is essential for proper patient selection. Pregnancy, systemic, or topical hormone therapy (currently or within 6 weeks prior to the procedure), active or recurrent genital and urinary infection (e.g., genital herpes, candidiasis, bacterial vaginosis), patients with human immunodeficiency virus, pelvic radiation therapy or brachytherapy, reconstructive pelvic surgery, previous vaginal treatment with energy-based devices, hyaluronic acid fillers, autologous therapy with plasma-derived products [platelet-rich plasma (PRP), platelet-rich fibrin (PRF)], or fat transfer are contraindications for the procedure.

COMPLICATIONS

High intensity focused ultrasound is a relatively safe technology as it is nonablative and nonionizing. As the ultrasound waves converge at a specific depth which is preprogrammed based on the transducer used, there is

BOX 1: Pros of treatment with high intensity focused ultrasound (HIFU).

Merits of HIFU treatment

- Noninvasive
- Good safety profile
- "Lunch-break" procedure
- No downtime
- Painless
- Avoids need for surgery in mild-to-moderate cases
- Can be performed in clinics

no thermal effect on the superficial mucosa or epidermis. However, there is always a theoretical risk of burns, scarring, and fistula. Since, HIFU is a robust technology with the greatest depth of penetration, it has to be used with caution in menopausal women with severe atrophy.

CONCLUSION

High intensity focused ultrasound is an effective and promising treatment modality for various concerns of woman in terms of intimate wellness. However, currently there are no guidelines or standardized protocols for the use of HIFU in gynecology. Also, randomized controlled trials are necessary to confirm the positive results of HIFU with highest level of clinical evidence. The follow-up of women treated with HIFU is still short, nonetheless, the results of various studies are encouraging.

As medicine advances and the longevity improves, the focus shifts from treatment of diseases to enhancing the functionality and well-being. HIFU is a safe, innovative, and cost-effective technology. Its versatility in being able to treat multiple gynecological conditions such as GSM, SUI, and FSD, makes it a great treatment modality. With many studies coming up in favor of HIFU for aesthetic and functional gynecological uses; HIFU is slowly but surely getting a foothold in our cosmetic gynecology practice.

REFERENCES

1. White WM, Makin IR, Barthe PG, Slayton MH, Gliklich RE. Selective creation of thermal injury zones in the superficial musculoaponeurotic system using intense ultrasound therapy: a new target for noninvasive facial rejuvenation. Arch Facial Plast Surg. 2007; 9:22-9.
2. Suh DH, Shin MK, Lee SJ, Rho JH, Lee MH, Kim NI, et al. Intense focused ultrasound tightening in Asian skin: clinical and pathologic results. Dermatol Surg. 2011;37:1595-1602.
3. Chan NP, Shek SY, Yu CS, Ho SG, Yeung CK, Chan HH. Safety study of transcutaneous focused ultrasound for noninvasive skin tightening in Asians. Lasers Surg Med. 2011;43:366-75.
4. Palma F, Volpe A, Villa P, Cagnacci A. Vaginal atrophy of women in postmenopause. Results from a multicentric observational study: The AGATA study. Maturitas. 2016;83:40-44.
5. Allahdadi KJ, Tostes RC, Webb RC. Female sexual dysfunction: therapeutic options and experimental challenges. Cardiovasc Hematol Agents Med Chem. 2009; 7(4):260-9.
6. Berek, Jonathan S (Ed). Berek & Novak's gynecology. 16th edition. Philadelphia, Wolters Kluwer; 2020.
7. Elrashidy RA. High Intensity Focal Ultrasound (HIFU) for Management of Vaginal Laxity with Impact on Sexual Satisfaction. Int J Sci Develop Res. 2022;7:308-311.
8. Alam M, White LE, Martin N, Witherspoon J, Yoo S, West DP. Ultrasound tightening of facial and neck skin: A rater-blinded prospective cohort study. J Am Acad Derm. 2010;62:262-9.
9. Hayashi K, Thabit G, Massa KL, Bogdanske JJ, Cooley A, Orwin JF, et al. The effect of thermal heating on the length and histologic properties of the glenohumeral joint capsule. Am J Sport Med. 1997;25:107-12.
10. Laubach HJ, Makin IRS, Barthe PG, Slayton MH, Manstein D. Intense focused ultrasound: Evaluation of a new treatment modality for precise microcoagulation within the skin. Dermatol Surg. 2008;34:727-34.
11. Meyer P, Meleck M, Borges F, Fortuny E, Farias S, Afonso F, et al. Effect of microfocused ultrasound on facial rejuvenation: clinical and histological evaluation. J Biosci Med. 2021;9:112-25.
12. Borges F, Carvalho M, Cerqueira C, Monteiro T, Almeida I, Benevides E, et al. Vulvar rejuvenation using high-intensity focused ultrasound (HIFU): fundamentals and technique journal of biosciences and medicines. 2022;10:239-52.
13. Oni G, Hoxworth R, Teotia S, Brown S, Kenkel M. Evaluation of a microfocused ultrasound system for improving skin laxity and tightening in the lower face. Aesthet Surg J. 2014;34:1099-110.
14. Jeon H, Kim T, Kim H, Cho B. Multimodal approach for treating horizontal neck wrinkles using intensity focused ultrasound, cohesive polydensified matrix hyaluronic acid, and incobotulinumtoxin A. Dermatolc Surg. 2018;44:421-31.
15. Bachmann GA, Nevadunsky NS. Diagnosis and treatment of atrophic vaginitis. Am Fam Physician. 2000;61:3090-6.
16. Bachmann G. Urogenital ageing: An old problem newly recognized. Maturitas. 1995;22:S1-S5.
17. Kolczewski P, Kozłowski M, Cymbaluk-Płoska A. Micro-Focused Ultrasound Therapy in Patients with Urogenital Atrophy and Vaginal Laxity. J Clin Med. 2022;11(23):6980.
18. Campbell P, Krychman M, Gray T, Vickers H, Money-Taylor J, Li W, et al. Self-reported vaginal laxity—prevalence, impact, and associated symptoms in women attending a urogynecology clinic. J Sex Med. 2018;15:1515-7.
19. Qureshi AA, Sharma K, Thornton M, Myckatyn TM, Tenenbaum MM. Vaginal laxity, sexual distress, and sexual dysfunction: a cross-sectional study in a plastic surgery practice. Aesthet Surg J. 2018;38:873-80.

CHAPTER 10

High Intensity Focused Electromagnetic Technology

Preeti Jindal, Ridhi Kalra

INTRODUCTION

High intensity focused electromagnetic (HIFEM) technology is a revolutionary, United States Food and Drug Administration (US-FDA) approved, noninvasive energy-based medical technology used for muscle stimulation and muscle strengthening. It uses HIFEM pulses as well as biofeedback mechanism for this purpose.

MECHANISM OF ACTION

High intensity focused electromagnetic technology generates high intensity electromagnetic pulses inducing supramaximal contractions in the muscles of pelvic area. It targets neuromuscular tissue and induces electric currents. Electric currents depolarize neurons resulting in concentric contractions and lift up of all pelvic floor muscles (PFM). Key effectiveness is based on focused electromagnetic energy, in-depth penetration, and stimulation of the entire pelvic floor area. This directly modifies the muscle structure, inducing a more efficient growth of myofibrils—muscle fiber hypertrophy, the creation of new protein strands and muscle fibers—muscle fiber hyperplasia. HIFEM technology causes deep PFM stimulation.

Supramaximal PFM contractions maximal voluntary contraction (MVC) is the greatest amount of tension that could be developed and held physiologically by the muscle, but usually only for a split second **(Fig. 1)**. Contractions with a tension higher than MVC are defined as supramaximal. HIFEM technology is able to create supramaximal PFM contractions and hold them for a couple of seconds. These contractions are independent of brain function and target directly the peripheral nerves in the pelvic floor area. These contractions are stronger than what the body can achieve through voluntary muscle contractions. Repetitive contractions can lead to muscle growth, increased strength, and improved tone.

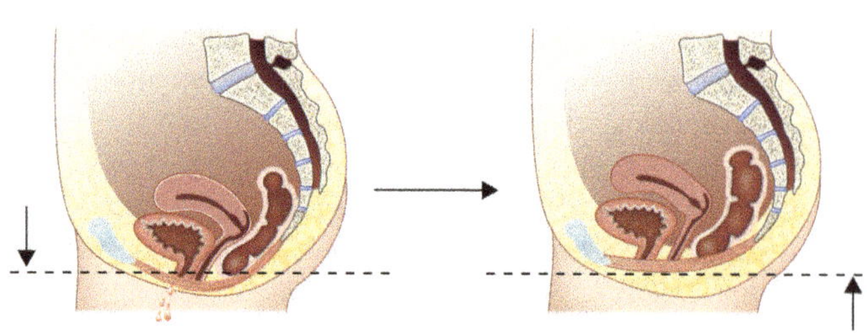

Fig. 1: Supramaximal pelvic floor muscle contractions, maximal voluntary contraction.

Key effectiveness is based on focused electromagnetic energy, in-depth penetration, and stimulation of the entire pelvic floor area. HIFEM technology effectiveness is in the gradually increasing intensity of the focused electromagnetic fields and frequency of pulses, which result in unique vigorousness of the contractions.[1-11]

In this device, a coil generates pulsed electromagnetic fields that penetrate deep into the PFM when a person sits on the chair inducing stimulation of the pelvic muscles and contracting them rhythmically in order to strengthen them. The device generates a focused electromagnetic field with intensities of up to 2.5 T and penetration up to a depth of 10 cm. The electromagnetic energy produced is directed vertically upward from the center of the seat. The chair design ensures that the patient's perineum is centered when he/she is sitting upright on the chair.[12,13]

This method is extremely important to PFM re-education as the patients are not able to perform this high-repetition rate pattern due to PFM weakness. Such effect cannot be achieved through common exercise (e.g., Kegel) **(Figs. 2 and 3)**.

TREATMENT PROTOCOL

Six sittings are recommended at a frequency of 2–3 sessions per week.

Each sitting is 28-minute treatment session, during which the patient sits in the center of HIFEM chair.

To ensure adequate PFM stimulation, the operator confirms the patient's chair posture throughout the session and adjusts the intensity of stimulus as high as tolerated

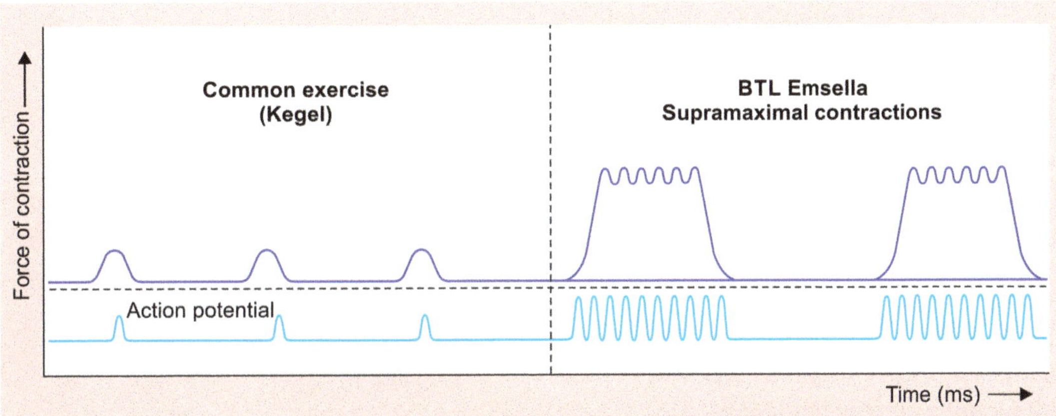

Fig. 2: Pelvic floor muscle (PFM) activation using high intensity focused electromagnetic (HIFEM) technology compared to common exercise (e.g., Kegel).

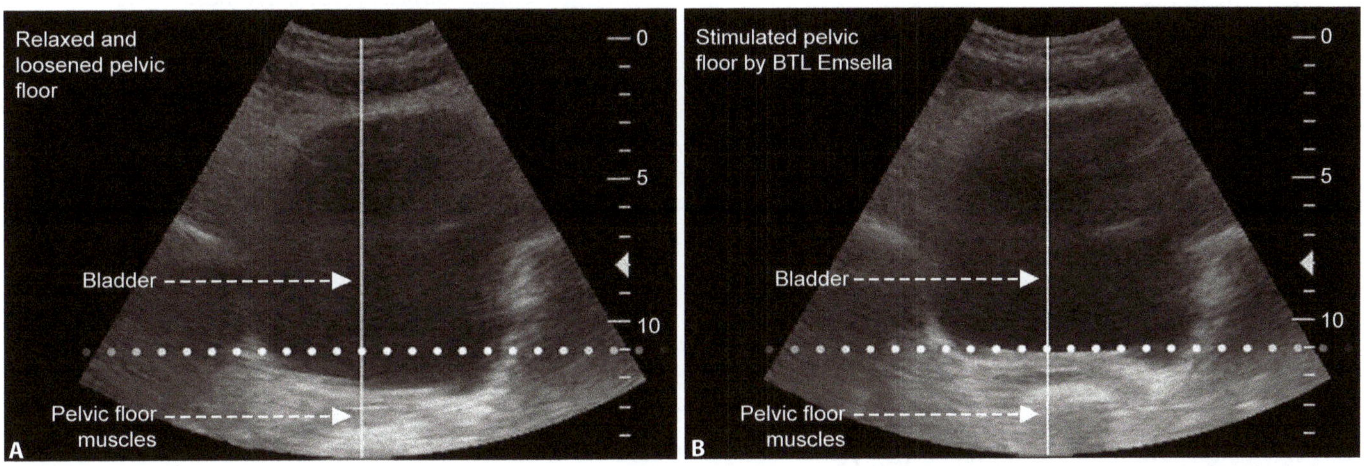

Figs. 3A and B: A frontal view of the pelvic floor muscles and bladder using medical ultrasound. Relaxed and loosened pelvic floor muscles and bladder (A). Stimulated and lifted pelvic floor muscles and bladder using high intensity focused electromagnetic (HIFEM) technology (B).

by patient ranging from (0–100).[12] During this duration, patients may experience contraction and relaxation of muscles throughout the session without any pain.[12] Emsella Chair delivers the equivalent of approximately 11,200 Kegel exercises in just one session.

INDICATIONS OF USE OF EMSELLA CHAIR

- *Stress incontinence:* It is the most common form of incontinence among women and is usually associated with menopause, aging, and/or childbirth. Emsella chair can help these women with stress incontinence without the risk of infection and complications associated with a surgery as it is noninvasive.[12,14]
- *Sexual rejuvenation:* As Emsella helps to regenerate and rejuvenate the PFM and vaginal canal, thus in turn it helps to treat sexual dysfunction caused by loss of muscle tone.
- *Urge incontinence:* Urge incontinence occurs when one has a sudden urge to urinate and cannot hold the urine. Emsella chair can rehabilitate the pelvic floor by contracting and relaxing the muscles of the pelvic floor, thus helping in treatment of urge incontinence.[15]
- *Erectile dysfunction:* Emsella treatment regulates training of the muscles of the pelvic floor to improve sexual function in males and in turn helps in treatment of erectile dysfunction.
- Pelvic organ prolapse[12]
- Vault prolapse
- Coccydynia
- Sports medicine—used to improve athletic performance and endurance

- Rehabilitation—used in rehabilitation programs to help recovery from muscle atrophy or injury.

CONTRAINDICATIONS[16]

- Pregnancy
- Implanted neurostimulators or defibrillators
- Cardiac pacemakers
- Hemorrhagic conditions
- Anticoagulation therapy
- Drug pumps
- Metal implants—hip/knee implants (relative contra-indication depending on type implant used)
- Malignant tumor
- Copper-based intrauterine devices
- Heart disorders

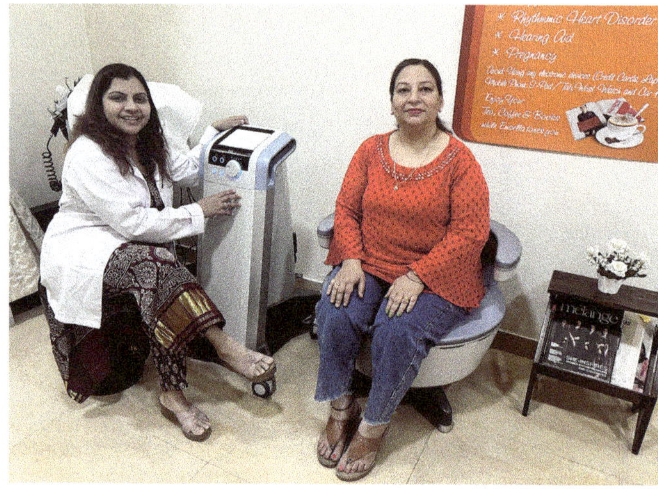

Fig. 4: Emsella device in Touch, Advanced Obstetrics, IVF and Cosmetic Gynae Centre.

PRECAUTIONS

- Patient should dress comfortably (preferably light fabric bottoms without zippers) on the treatment days.
- Patients should take off jewelry.
- Patients should not wear jeans or thick clothing as it may hamper optimal muscle stimulation.
- One should take out credit cards and coins from the pockets.
- Patient should take out iPads, watches, or phones as electromagnetic energy may harm the devices.

ADVANTAGES OF HIGH INTENSITY FOCUSED ELECTROMAGNETIC CHAIR

- It is painless, noninvasive, and safe 28-minute outpatient department (OPD) treatment procedure
- No recovery or healing time involved
- One may remain fully clothed during the treatment
- Significant improvements after a single session
- FDA approved

CONCLUSION

High intensity focused electromagnetic chair is a completely noninvasive and safe procedure. In treatment of non-neurological urinary incontinence, single session lasts for about 28 minutes and the most of the patients experience improvements after six sessions. The treatment improvement is subjective with varying results in different patients. There is no pain associated with this treatment and there is no requirement of anesthetics. Patients can resume normal activities on a daily basis immediately after the treatment. In a study conducted by Jindal et al. preventive exercises such as Kegel exercises are not very effective but nowadays noninvasive treatment such as HIFEM, laser, radiofrequency, platelet-rich plasma (PRP), and HIFU are more lucrative options because of better patient compliance and lesser side effects.[12]

Emsella device was introduced for the first time in India at "The Touch, Advanced Obstetrics, IVF and cosmetic Gynae Centre" Mohali by the editor. Note the ease patient is in while taking therapy **(Fig. 4)**.[17]

REFERENCES

1. Abrams P, Blaivas JG, Stanton SL, Andersen JT. The standardisation of terminology of lower urinary tract function. The International Continence Society Committee on Standardisation of Terminology. Scand J Urol Nephrol Suppl. 1998;114:5-19.
2. Wallis M, Davies E, Thalib L, Griffiths S. Pelvic static magnetic stimulation to control urinary incontinence in older women: a randomized controlled trial. Clin Med Res. 2011;10(1):7-14.
3. Yamanishi T, Yasuda K, Sakakibara R, Hattori T, Ito H, Murakami S, et al. Pelvic floor electrical stimulation in the treatment of stress incontinence: an investigational study and a placebo controlled double-blind trial. J Urol. 1997;158:2127-31.
4. Haylen BT, de Ridder D, Freeman RM, Swift SE, Berghmans B, Lee J. An International Urogynecological Association (IUGA)/International Continence Society (ICS) Joint Report on the Terminology for Female Pelvic Floor Dysfunction. Neurourol Urodyn. 2010;29(1):4-20.

5. Almeida FG, Bruschini H, Srougi M. Urodynamic and clinical evaluation of 91 female patients with urinary incontinence treated with perineal magnetic stimulation: 1-year follow-up. J Urol. 2004;171(4):1571-4.
6. Bickford R, Guidi M, Fortesque P, Swenson M. Magnetic stimulation of human peripheral nerve and brain. Neurosurgery. 1987;20(1):110-6.
7. Coletti D, Teodori L, Albertini M, Rocchi M, Pristerà A, Fini M, et al. Static magnetic fields enhance skeletal muscle differentiation in vitro by improving myoblast alignment. Cytometry A. 2007;71A(10):846-56.
8. Ishikawa N, Suda S, Sasaki T, Yamanishi T, Hosaka H, Yasuda K, et al. Development of a non-invasive treatment system for urinary incontinence using a functional continuous magnetic stimulator (FCMS). Med Biol Eng Comput. 1998;36(6):704-10.
9. Ostrovidov S, Hosseini V, Ahadian S, Fujie T, Parthiban S, Ramalingam M, et al. Skeletal muscle tissue engineering: methods to form skeletal myotubes and their applications. Tissue Eng Part B Rev. 2014;20(5):403-36.
10. Stölting M, Arnold A, Haralampieva D, Handschin C, Sulser T, Eberli D. Magnetic stimulation supports muscle and nerve regeneration after trauma in mice. Muscle Nerve. 2016;53(4):598-607.
11. Wallis M, Davies E, Thalib L, Griffiths S. Pelvic static magnetic stimulation to control urinary incontinence in older women: a randomized controlled trial. Clin Med Res. 2011;10(1):.7-14.
12. Jindal P, Sahdev S, Gulati R, Kundal I. Nonsurgical management of stress urinary incontinence (SUI). Acta Sci Women's Health. 2020;2(11):51-4.
13. Samuels JB, Pezzela A, Berenholz J, Alinsod R. Safety and efficacy of a non-invasive high-intensity focused electromagnetic field (HIFEM) device for treatment of urinary incontinence and enhancement of quality of life. Lasers Surg Med. 2019;51(9):760-6.
14. Preeti J, Madhu G, Isha K, Mittal M, Ridhi G, Cherry M, et al. Female urinary incontinence: a revisit on prevalence of this problem in today's society, which is increasing due to increase in average life span. Acta Sci Womens Health. 2021;3(9):27-33.
15. Goldstein S, Williams J, Kim N, Goldstein I. A Double-Blind, Sham Controlled Prospective Pilot Study of Urinary Stress Incontinence and Sexual function in women after 6 treatments with HIFEM Technology (Emsella): Interim Analysis. https://doi.org/10.1016/j.jsxm.2020.04.285
16. Deshpande J, Singh CK. Emsella: a breakthrough, noninvasive technology for treatment of incontinence. Indian J Obstet Gynecol Res. 2023;10(2):224-6.
17. Prasad AJR, Pai GS, Pai AH. Laser in aesthetic and regenerative gynecology: physics, types, applications, safety profiles. In: Jindal P, Malhotra N, Joshi S (Eds). Aesthetic and Regenerative Gynaecology. Springer; 2022. pp. 53-66.

CHAPTER 11

Carboxy Therapy in Cosmetic Gynecology

Poonam Mishra

INTRODUCTION

Carboxytherapy emerges as an impressive advancement in the realms of cosmetology and cosmetic gynecology.[1]

CHARACTERISTICS

It stands as colorless, scentless, the body's natural metabolite, nontoxic, nonembolic, with a remarkably high diffusibility (25 times that of O_2).

Employing heated medical gas, specifically carbon dioxide, the flow of gas per minute is meticulously regulated toward the targeted tissue.

CARBON DIOXIDE'S MECHANISM OF ACTION IN TISSUES

Effects manifest as both direct and indirect.

Carbon dioxide interacts with water molecules, forming molecular carbonic acid. This acid lowers tissue pH, invoking the Bohr effect—wherein a lower pH weakens the bond between hemoglobin and oxygen. During carboxytherapy, this results in increased oxygen release from hemoglobin. Furthermore, at pH levels of 6.8 and lower, capillary wall permeability increases. At pH levels of 6.5 and lower, collagen fiber flexibility increases while their firmness decreases. Other chemical reactions involve the reduction of divalent calcium ions and the splitting of carbonic acid into H^+ and HCO_3^-, yielding calcium hydrogen carbonate—$Ca(HCO_3)_2$, sodium hydrogen carbonate, and potassium hydrogen carbonate ($NaHCO_3$ and $KHCO_3$).

As a consequence, pH shifts to alkaline, ultimately inducing an analgesic and spasmolytic effect. Arteries' and capillaries' tonus diminishes while skin temperature elevates by 1°C. This, combined with altered nerve ending activity, enhances the trophicity of treated areas. Simultaneously, fat oxidation within adipose cells is stimulated. Any residual CO_2 is exhaled via the lungs.

Resulting effects include: Vasodilation, neoangiogenesis, collagen reorganization, lipolysis, and hypopigmentation (due to neoangiogenesis). These effects become apparent quite early, often after two sessions, within 7–14 days. Skin tonus and aesthetic parameters visibly improve.[2]

Carboxytherapy serves as a therapeutic option for patients with poorly healing leg ulcers, peripheral diabetic complications, hypertrophic and keloid scars, slow-healing surgical wounds, Raynaud's disease, Morbus Buerger, acrocyanosis, lymphedema, and for skin healing post-skin implant application.[1]

In aesthetics, carbon dioxide is utilized for treating—double chin, neck, décolleté, lax abdominal skin, arms, inner thighs (as part of body contouring), postliposuction conditions, lipomatosis, stretch marks, skin around the glabella, crow's feet, fine eye wrinkles, lower lids, and in cosmetic gynecology for abdominal fat reduction, scar correction (cesarean and episiotomy scars), monsoplasty, as part of genital bleaching, vulvovaginal rejuvenation, and G-spot augmentation—yet, the latter necessitates substantial expertise.[3]

SIDE EFFECTS

Pain, bruising (solely due to needle pricks), and transient emphysematous sensations (which dissipate within 15–30 minutes).

CONTRAINDICATIONS

Severe ischemic heart disease, acute embolism, thrombophlebitis, phlebothrombosis, gangrene, renal failure, untreated hypertension, stroke, pregnancy, lactation, severe obesity (following body contouring), acute infectious diseases, fever, and blood clotting disorders.

Unrealistic patient expectations and advanced age also serve as contraindications.

Gas is administered under pressures of 2.5–3.5 bar (i.e., 250,000–350,000 per annum). Parameters for application [gas flow in milliliter (mL)/minute, total volume in mL] are individually selected based on indication and site. Injections are delivered using a 30G mesotherapy needle, which may range from 4 to 13 mm in length. Gas instillation is controlled via a foot pedal.[4]

Injection angle: This holds significant importance. A 30° angle is used for superficial subcutaneous applications, visibly elevating tissue, useful for treating facial and décolleté skin issues and improving stretch marks' appearance. For deeper intradermal gas applications, a 45° injection angle is employed, particularly for reducing fatty tissue.[5]

The total carbon dioxide volume applied ranges from 25 to 50 mL for the face and 200–1,000 mL for the trunk and extremities.

NUMBER AND FREQUENCY OF SESSIONS

The number of sessions varies greatly based on indication and treated area. Patients must understand that optimal results may not be immediately apparent after a single session. Typically, applications are repeated once or twice weekly. However, many patients notice positive effects and improved skin aesthetics after just one or two sessions. In body shaping for the trunk, abdomen, arms, and thighs, visible effects typically arise after 6–8 sessions. The total number of sessions depends on achieved and desired effects.[6]

CONCLUSION

Carboxytherapy stands as a remarkable tool in gynecological aesthetics, devoid of side effects when performed skillfully. It can be combined with other therapies such as platelet-rich plasma (PRP), hyaluronic acid (HA), toxins, and energy based devices (EBDs). Much exploration remains to be done for its full potential."[7]

REFERENCES

1. Lee GSK. Carbon dioxide therapy in the treatment of cellulite: An audit of clinical practice. Aesthetic Plast Surg. 2010;34(2):239-43.
2. Brandi C, D'Aniello C, Grimaldi L, Caiazzo E, Stanghellini E. Carbon dioxide therapy: effects on skin irregularity and its use as a complement to liposuction. Aesthetic Plast Surg. 2004;28(4):222-5.
3. Sinozic T, Kovacevic J. Carboxytherapy - supportive therapy in chronic wound treatment. Acta Med Croatica. 2013;67(Suppl 1):137-41.
4. Koutna N. Carboxytherapy - a new non-invasive method in aesthetic medicine. Cas Lek Cesk. 2006;145:841-3.
5. Ferreira JCT, Haddad A, Tavares SAN. Increase in collagen turnover induced by intradermal injection of carbon dioxide in rats. J Drugs Dermatol. 2008;7:25-30.
6. Paolo F, Nefer F, Paola P, Nicolò S. Periorbital area rejuvenation using carbon dioxide therapy. J Cosmet Dermatol. 2012;11:223- 8.
7. Brandi C, D'Aniello C, Grimaldi L, Bosi B, Dei I, Lattarulo P, et al. Carbon dioxide therapy in the treatment of localized adiposities: clinical study and histopathological correlations. Aesthetic Plast Surg. 2001;25:170-4.

CHAPTER 12

Intimate Thread Lifting

Doaa Saleh, Salwa Bahkali

INTRODUCTION

Thread lifting, once solely focused on facial rejuvenation, has become a topic of interest in aesthetic gynecology. This minimally invasive procedure, known as intimate thread lifting, promises a nonsurgical solution for concerns like laxity in the labia or vaginal tightening. While it offers the attraction of rejuvenation through lifting, filling, and overall vulvovaginal improvement, important considerations exist. This chapter will explore the science behind intimate thread lifting, its applications, and the crucial factors to weigh before deciding if this approach is right for the patient or not.[1]

HISTORY OF THREAD LIFTS: FROM POLYDIOXANONE TO POLYCAPROLACTONE

The history of thread lifts traces back to the early days of facial rejuvenation. While the initial methods in the 1910s involved simply pulling the skin tense, the concept evolved in the late 1990s with the introduction of absorbable polydioxanone (PDO) sutures for lifting facial tissues. Over the years, the technology continued to develop, then poly-l-lactic acid (PLLA) threads emerging as an option offering longer-lasting results. Today, thread lifting remains a popular minimally invasive technique, with various thread types and designs catering to specific needs and areas of concern.[2]

Polydioxanone Threads (Strong in Lifting)

Polydioxanone threads are biocompatible and absorbable synthetic polymer have been the pillar of thread lifts for many years. Used in surgeries for their biocompatibility, they dissolve naturally within 6 months. PDO threads are absorbed into the body over 6 months by hydrolysis. PDO threads offer an immediate lifting effect and trigger neovascularization and collagen production in the targeted area by triggering fibroblasts.[3,4]

Poly-L-Lactic Acid Threads (Longer-lasting Lift)

Following PDO, polylactic acid (PLA) threads emerged. Made from a safe, dissolvable polymer derived from lactic acid, PLA threads offer a longer-lasting solution, but they have less tensile strength compared to PDO. PLA threads stimulate collagen production for a more extended period compared to PDO, potentially leading to results lasting for several years.

Polycaprolactone Threads (The Newcomer)

Polycaprolactone (PCL) threads are the latest addition to the thread lift family. These bio-absorbable threads are not currently used in the intimate area due to potential stiffness. Like PLA, they boast a lengthy dissolving time and promote collagen regeneration over an extended period. This leaves behind a collagen structure that provides long-term support and helps prevent sagging skin.[5]

UNDERSTANDING THE SCIENCE OF THREAD LIFTING

The cornerstone of this procedure is the use of biocompatible and absorbable synthetic threads to produce mechanical and stimulatory actions. The mechanism of action of threads used in thread lifts involves two key aspects:

Immediate Lifting

Mechanical lifting: The term "mechanical lifting" in thread lifting does not directly refer to a specific technique. However, it can be understood as the immediate lifting effect achieved by the physical structure of the threads themselves. The threads themselves provide immediate lifting by acting like tiny anchors or scaffolding within the tissue. Depending on the thread design (barbed, smooth, etc.), they physically reposition sagging skin to create a lifting effect (physical support).[6]

Collagen Stimulation

Beyond the immediate lifting effect achieved by the physical structure of the threads, the following collagen stimulation takes place:[7,8]

Foreign Body Response

The presence of the threads in the tissue triggers the body's natural "foreign body response." This response involves the activation of fibroblasts, cells responsible for producing collagen, the building block of skin firmness and elasticity.

Increased Collagen Production

As fibroblasts are stimulated by the threads, they start producing more collagen. This new collagen production creates a denser network within the skin, providing better support and structure and strengthen the skin. Moreover, collagen helps to fill in fine lines and wrinkles, leading to a smoother and more youthful appearance, and improve skin texture.

Long-term Effect

While the threads themselves eventually dissolve (depending on the material), the newly produced collagen provides a long-lasting improvement in skin tightness and elasticity.

POLYDIOXANONE VERSUS POLY-L-LACTIC ACID THREADS

Although both PDO and PLLA threads can be used for the same indication, the choice of material plays a crucial role in the results and experience. The following **Table 1** demonstrates the key differences between the two most common thread types used in aesthetic gynecology (considered off-label use).

TABLE 1: Comparison between polydioxanone (PDO) and poly-l-lactic acid (PLLA) threads.

Feature	*PDO threads*	*PLLA threads*
Material	Polydioxanone	Poly-l-lactic acid (partially synthetic polymer)
Dissolution rate	Fastest (6–12 months)	Slower (up to 2 years)
Tensile strength	High	Low–Moderate
Collagen stimulation	Yes	Yes
Initial results	Immediate lifting effect	Gradual lifting over weeks
Results duration	Short (6–12 months)	Longer lasting (2 years)
Suitability for intimate areas	Fine lines, mild sagging	Moderate lines, sagging
Cost	Less expensive	More expensive
Stiffness	Less likely	May feel slightly stiffer
Infection risk	Lower	Potentially slightly higher due to longer presence in tissue

TYPES OF THREADS

Thread lifting utilizes various thread designs, come in various lengths, thicknesses, to achieve different aesthetic goals. There are three main types of threads:

Mono Threads (Smooth)

Mono threads are single filaments, devoid of barbs or cogs. They offer a smooth surface for minimal tissue disruption. Primarily focused on stimulating collagen production, mono threads provide a subtle tightening effect. As the body responds to the presence of the threads, collagen synthesis increases, leading to improved skin texture and elasticity. They are ideal for general skin tightening and rejuvenation **(Fig. 1)**.

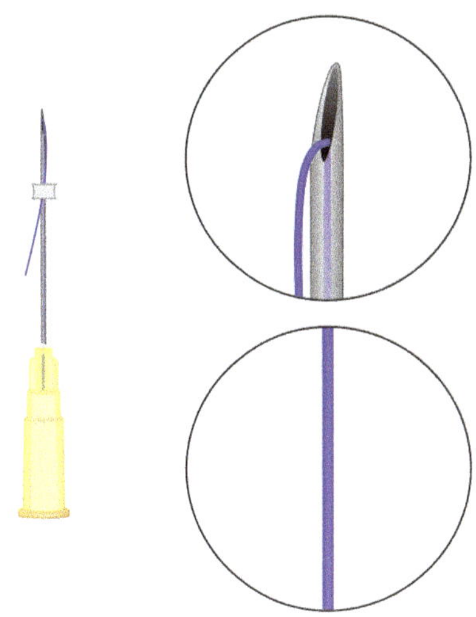

Fig. 1: Mono threads.

Spring Threads (Screw Threads)

Spring threads, also known as screw threads, feature a tightly coiled design with a spiral or screw-like structure resembling a spring. These threads screw into the skin

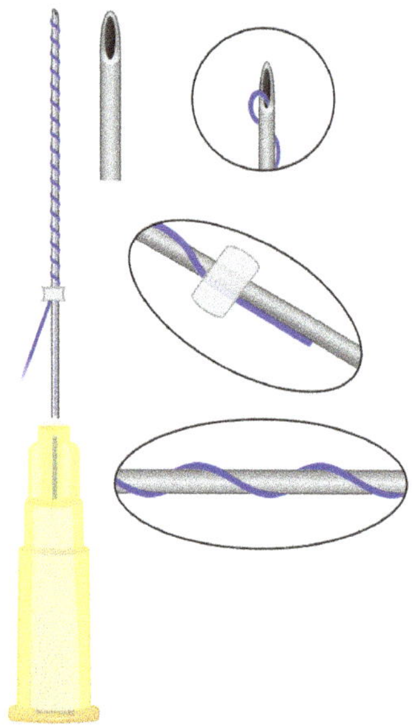

Fig. 2: Spring threads.

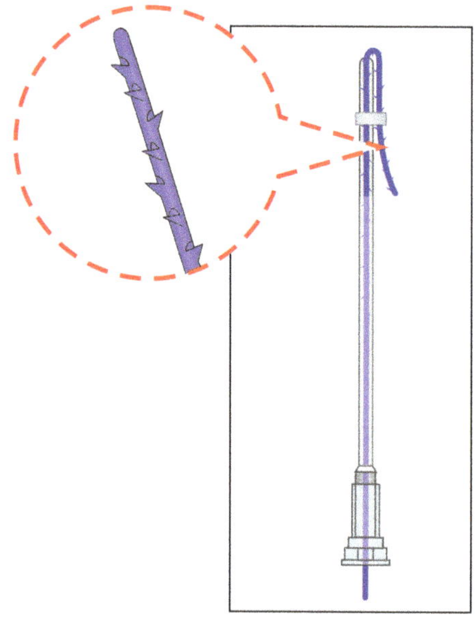

Fig. 3: Cog thread.

tissue, allows for better tissue engagement compared to mono threads, offering a filling and tightening effect. This makes them a good option for addressing moderate laxity and creating a smoother pluming appearance **(Fig. 2)**.

Cog Threads (Barbed Threads)

Cog threads are distinguished by the presence of tiny barbs or cogs along their length **(Fig. 3)**. Cog threads boast the strongest lifting effect among the three types. The barbs act like anchors, effectively grabbing onto the underlying tissue and pulling it upward. This results in a significant lifting effect and improved definition in the treated area. They come in two variations—(1) sharper barbs for a more pronounced lift and (2) duller barbs for a gentler approach. Cog threads are ideal for addressing sagging skin and creating well-defined contours **(Fig. 4)**. However, it is important to remember their strength also translates to potentially more aggressive placement and potential discomfort compared to other thread types.

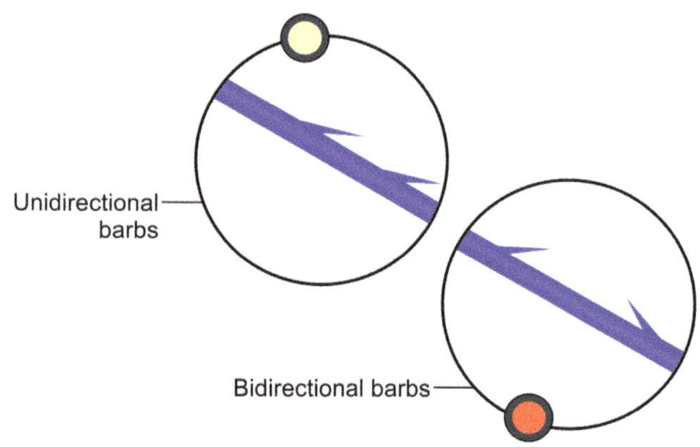

Fig. 4: Difference between unidirectional and bidirectional barbs.

TYPE OF NEEDLE

In thread lifting procedures, the threads are typically inserted using a *blunt-tipped cannula* or sharp needle **(Fig. 5)**.

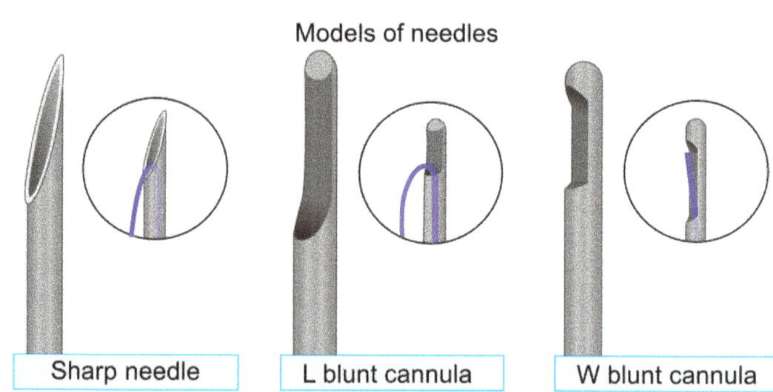

Fig. 5: Types of needles.

Sharp Needle

This is a traditional needle with a pointed tip that pierces the skin to create a pathway for insertion. They are used with the mono and spring threads. They are less commonly used with the cogged threads due to the potential for increased tissue trauma and bleeding.

Blunt-tip Cannula

This is a thin, flexible tube with a blunt, rounded end. It allows for smoother insertion beneath the skin's surface, minimizing tissue disruption, and reduced risk of bleeding and trauma. There are specific cannula size and design vary depending on the type of thread and treatment area.

ADVANTAGES OF INTIMATE THREAD LIFTING

Thread lifting has recently sparked interest in aesthetic gynecology as a potential solution for many intimate concerns. However, offering this service necessitates a cautious approach. So, it is crucial to weigh these significant considerations and prioritize a thorough discussion with patient to determine if this approach aligns with her well-being and desired outcomes.

- *Minimally invasive:* Compared to traditional surgical labia majora lifts, thread lifting is a minimally invasive procedure with shorter recovery times.
- *Natural-looking results:* Threads offer a delicate lifting effect, avoiding the "overdone" appearance sometimes associated with surgical procedures.
- *Minimal downtime:* Most patients experience minimal downtime after thread lifting, allowing for a quick return to daily activities.
- *Stimulates collagen production:* Thread lifting not only provides immediate lifting but also promotes collagen production for long-term skin improvement.

SIDE EFFECTS OF INTIMATE THREAD LIFTING

Intimate thread lifting, while marketed for intimate rejuvenation, is an off-label use with limited research on its safety and efficacy. Here is a breakdown of potential side effects to consider:

Immediate Side Effects

While minimally invasive procedures generally have fewer side effects, intimate thread lifting carries also the possibility of temporary side effects. The most common side effect associated with intimate thread lifting are:

- *Bruising and swelling:* These are common after the procedure and typically resolve within a few days.
- *Pain and discomfort:* The insertion of threads might cause some discomfort, although numbing agents can be used to minimize pain.
- *Bleeding:* Minor bleeding at the insertion site is possible especially if we use sharp needle or increase the number of threads.

Potential Complications

Adverse effects can vary for each patient, depending on their age, general health, lifestyle, and quality of the treated area. They can be mild, moderate, or severe.[9]

- *Infection:* The genital area is more prone to infection compared to the face. The introduction of foreign material such as lifting threads increases the risk of infection, especially in a moist environment such as the genitals. There is always risk of infection if sterile technique is not strictly followed during the procedure, or if patient had local infection at the treated area.
- *Nerve damage:* Improper thread placement at dangerous zones could potentially damage nerves in the delicate intimate area, leading to numbness, tingling, or altered sexual function.
- *Scarring:* Thread migration, infection, or improper insertion might increase the risk of scarring, potentially worsening the cosmetic appearance.
- *Thread migration:* Over time, the threads might move from their original position, causing visible bumps or irregularities.
- *Discomfort during intercourse:* The presence of threads could lead to discomfort during sexual activity.
- *Allergic reaction:* While rare, an allergic reaction to the thread material is possible.
- *Unsatisfactory results:* The results might not meet patient's expectations, and the lifting effect might be temporary.

CONSIDERATIONS AND CAUTIONS SURROUNDING INTIMATE THREAD LIFTING

While thread lifting for the intimate area is advertised as minimally invasive and promises benefits such as improved labial definition and vaginal tightening, it is crucial to address the significant considerations and cautions surrounding this procedure to minimize the risk of complications.

- *Anatomic considerations:* The genital area is a delicate region with unique anatomical features. Skin in this area is often thinner, loose, and more sensitive compared to the face. Additionally, the presence of muscles, blood vessels, and nerves necessitates a thorough understanding of the anatomy to minimize risks during the procedure.

- *Limited research:* Research on thread lifting in aesthetic gynecology is scarce compared to facial applications. Long-term safety and efficacy data are limited.
- *Off-label use:* Thread lifting for the genital area is considered off-label use, meaning it has not been specifically approved for this purpose by regulatory bodies.
- *Psychological impact:* Unsatisfactory results or complications could lead to psychological distress and impact self-esteem.
- *Considerations before thread lifting:* Intimate thread lifting has emerged as an alternative to surgery for intimate rejuvenation. However, it is important to approach this procedure with caution. Thread lifting for the intimate area is considered "off-label use," meaning it has not been specifically approved for this purpose by regulatory bodies. Additionally, extensive research on its safety and efficacy is lacking. Therefore, a qualified physician must assess patient's needs and recommend the most appropriate thread type for optimal results. The choice of thread design will depend on patient's specific aesthetic goals, the degree of laxity, and the quality of the treated area. Before considering intimate thread lifting, there are several factors to carefully weigh. These include:
  - *Realistic expectations:* Patient should not expect dramatic or permanent changes. She should know that thread lifting offers a subtle and temporary approach and her goal might be to achieve a slight improvement, not a dramatic transformation.
  - *Prioritize safety over aesthetics:* Discuss all risks and alternative options with the patient before proceeding.
  - *Patient selection:* This procedure is not suitable for severe skin sagging which need surgical intervention. Ideal candidates have mild-to-moderate skin laxity and good skin elasticity.
  - *Postprocedure instructions:* Patient should be ready to follow the postprocedure instructions and avoid heat, massage at the treated area, intercourse, and strenuous exercise for 1 week or as instructed.

APPLICATIONS OF INTIMATE THREAD LIFTING

While research is limited, some propose that intimate thread lifting might offer solutions for concerns related to intimate aging and vaginal laxity. However, the choice of thread type depends heavily on individual needs and should be determined by a qualified physician. The potential thread applications:

- *Smooth mono thread for skin tightening:* Smooth threads might provide a subtle tightening effect for overall skin texture improvement in the intimate area and reducing the appearance of fine lines.
- *Spring/screw threads for fold reduction:* For concerns such as minor folds or wrinkles, spring threads could potentially offer a delicate lifting effect to minimize their appearance. It can also give a filling effect and volumizing the treated area.
- *Cog/barbed threads for lifting:* It is crucial to exercise caution with cog threads in the intimate area due to their aggressive nature. While they might be used to elevate the mons pubis or labia majora for a more defined shape (off-label use), the potential for discomfort, and complications is significant.

THE THREAD LIFTING PROCEDURE

The thread lifting procedure is typically performed on an outpatient basis in the following steps:

- *Consultation:* During the consultation, the physician will assess patient's concerns, medical history, and patient's suitability for the procedure.
- *Local anesthetic:* In case of mono and spring threads, numbing cream is applied to the treatment area to minimize discomfort. But in case of using cog threads, lidocaine 1–2% could be used in the insertion points and along the thread path.
- *Thread insertion:* In case of using sharp needle, thread inserted directly into specific level and locations according to the our goal. However, if we use blunt canula we must create an opining to insert the canula with threads.
- *Positioning:* The threads are then carefully positioned and secured to achieve the desired firming, volumizing, or lifting effect. Threads could be inserted in serial, parallel; fanning or crosshatch pattern according to our aim **(Figs. 6A to C)**.
- *Number of threads:* Number will depend on the case. An adequate number of threads will give better results if done appropriately.
- *Recovery:* There might be some initial swelling or bruising, but most patients recover quickly and can resume normal activities within a few days.

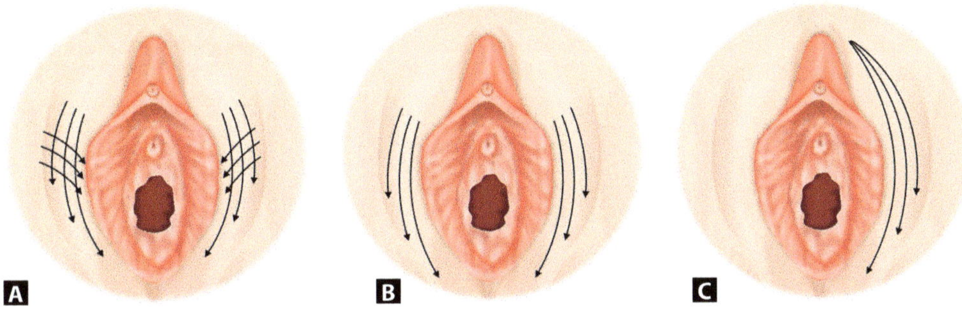

Figs. 6A to C: Positioning of threads.

CONCLUSION

Intimate thread lifting is a controversial topic with limited research and significant potential risks. It is crucial to prioritize safety and explore alternative options with a proven track record. If you are considering this procedure, you have to be expert in both thread lifting and genital anatomy. Discussion of the risks and benefits thoroughly with the patient will help in making an informed decision based on patient's individual needs and expectations.[10]

REFERENCES

1. Adam A, Karypidis D, Ghanem A. Thread lifts: a critical analysis of treatment modalities. J Drugs Dermatol. 2020;19(4):413-7.
2. Albucker SJ, Lipner SR. "Weekend Facelifts" Gone Wrong: Retrospective Analysis of the MAUDE Database on Thread-Lifting Complications From 2003-2023. J Cutan Med Surg. 2023;27(6):647-8.
3. Ali YH. Two years' outcome of thread lifting with absorbable barbed PDO threads: Innovative score for objective and subjective assessment. J Cosmet Laser Ther. 2018;20(1):41-9.
4. Bernardini FP. Is there a role for a noninvasive alternative to face and neck lifting? The polydioxanone thread lift. Aesthet Surg J. 2019;39(8):362-3.
5. Chen Y, Niu Z, Jin R, Lei Y, Han Y. Treatment of complications following facial thread-lifting. Plast Reconstr Surg. 2021;148(1):159e-61e.
6. Fukaya M. Two mechanisms of rejuvenation using thread lifting. Plast Reconstr Surg Glob Open. 2018;6(12):e2068.
7. Halepas S, Chen XJ, Ferneini EM. Thread-lift sutures: anatomy, technique, and review of current literature. J Oral Maxillofac Surg. 2020;78(5):813-20.
8. Hügül H, Özkoca D, Kutlubay Z. Thread lifting: Does patient satisfaction change according to age, type of threads used, number of threads used and treatment area? J Cosmet Dermatol. 2022;21(5):1936-9.
9. Niu Z, Zhang K, Yao W, Li Y, Jiang W, Zhang Q, et al. A meta-analysis and systematic review of the incidences of complications following facial thread-lifting. Aesthetic Plast Surg. 2021;45(5):2148-58.
10. Obourn CA, Williams EF 3rd. A decade of thread-lifting-what have we learned over the last 10 years? JAMA Facial Plast Surg. 2018;20(5):349-50.

CHAPTER 13

Liposuction and Its Use in Cosmetic Gynecology

Mohan Thomas, James Dsilva

INTRODUCTION

Liposuction is a cosmetic procedure to remove unwanted fat, which can be performed under local or general anesthesia. There are many terms used to refer to this procedure, such as suction-assisted lipectomy, suction lipoplasty, liposculpting, and liposculpture. The concept of liposuction, i.e., suctioning out unwanted fat, traces its origins back to the early 1900s, but it was not until 1970s that Illouz really popularized liposuction as we know it today. With the constantly growing body mass index (BMI) worldwide, and given the fact that apart from using implants, fat contouring is the only way to really sculpt the body, it is not surprising that liposuction continues to grow and has slowly become a major component, or an add-on to most procedures cosmetic surgeons perform today. It requires 3D understanding of the anatomy of the adipose tissue, precision of the surgeon, skill, and ability of the artist that is attained only with a hands-on experience.

The first and most important thing to know is that not all patients are candidates for liposuction as it is not a weight loss procedure rather is only for body contouring. The satisfaction of a good outcome for both the patient and the operating surgeon would come from selecting the right patient. Liposuction is most effective for treating localized adipose deposits, particularly combined with a targeted weight loss and lifestyle changes. The suction-based removal of excess fat—which is the most basic requirement of liposuction—is the simple part. The creative part includes determining how much fat to remove for an overall contouring, how much to leave behind for a smooth coverage, and how retractile the skin is.[1]

People have different body shapes, eye colors or hair, similarly there is also enormous variation in pelvic areas, vaginas, and vulvas, regardless of age. The tissues in the vagina and vulva lose volume and their color change from pink to a paler or darker hue. The labia deflates and the clitoris shrinks along with appearance of crinkly, inelastic thin skin in the majoras.

Aging and obstetric perineal trauma can be the cause of atrophy and dimensional problems such as dyspareunia and vaginal laxity and leading to postpartum sexual dysfunction.[2] This frequent condition has a negative impact on women's quality of life and sexual health. Vaginoplasty and a combination of a few noninvasive treatment options as well such as hyaluronic acid (HA) injection or fat transplantation alone enhances the women's quality of interpersonal relationship.

The aging process causes a diminished trophism of the vulvovaginal structures—reduction of fat deposits of labia majora, with has a "sagging bag" look, and reduced trophism of the labia minora; reduction of the fat pad of the ischiorectal fossa; and reduction of trophicity of the vaginal mucosa and lamina propria.[3,4]

Ever since the publication of the standardized technique for fat grafting by Coleman, lipofilling has become a very important and valuable tool in plastic surgery[5] as well as in cosmetic gynecology. Since then, much research into these multipotent mesenchymal-derived progenitor cells also called stem cells have been performed. Stem cells are well known for their regenerative potential and ability to differentiate into ectoderm, endoderm, and mesoderm lineages. In gynecological practice, liposuction is usually required to treat a prominent Mons or to harvest fat for augmentation of the labia majora.

Usually, fat is harvested in a sterile manner either under local anesthesia or general anesthesia. This fat is then processed by decantation and sometimes centrifuging of the harvested tissue. Fat obtained from liposuction can now be injected in areas where there is a deficiency such as the labia majora in a female.

Awareness of the genital appearance in today's society is because of the hairless appearance as well as more open discussion about the genital appearance and the available corrective options. Women consider prominent labia majora as the sign of youthfulness, hence, knowledge about techniques to return fullness to the genitalia is an important part of the cosmetic surgeon's armamentarium. Autologous fat grafting from fat samples is a technique for improving the appearance of the inner lips and is an important procedure in vulvar plastic surgery.

ANATOMY OF SUBCUTANEOUS TISSUE

It is very important to understand the structure of subcutaneous fat before operating on it. Subcutaneous fatty layer is divided into superficial and deep layers with a fascial tissue such as Scarpa's fascia in the abdomen or superficial musculoaponeurotic system (SMAS) layer of the face. Taking out fat from the deeper layer is much safer as the risk of contour irregularities or damage to the vasculature of the overlying skin is significantly reduced.

The consistency of fatty tissue can be divided into two groups:

1. Fibrofatty tissue is not suitable for liposuction procedures and is usually found in the outer layer.
2. Areola fat is deep in the fat layer, the tissue is looser and the fiber matrix component of the fat is less, so it is sensitive to liposuction.

   To reduce the risk of contour irregularities, areas of adhesion (ZOA) where subcutaneous tissue adheres to the fascia of the central muscle should be avoided during liposuction.

Liposuction Indications

- The patient must demonstrate deviations from normal body contour caused by excess adiposity in the region.
- The patient should be within 30% of their normal BMI.
- An ideal candidate is nonobese, with minimal skin laxity, and minimal to moderately excess adipose tissue.

Contraindications

- People with body dysmorphic disorder (BDD), or those with unrealistic expectations and a tenuous understanding of the procedure at hand should not proceed with surgery until proper evaluation has been obtained.
- People with BMI of >33 where weight loss rather than improvement in body shape is a priority.
- Relative contraindications include abdominal scars, clinical hernias, patients on blood thinners, those with cardiac insufficiency, etc.

EQUIPMENT

Since the inception of liposuction, the cannulas used have evolved over time. What was once a sharp, single-hole cannula has now become a blunt cannula with several holes near the tip. Blunt-ended cannula helps reduce the risk of inadvertent puncture of the pleura, peritoneum, or deep structures and also helps reduce intraoperative bleeding.

The cannula works by aspirating fat cells through the fibrous matrix that separates the fat pockets, allowing the fat to enter the vacuum tube. Therefore, a larger diameter (and surface area) cannula causes more damage and more fat avulsion; however, large diameter cannulas can also cause more injuries and blood loss than small diameter cannulas.

The choice of liposuction aspiration device (manual syringe or suction machine) depends on how much fat needs to be removed and whether the aspirated fat is intended for autologous grafting in which case manual liposuction will get the best yield of fat cells. Use of a wetting solution (i.e., tumescent solution) composed of a mixture of diluted lidocaine and epinephrine and infiltrated subcutaneously prior to the actual liposuction being performed gives a bloodless collection of fatty aspirate.

FAT AS A VOLUME ENHANCER

Pros

- Autologous fat (from your own body), as opposed to dermal fillers, replaces "like with like".
- Fat transfer results are natural, long lasting, and safe.
- Fat transfer is a noninvasive method for achieving facial rejuvenation.
- It improves the vascularity of the area.
- The skin overlying fat graft has improved glow.

Cons

- It is time consuming to prepare fat tissue before transferring it, compared to dermal fillers, which are pre-packaged. Anesthesia may be required.
- Though longer lasting than dermal fillers, fat transfer costs more.
- For augmentation, you may require multiple sessions to achieve the desired look.
- Once injected, it is almost impossible to remove completely if over filled.
- Can cause vascular compromise if injected directly into a vein.

INDICATIONS OF FAT TRANSFER TO THE GENITAL AREA

The genital area is highly vascular with a network of vessels supplying the area. The skin in the genital area is thin, sensitive as well as shows signs of aging with weight loss as well as hormonal changes. The availability of this highly vascular tissue scaffold makes it an ideal recipient area for the transferred fat with a minimal resorption rate.

Indications of fat grafting in functional gynecology:

- Treatment of depressed scars
- Atrophy or dystrophy of the vagina with or without pain
- Postradiation dermatitis of the genital area

Indications of fat grafting in aesthetic gynecology:

- Volume replacement of the labia majora
- Plumping of the labia minora
- Augmentation of the "G" spot
- Peri vulvar areas and vaginal walls to improve vaginal laxity.

Mechanism of Action of Adipose-derived Stem Cells[6]

- Adipose-derived stem cells (ADSCs) stimulate the recruitment of endogenous stem cells and promote their differentiation into specific tissues.
- They increase the secretion of growth factors, vascular endothelial growth factor (VEGF), hepatocyte growth factor, and insulin like growth factor and thus improve the vascularity of the overlying skin.
- Antioxidant capabilities of ADSCs mitigate inflammation.
- Cultured ADSCs have also been found to reduce wrinkles through collagen and elastic fiber production and other antiaging effects in the skin through glycation suppression, antioxidation, and trophic effects.

This leads to:

- Enhanced collagen deposition and skin elasticity
- Formation of new blood vessels
- Tissue remodeling,
- Thickening of the dermis
- Down regulation of melanogenic activity

WHY PERFORM AUGMENTATION OF THE LABIA MAJORA?

The main indications for augmentation of the labia majora are:

- *Labia majora hypoplasia:* May be normal but may be perceived as hypoplastic due to the perceived ideal of a fuller labia majora.
- *Laxity of the labia majora skin:* This has several causes, and these may be acquired such as secondary to massive weight loss, trauma, or tumors but also physiologic causes such as aging and those associated with menopause or changes during pregnancy.
- After surgical reduction of the labia majora, for a fuller look.

LIPOSUCTION AND FAT GRAFTING PROCEDURE

Photographs and Marking

The areas to be treated are always marked with the patient in a standing position.

- Areas to be liposuctioned are marked with blue and the areas that have to be left untouched or have deformities are marked with red color, as seen in **Figures 1A and B**.
- Any previous scars or adhesions are marked and checked for hernias.
- The treatment plan is thoroughly discussed with the patient one last time on the day of surgery. A video consent along with a written consent is taken and confirmed. Patient is asked to examine himself/herself in a full-length mirror to verify areas to be treated.

The examination of the genital area should also be performed in the standing position as well as in a lithotomy position preferably with a mirror as in **Figures 2A and B** so that the patient can explain her concerns clearly. Careful

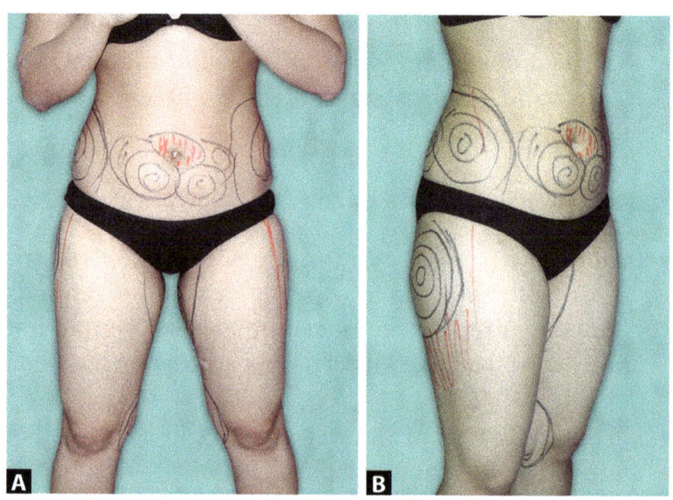

Figs. 1A and B: Patient being marked in the standing position so that the elevations and depressions are well established according to topography.

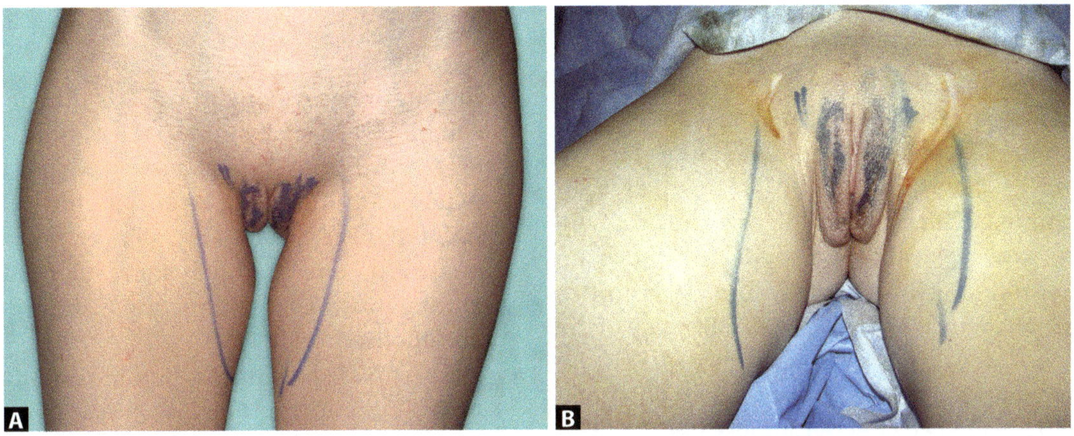

Figs. 2A and B: Deflated labia majora of a 45-year-old lady who underwent a 15 kg weight loss over 6 months.

documentation of the anatomy, including any variations, has to be brought to the patient's notice as well as recorded for medicolegal purposes.

If the labia majora are very "baggy" with significant excess skin, then excisional labia majora reduction (majoraplasty) should also be considered. The discussion should include the extent of fat grafting and the need for touch up procedures at a later date.

Anesthesia

Liposuction may be performed under local, regional, or general anesthesia. The anesthetic technique will vary according to the areas being operated upon; arms, thighs, abdomen, or buttocks and the volume of liposuction being performed.

- General anesthesia is recommended for large volume liposuction or if the patient desires it and an orotracheal tube is used for intubation.
- Wetting solution (containing lignocaine and adrenaline) is then administered, allowing 15–30 minutes to pass for maximal vasoconstriction and anesthesia.

Painting and Draping of Patient

- The surgical procedure begins with the cleaning and painting of the areas to be operated. We only use povidone iodine 5% or 10% solution for painting the area.
- Access points which can be 3–4 mm in size made with a stab knife or a skin punch are usually placed in such a way that they are hidden as well as provide easy access to all areas of fat removal as seen in **Figure 3.**

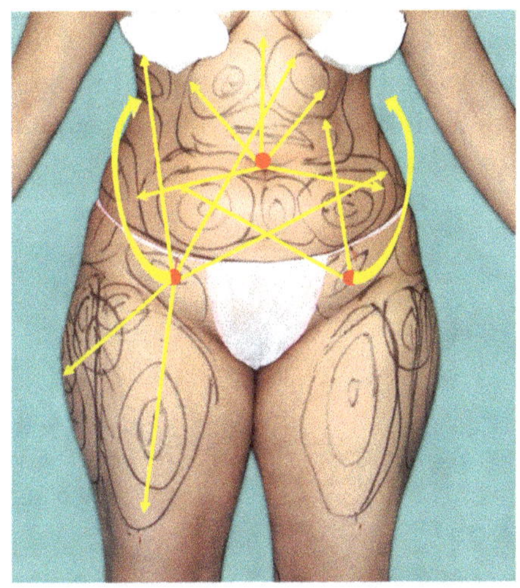

Fig. 3: Access points marked in red are placed in hidden areas from which different areas can be accessed for liposuction as marked by yellow arrows.

- The areas to be treated which have been pre-marked are selectively infiltrated. The dominant hand controls the cannula or the syringe (if manual suction is employed), while the nondominant hand is spread wide on the skin, constantly feeling the presence of the distal cannula. The nondominant hand provides two important functions, to lightly palpate for areas of adiposity and to constantly monitor the depth of the cannula.
- Suction should occur just beneath the superficial fat layer. The presence of skin dimpling is an indicator that the cannula resides in a too superficial of a location, which can lead to obvious contour irregularities.

Traditional suction-assisted liposuction (SAL) with cannulas is the most widely used technique; however, there are recent technological advancements that have led to new techniques that deserve discussing.

Power-assisted liposuction (PAL) utilizes a cannula that has a small motor which oscillates the cannula back and forth and is thought to make the process more efficient.

Ultrasound-assisted liposuction (UAL) utilizes an ultrasound cannula, which causes the breakdown of the adipose cells, which can then be suctioned out using a standard cannula, again with the effort in mind to alleviate surgeon fatigue and increase the efficiency of the procedure.

Laser-assisted liposuction (LAL) uses a laser-equipped cannula to help breakdown targeted adipose tissue, which can then be suctioned out, also demonstrates higher efficiency in terms of fat reduction.

Regardless of the technology employed, the endpoint of liposuction is based on the clinical judgment of the surgeon taking into account the lack of palpable adipose tissue in the targeted area.

Harvest of Fat

- Usually, about 100–150 cc of fat is obtained by liposuction through a 1.8–2.0 mm fat extraction cannula. We usually undertake lipocontouring of the area at the same time as a result we use a liposuction machine and harvest larger quantities of fat. After infiltration, 15 minutes are allowed to pass for proper anesthesia and the hemostatic effect of adrenaline. During this time, recipient areas for injection can be anesthetized.
- Harvest is done with multihole cannula with 1 mm holes (Tulip Corp, USA). We prefer using a Luer lock 20 cc syringe for small fat harvest or liposuction machine and a sterile vacuum system for larger volume of fat aspirate as this maintains a closed system for the entire procedure **(Figs. 4A to C)**.

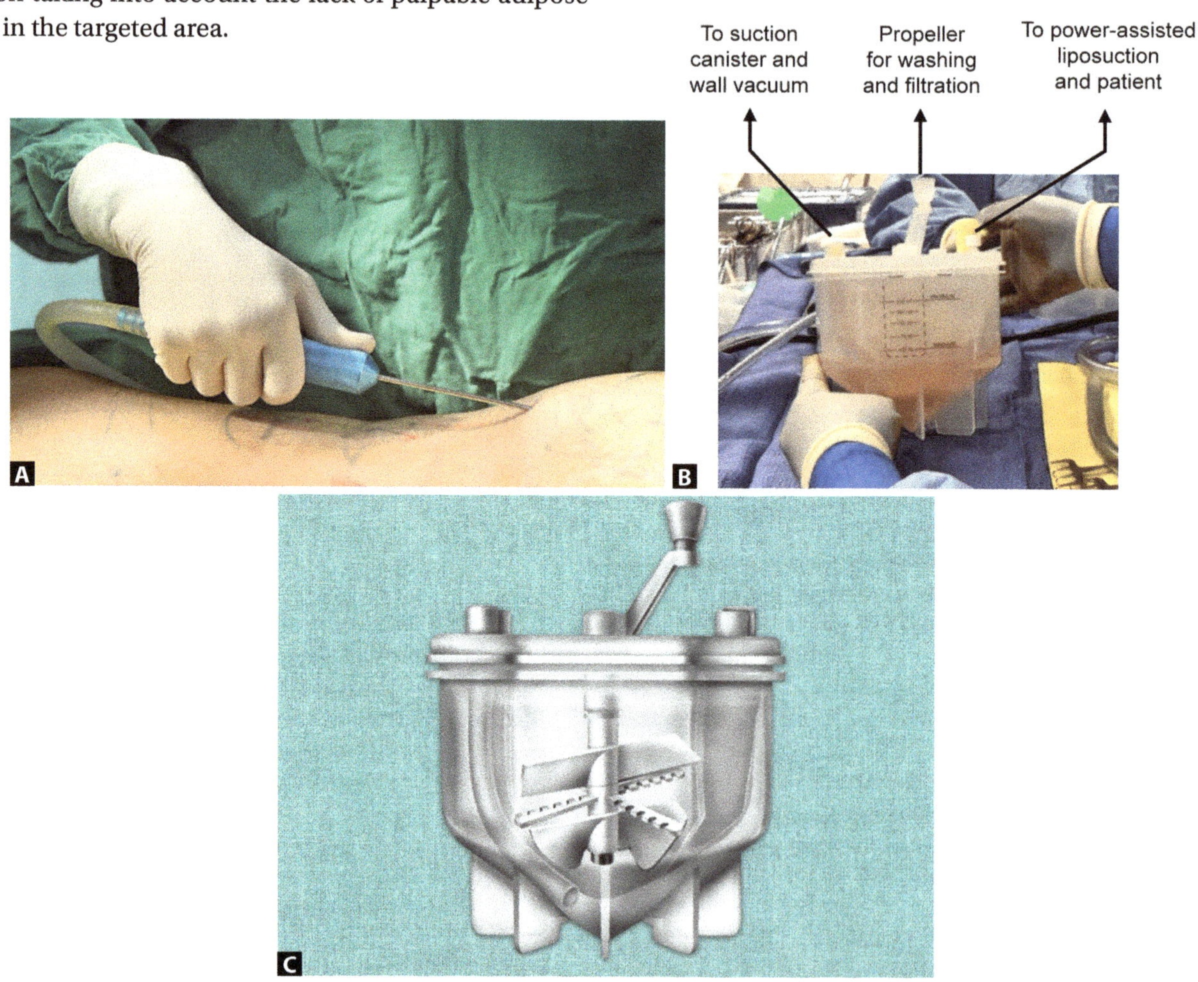

Figs. 4A to C: (A) Fat harvest from the abdomen; (B) Closed resolve system for fat washing and harvest; (C) Resolve system as close-up.

- After harvest the donor area is dressed with a pressure dressing that is opened by the patient himself/herself the next day. Compression garment is used for about 3 weeks to prevent excess swelling and hematomas.

Nanofat Preparation

Several techniques have been described to harvest and process the fat such as centrifuging, washing and straining, and decantation. The fat is first sedimented allowing the fat to settle by gravity to separate the aqueous and fatty layers. The aqueous layer is discarded while the supernatant fat is taken and washed multiple times with saline to remove the blood impurities.

This supernatant washed fat is then taken in test tubes and centrifuged at 3,000 rpm for 3 minutes.[7] This separates the oil, blood, and fluid from the adipocytes and stromal vascular fraction (SVF) **(Figs. 5 A to C)**.

- The collected fat and SVF is then further processed by emulsification using the Tulip nanofat filtration system:
    - The fat is transferred to 1 mL/5 mL syringes having a Luer lock.
    - One full syringe and one empty syringe are connected using a Tulip connector.
    - This aspirate is passed through a 1.4 mm followed by a 1.2 mm connector 20 times respectively.
    - The broken-down fat is then passed through a 0.8 mm connector 20 times to further break it down into a liquefied state **(Figs. 6A to C)**.
- Finally, the emulsified material is filtered by passing through a Nanofat filter. This filter captures large collagen particles which can be an impediment to injection at a cutaneous level through thin needles. This is generally required only for the difficult areas on the face such as the lids or infraorbital regions.

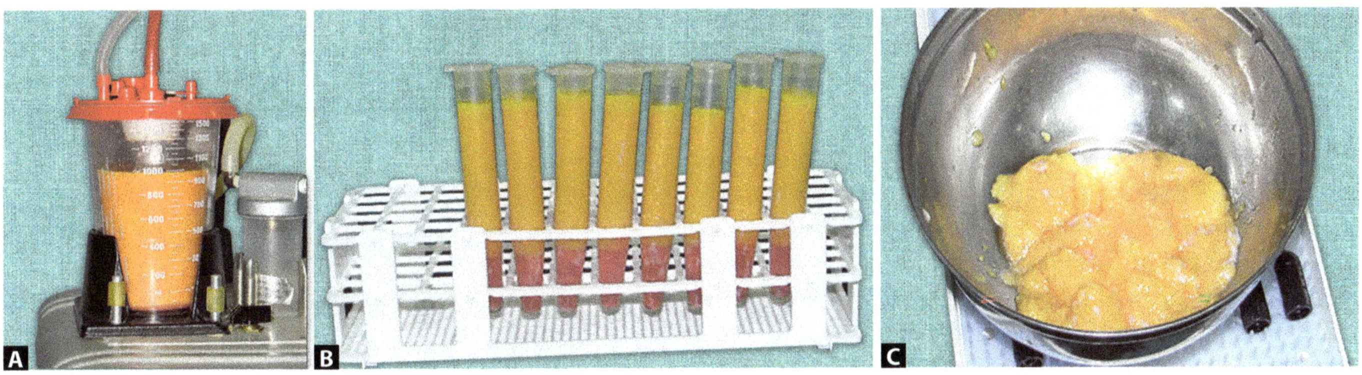

Figs. 5A to C: Fat separation. (A) Harvested fat being allowed to stand to separate the fat from the fluid. (B) The supernatant after being centrifuged; (C) The fat is now ready for grafting as a macro and micro fat grafts.

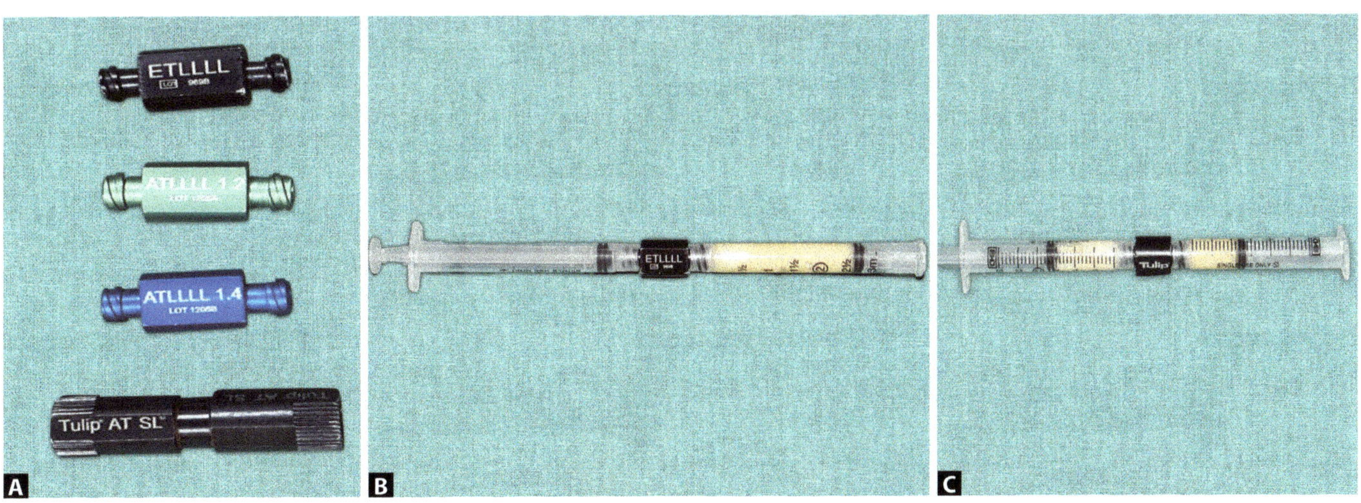

Figs. 6A to C: Nano fat preparation. (A) Different Tulip connectors used to breakdown fat cells; (B) A 3-cc syringe having filtered and separated fat connected to an empty syringe; (C) The fat after being broken down and passed through the narrowest connector. The color and consistency of the tissue changes.

Injection

For the genital area use of Emla followed by a field block will provide adequate anesthesia. Pudendal block can be utilized when Nano fat transfer is considered in the introitus.

- Injection is done through cannulas of 26/27G needles using 1 mL syringes **(Fig. 7).**
- Injection is done into the dermis till a blanching is seen. This process usually follows volume addition of normal fat into the deeper layers.
- The entire area is covered with Nano fat. Typically, 1 mL of Nanofat can cover 1 cm^2. It is generally used to improve the fine lines.

MARKING OF THE DEFLATED GENITAL AREAS

If fat grafting alone is performed, then we mark the areas requiring fat grafting with the patient in the lithotomy position. Long, oval-shaped outlines are drawn on each labia majora, starting at the level of the outer introitus from the interlabial sulcus medially to the labial-thigh sulcus laterally. Posteriorly the oval marking (marked in solid blue in **Figure 8**) extends from the posterior fourchette to the level of the pubic prominence (2–3 cm above the distal upper part of the clitoral hood) anteriorly. This is the area for transfer of normal fat grafts which are injected in a retrograde manner using 2 mm Coleman tips. A rhomboid area is marked above the pubic symphysis (marked in red in **Figure 8**) specially in people who have lost the prominence of the pubic pad of fat which may need fat augmentation. A triangular area of the labia on outer side of the oval marking is marked (marked in green in **Figure 8**) which will need micro and nano fat grafts.

Incisions are placed, one on each side above the labia majora and if required at the lower end of labia majora. Placement of these incisions is crucial to ensure that the whole length of the labia is uniformly injected with fat graft. Placing these too low or too high may sometimes lead to deficiencies in fat filling as crisscrossing of the cannula tracks is important for uniform and adequate fill. **Figure 9** shows points of insertion of the cannula.

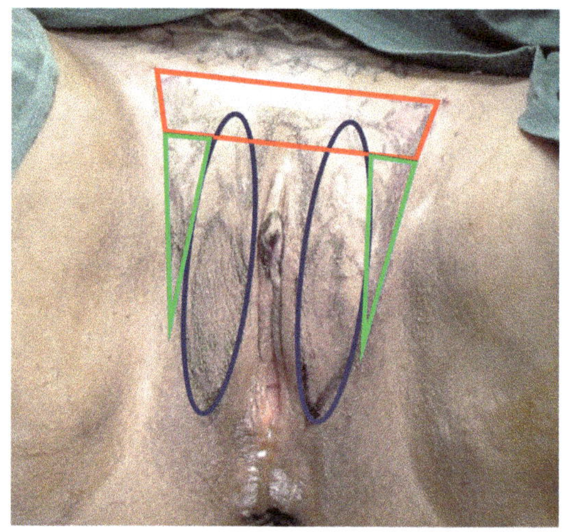

Fig. 8: Marking of the areas for fat grafting. Blue areas will need normal, concentrated fat while the red and green areas will require injection of micro and nano fat.

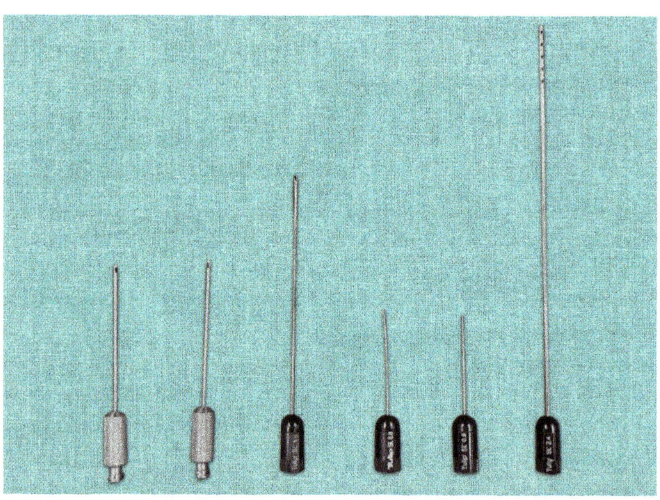

Fig. 7: Various types of cannulas used for Macro, Micro and Nano fat transfer to the face and genital areas.

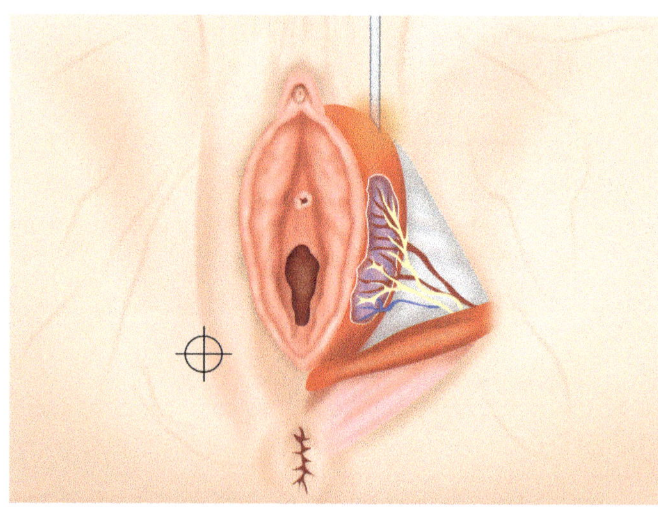

Fig. 9: Placement of access for fat grafting.

Injection technique is crucial to prevent fat necrosis causing fat lakes and cyst formation. A layered deposition of small aliquots more like a "spaghetti" into the deep and superficial layers is essential to prevent these issues.

When fat is introduced, one hand is placed on the syringe itself and softly pushes the syringe plunger, while the other hand is in the marked area guiding the fat to where it needs to stay as it is actively introduced.

If the fat is injected without moving the cannula, then a large blob of fat is deposited. If, on the other hand, the syringe is withdrawn too fast and over a long distance while injecting the fat the result is deposition of a thin ribbon of fat. Based on calculations it has been deduced that for each 1,000 mm^3 (1 mL) of fat delivered, the cannula has to retract in its channel for 100 mm or 10 cm. Note that this rule applies regardless of the cannula diameter, the size of its hole, the pressure of injection, or the rate of injection in mL/second (milliliter per second) **(Figs. 10A and B)**.

Once sufficient fullness of the areas has been achieved, the surgeon molds the fat between his thumb and fingers so that there are no lumps and the augmentation is uniform. In the presence of crinkly skin "Nano fat" created by passing normal fat a few times through a filter till it becomes a pale color and liquidy, is injected at a superficial level **(Figs. 11A and B)**. This also improves the skin quality. Finally sterile tapes are placed on the access points to prevent tracking out of fat.

Postoperative Care

Swelling and tenderness are expected for up to 4 weeks. No special recommendations are given to patients other than to avoid strenuous exercise and sexual intercourse for 4–6 weeks. Broad spectrum antibiotics specially those covering gram-negative and anaerobic organisms are prescribed for 3–5 days **(Figs. 12 and 13)**.

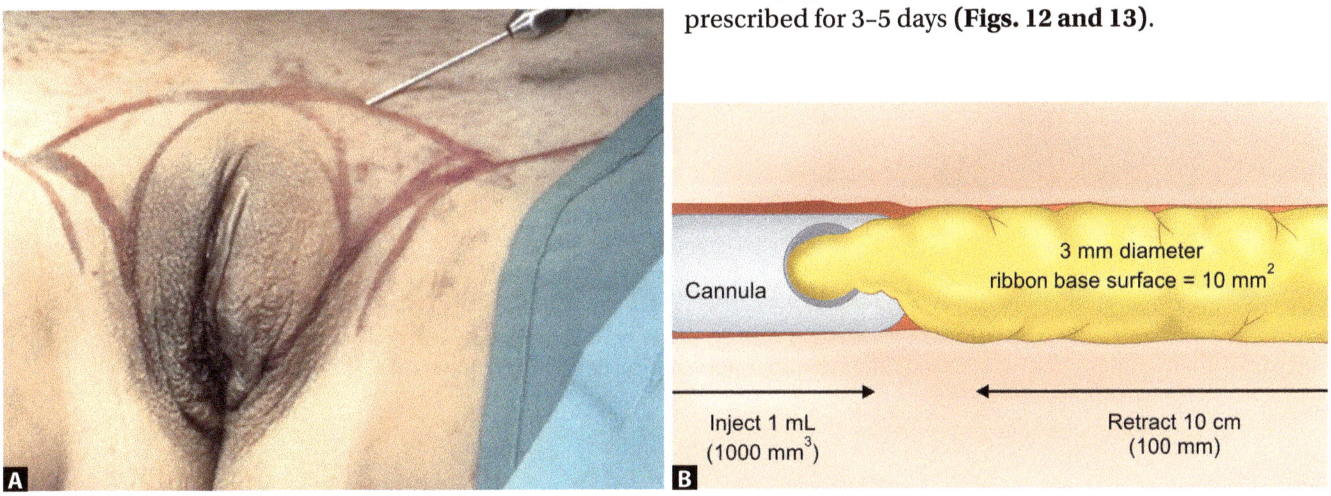

Figs. 10A and B: (A) Placement of fat from the superior access point; (B) Placement of fat graft as a ribbon with uniform thickness for vascularization at its best.

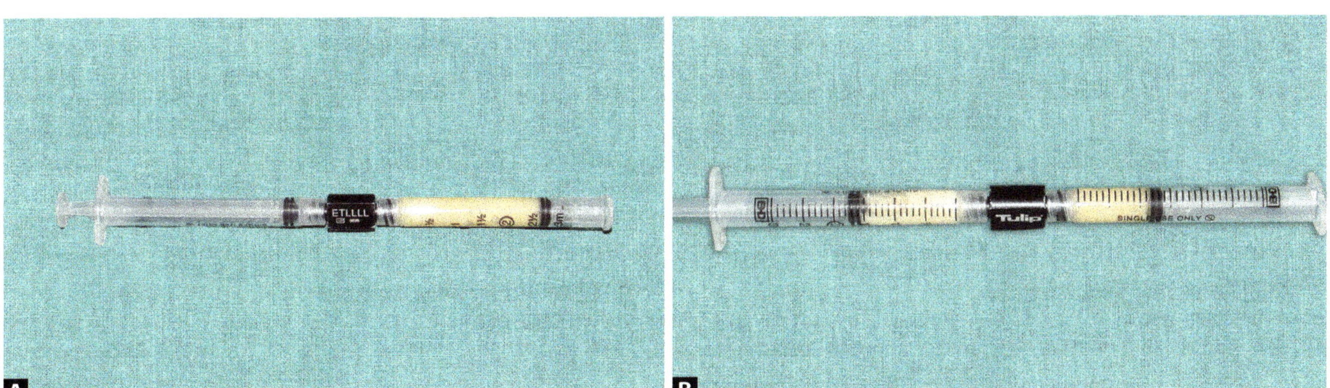

Figs. 11A and B: (A) Normal fat; (B) Nano fat formed after passing through the filter.

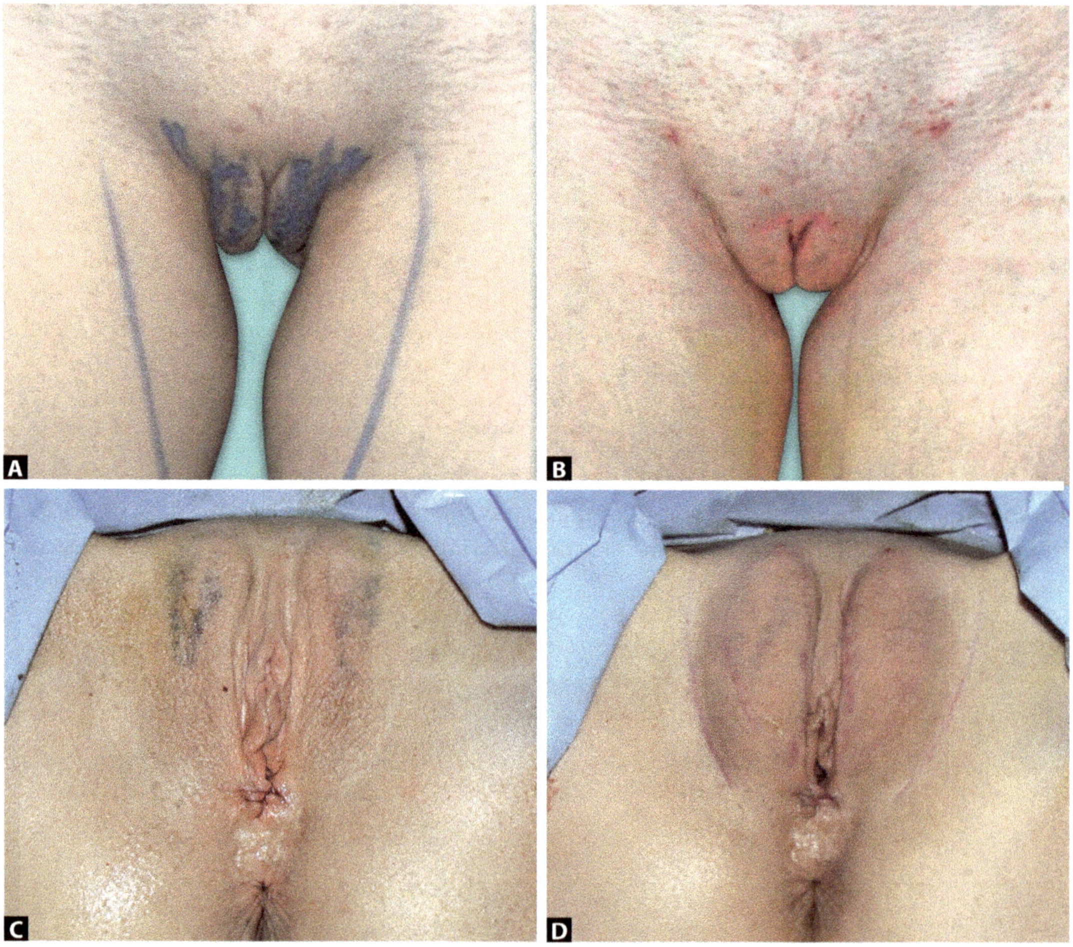

Figs. 12A to D: A 45-year-old woman underwent vaginoplasty with lipomodeling. (A and C) Preoperative appearance; (B and D) Postoperative.

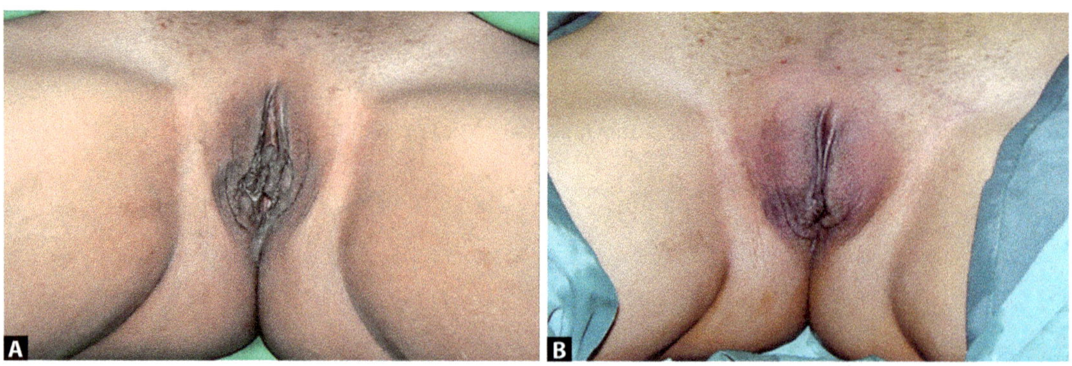

Figs. 13A and B: A 27-year-old female who has a genetically deflated labia majora. (A and B) Pre- and postoperative photographs.

COMPLICATIONS

Patients must be counseled before the procedure that some complications are definitely expected, such as postoperative bruising. The following are some common complications that the patient and the team should be mindful about:

Complication of liposuction—is the presence of bruising and contour deformities. Patients should know that postoperative bruising is certainly expected and may take 1–2 weeks to resolve; however, postprocedural edema may take up to several weeks to dissipate, and thus the final shape and contour may not be evident until such swelling has resolved.

- Seroma
- Temporary weight gain
- Paresthesias
- Lidocaine toxicity

The most disastrous but also least common complications of liposuction include fat emboli (present with shortness of breath and dyspnea), DVT (pain in the calf area and swelling of the legs), and pulmonary embolism (signs of dyspnea and tachycardia).

Complications of Nanofat include:

- Unevenness
- Infection of the injected fat
- Fat cysts
- Bruising and hematoma

CONCLUSION

Liposuction for fat grafting or autologous fat transfer in a Gynecological setting is a minimalistic procedure and is usually confined to volumizing the Labia which can be mastered by a surgeon well versed with the anatomy of the abdomen and the lower body. Achieving an outstanding aesthetic result requires experience and an artistic eye. As with any cosmetic procedure, the dictum of 'less is more, less is better' holds especially true with fat grafting to the genital area.

REFERENCES

1. Thomas M, D'silva J, Abraham A. Use of technologies to improve the liposuction outcome including skin texture and form. Enhanced Liposuction-New Perspectives and Techniques. Intech Open; 2022.
2. Signorello LB, Harlow BL, Chekos AK, Repke JT. Postpartum sexual functioning and its relationship to perineal trauma: a retrospective cohort study of primiparous women. Am J Obstet Gynecol. 2001;184(5):881-90.
3. Jelovsek JE, Maher C, Barber MD. Pelvic organ prolapse. Lancet. 2007;369(9566):1027.
4. Garagiola DM, Tarver RD, Gibson L, Rogers RE, Wass JL. Anatomic changes in the pelvis after uncomplicated vaginal delivery: a CT study on 14 women. AJR Am J Roentgenol. 1989;153(6):1239-41.
5. Coleman SR. Structural fat grafts: The ideal filler? Clin Plast Surg. 2001;28:111-9.
6. Banyard DA, Sarantopoulos CN, Borovikova AA, Qiu X, Wirth GA, Paydar KZ, et al. Phenotypic analysis of stromal vascular fraction after mechanical shear reveals stress-induced progenitor populations. Plast Reconstr Surg. 2016;138(2):237e-47e.
7. Zhu M, Zhou Z, Chen Y, Schreiber R, Ransom JT, Fraser JK, et al. Supplementation of fat grafts with adipose-derived regenerative cells improves long-term graft retention. Ann Plast Surg. 2010;64:222-8.

CHAPTER 14

Botulinum Toxin for Vaginismus

Ayman El Attar

INTRODUCTION

Women who suffer from this physical and psychological disorder may experience pain during sexual intercourse, gynecological examinations, or while inserting tampons. They tend to experience fear and anxiety that causes them to panic and withdraw from these situations. Vaginal penetration disorder is a major sexual problem with a negative impact on the patient, her partner, and even their family. Treatment of vaginismus is still a big challenge and often without success.

The successful treatment of vaginismus in our center started in 2018 using our protocol of injecting botulinum toxin in the bulbospongiosus muscle 50–200 units according to the severity of the case.

In 1862, the father of modern gynecology James Marion Sims **(Fig. 1)** coined the term vaginismus to describe recurrent and persistent involuntary contractions of perineal muscles during penetration, resulting in anxiety, fear, and pain.[1] The prevalence of vaginismus varies significantly between developed and developing countries. This could be attributed to cultural differences and ranges. The great variation of reporting the prevalence ranged from 1 to 60%.[2-4] The American Psychiatric Society has defined vaginismus as "an uncontrollable contraction of the muscle of one-third of the external vagina that prevents intercourse."[5] According to the Diagnostic and Statistical Manual of Mental Disorders, fifth edition (DSM-5), vaginismus is under the category of genitopelvic pain/penetration disorder.[5,6] The World Health Organization has emphasized the pain associated with vaginismus and categorized it as a disorder of female sexual penetration pain in its International Statistical Classification of Diseases and Related Health Problems, 11th edition (ICD-11).[7]

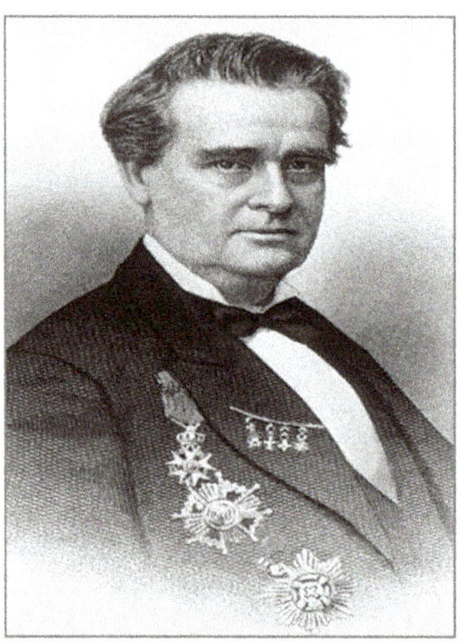

Fig. 1: James Marion Sims (January 25, 1813 to November 13, 1883).

The term "vaginism" describes an involuntary, recurrent, or persistent contraction of the perineal muscles surrounding the lower third of the vagina or the orgasmic plateau. It occurs during sexual intercourse and/or penetration or during a gynecological examination with a speculum.

A controversial American physician is considered the "Father of modern gynecology," who developed a surgical technique for the repair of vesicovaginal fistula and used enslaved African-American women, without consent or anesthesia, as experimental subjects. He was regarded by many modern historians as highly unethical. He described it as "a prime example of progress in the medical profession made at the expense of a vulnerable population."

In 1862, he described vaginismus as a reflex-like contraction of circumvaginal musculature, resulting in nonconsummation of marriage. This condition is characterized by spastic, painful, and uncontrollable contractions of the vaginal muscles, which makes any attempt at penetration feel as if there is a wall or barrier to the vaginal canal. Theories behind vaginismus.

PREVALENCE

Half the world's female population suffers from some kind of sexual dysfunction. Vaginismus affects up to 7% of women, a figure that may represent an underestimation.

PATHOGENESIS OF VAGINISMUS

The exact etiology of vaginismus remains elusive. Multiple theories and various predisposing factors for vaginismus have been proposed. Strict religious prejudice and upbringing in a sexually sinful context with a negative psychological outlook on sex. This will predispose the female to apprehension toward first-time sex, sexual myths, and anxiety during gynecological examinations. Other theories postulated are the impact of the history of sexual and physical abuse, upbringing in a conflicting family, cultural taboos, and lack of sex education.

Many other factors have been found to predispose to vaginismus including sexually transmitted diseases, vaginal atrophy, pelvic inflammatory disease (PID), and endometriosis. Congenital abnormalities, such as hymen anomaly, scarring from trauma, and cancer, may also induce vaginismus.

ETIOLOGY

- Strict religious beliefs
- *Strict sexual beliefs:* Pain, bleeding, and injury
- History of sexual abuse at a young age (two times more common in vaginismus patients)
- *Organic causes:*
  - Sexually transmitted disease (STD)
  - Endometriosis
  - Hymenal abnormalities
  - Trauma associated with genital surgery
  - Radiotherapy
  - Vaginal atrophy
  - Pudendal neuralgia
  - Pelvic inflammatory disease
  - Pelvic organ prolapse
  - Vaginal lesions
  - Vaginal tumors
  - Diabetes mellitus
  - Multiple sclerosis
  - Spinal cord injury

DIAGNOSIS

Take a detailed history of each patient keeping in mind the previous causes. Stage the degree of vaginismus, i.e., mild to severe. Differentiate between psychological causes and true vaginismus.

CLASSIFICATIONS OF VAGINISMUS

According to the ICD-11 and the DSM-5, vaginismus can be classified as either primary, when a woman has never had intercourse or acquired, or secondary, when a woman loses the ability to have penetration, usually as a result of acquired dyspareunia secondary to physical events, mental and psychological factors, and infection or menopausal changes. Furthermore, vaginismus is classified as total vaginismus, where intercourse is not possible, and partial vaginismus, in which intercourse is possible but causes genital pain.[5,7-9]

Vaginismus was first described in 1978 by Lamont, who divided the pathology into four degrees according to the severity of the condition:

1st degree	• Levator and perineal spasm relieved with reassurance • Able to tolerate vaginal examination
2nd degree	• The perineal spasm is maintained through the gynecology examination • Unable to relax for the pelvic examination
3rd degree	• Spasm of the levator muscle • Guarding by elevation of buttocks during a pelvic examination
4th degree	• Perineal and levator spasm • Adduction of thighs, elevation of buttocks, and unable to tolerate the pelvic examination

DEVELOPMENT OF VAGINISMUS TREATMENT

As procreation defines marriage and a healthy sexual life, vaginismus affects a couple's emotional health within their marriage; thus, the treatment and improvement of vaginismus are of chief importance.[3,10]

Repeated episodes of vaginismus and failed intercourse may affect the sexual health of a woman, decreasing her self-esteem and adversely impacting her marital relationships leading to marital discourse, infidelity, and ultimately separation or divorce. Currently, due to the variable efficacies of different current therapeutic interventions, no standard approach has been proposed to date.[4,6,9]

Vaginismus also contributes to vaginal atrophy and dyspareunia. Treating these problems can help to ameliorate coital pain.

Considering the physical and behavioral factors, various treatment modalities include cognitive and behavioral therapies, relaxation methods, sex education, local anesthetic agents, psychotherapy or sex therapy, and physiotherapy of pelvic muscles.

While mild vaginismus may respond to modalities and conventional therapies, severe forms require interventional therapies, such as botulinum toxin injections.

Botulinum neurotoxin type-A (BoNT-A) is a polypeptide produced by gram-positive anaerobic bacillus *Clostridium botulinum*. It is made of a zinc-dependent endopeptidase 50 kDa short chain and 100 kDa long chain which attach to the high-affinity motor never vending cell membrane receptors. The short chain will cleave the membrane-associated 25-SNAP protein rendering the release of acetylcholine from vesicles in the nerve-ending cytoplasm impossible. Following its use in vaginismus in 1997, many researchers have explored the use of botulinum toxin in the treatment of vaginismus and have conferred that treatment with botulinum toxin is a safe and effective modality that inhibits vaginal muscle spasm and helps to achieve painless intercourse.[11]

However, limited studies are available comparing the efficacy of different Botox doses in the treatment of vaginismus; thus, we proposed a dosing regimen based on the severity of symptoms as explained in the treatment section.

Muscles of the lower one third of the vagina, circumvaginal muscles according to a publication by Van de Wiel in 1990. Lamont in 1994 published that the main muscles involved are bulbocavernosus, levator ani, and pubococcygeus.

WHY IS BOTULINUM TOXIN USED FOR VAGINISMUS?

It was first described by Brin and Vapnik in 1997. Botulinum toxin is a muscle relaxant that can weaken or stop any muscle's ability to contract, including the vaginal muscles. Botulinum toxin doses are administered according to the size of the target muscle, so larger muscles require larger doses.

In the treatment of vaginismus, the procedure is done with an in-office nitrogen delivery system to suppress the fear and anxiety that vaginismus sufferers often experience during gynecological examinations or any form of general touch to the pelvic area.

This treatment protocol not only helps the patient remain relaxed and comfortable as the Botulinum toxin is injected, but also facilitates progressive dilation of the vagina for the insertion of the larger dilators.

Muscles contributing more to the vaginismus symptoms are determined at the time of examination. Botulinum toxin can be injected into one, a combination, or all of the three vaginal muscles responsible for the patient's uncontrollable vaginal spasms, with the dose being divided to inject a larger volume of Botulinum toxin into the more powerful muscles. The pubococcygeus muscle group as part of the pelvic floor muscles, often resembles a tightly drawn fist in the most severe vaginismus cases, and it is usually the muscle that receives the largest dose of the toxin.

BOTULINUM TOXIN RECONSTITUTION AND HANDLING

Before the treatment, one vial of frozen Botox containing 100 U was diluted with 2 mL of preservative-free saline without shaking to prevent foam formation. The procedure was conducted either under local or general anesthesia based on the patient's comfort. In the Botox 150 U group, Botox 50 U (1 mL) each was injected into the bulbospongiosus muscle and the lateral submucosal areas of the introitus, marked by the residual hymenal fragments, at 9 o'clock and 3 o'clock positions using a 1 mL insulin syringe. In the Botox 200 U group, 75 U (1 mL) was used and injected into the areas similar to the Botox 150 U group. In patients with persistent spasms and tightness of the levator ani muscle, an additional 50 U was injected subcutaneously into the perineal body in both groups. To avoid urinary and rectal incontinence, care was taken not to inject the solution anteriorly or posteriorly. In some patients, an additional hymenectomy was done. Following injections, a medium-sized plastic speculum was inserted into the vagina for 6 hours. The patients were initially followed up after 2 weeks, and the postoperative outcome was recorded using a similar preoperative questionnaire. All patients were followed up for a year over phone calls.

Keep the vial refrigerated (2–8°C). Xeomin does not require refrigeration. In nonreconstituted form may store for up to 24 months (do not use beyond expiration date). Reconstitute with 2.5 cc of 0.9% nonpreserved sodium chloride (NaCl) for 4 hours up to 6 weeks if refrigerated.

Store after reconstitution in the refrigerator between 2°C and 8°C. The toxin may be stored for 4–6 weeks (with 87% potency). Using the reconstitution needle 21G 1.5 inch, draw up the proper amount of saline.

The toxin should be clear, colorless, and free of particulate matter. Insert the needle straight into the vial, then tilt the vial at a 45° angle. Slowly inject the saline into the vial. Vacuum demonstrates that the sterility of the vial is intact. Do not use the vial if the vacuum does not pull the saline into the vial. Release the vacuum by disconnecting the syringe from the needle and allowing air to flow into the vial. Gently mix with the saline by moving the vial side to side or rotating the vial. Draw the fluid into the injection syringe by placing the needle into the bottom corner of the vial for full extraction.

Use a reconstitution sticker to record the date and time of reconstitution, the amount of diluent added, the resulting dose to be administered, and the filled syringes stored in a refrigerator.

INJECTION TECHNIQUE

Botulinum toxin is injected above the hymenal ring in the insensitive middle third of the vagina into the vaginal side walls in vaginismus patients; the urethra and rectum are carefully avoided to prevent urinary incontinence. The exact points should be as demonstrated in the **Figure 2** located at 2-3-4 o'clock and 8-9-10 o'clock while the patient is in the lithotomy position. The injection should be performed using 1 mL syringes attached to a 13-mm 34G needle. The entire needle should be inserted into the depth of the lateral vaginal wall with the needle hub touching the vaginal mucosa.

It is possible to treat grades 1–3 while patients are awake or using nitrous gas or oral sedation. In the case of grade 4, patients have to be treated under general anesthesia.

Once injected into the vaginal walls, Botulinum toxin begins to take effect in 2–5 days and reaches a maximal effect within 7 days. Weakening even a portion of the affected vaginal muscles blocks their ability to fully contract and eventually go into spasm, making the muscle more flexible and easier to stretch with dilators or during intercourse.

HOW OFTEN IS BOTULINUM TOXIN USED TO TREAT VAGINISMUS?

In most cases, a single treatment is sufficient. Once the vagina is progressively stretched, and the patient can experience pain-free penetration, a second round of injections is rarely necessary. Once the vagina remains relaxed and dilated for 12 months, the affected vaginal muscles are less likely to resume their spastic nature. Once the patient achieves pain-free penetration and intercourse with dilators, the neural response that previously triggered vaginal spasms, fear, and anxiety upon penetration gradually shuts down.

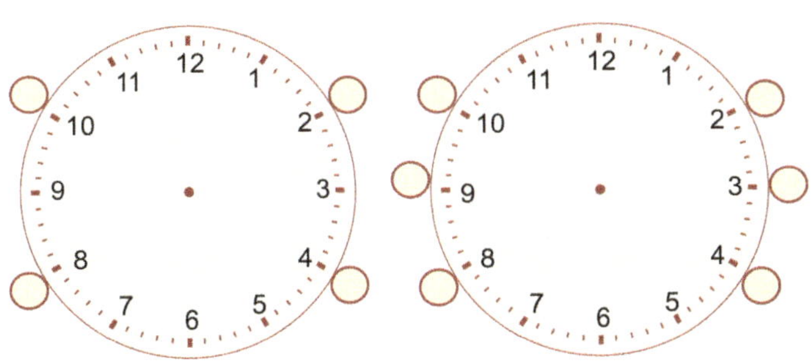

Fig. 2: Injection sites one cm above the hymenal ring in the lithotomy position.

Dose Recommendation

According to vaginismus, grade does vary. Most therapeutic failures happen because of the undertreatment of the patients. Botulinum toxin's lethal dose is 30 IU/kg, so it is a safe product to use even in large doses. The points of needle entry are demonstrated in **Figure 2**.

Vaginismus grade	*I*	*II*	*III*	*IV*	*V*
Dose (U)	25 × 2 = **50**	50 × 2 = **100**	75 × 2 = **150**		100 × 2 = **200**
Points	2 × 2			3 × 2	

Adjuvant Therapies

Platelet-rich plasma with its multitude of growth factors has been demonstrated to be of additive therapeutic value. It is the author's practice to administrate it in the same session. Tadalafil (Cialis) 2.5 mg per os (PO) daily for 30 days is also given to the patient.

Although there is no scientific evidence of any actual muscular fibrosis in vaginismus patients, the use of dilators by self-insertion 10 days after the treatment will help to alleviate the fear of pain in most patients. If patients can comfortably self-insert the dilator's place, intercourse should become simpler and painless. While the fear of penile penetration may initially remain in some patients, the anxiety surrounding penile penetration tends to subside rather quickly as they transition into intercourse. Daily use of vaginal dilators from day 10 post-treatment for 15 minutes every night.

No significant difference was found in comparing low-dose Botox (150 U) versus high-dose Botox injections (200 U) in vaginismus patients. However, it is estimated that it affected 57% of women in childbearing years in some studies.[12] Overall, the patients' mean [standard deviation (SD)] age in our study was 30.2 (8.3) and similar between both groups. The mean age of vaginismus patients was in accordance with a study by Yule[13] (28.8–30.8 years) and slightly higher than the mean age of patients (21–28 years) reported in the literature.[3,9,10] The difference could be due to late marriages and cultural taboos; women do not openly speak up about sexual problems. According to previous studies, the self-reported duration of vaginismus ranges from 3 months to 44 years.[3,14–16]

In our study, the mean duration of vaginismus was 19.3 months (range: <1–96 months). The shorter duration of our study could result from religious and cultural norms where procreation is considered an important aspect; many women approached marriage at an earlier stage.[15] Patients who never experienced nonpainful intercourse comprise the primary vaginismus group; those who acquired vaginismus later in life are categorized as secondary vaginismus. In our study, the frequency of primary vaginismus (88.9%) was higher than secondary vaginismus (11.1%). The findings are in accordance with previous studies.[14,16] Similar to the study by Velayati et al.,[17] (88.6%) approximately 90% of patients were nulliparous in our study.

Based on the Female Sexual Function Index (FSFI) questionnaire, more than half of patients had anxiety and pain scores of 10, suggesting severe anxiety and impossible or extremely painful, respectively. Sexual and reproductive health are considered the defining factors in the well-being of a person.[18] Inability to have intercourse negatively affects an individual's marital satisfaction, stability, overall health, and quality of life.[19,20] Therefore, treatment of vaginismus at earlier stages of marriage is the need of the hour. Various treatment modalities for vaginismus management include physical therapy, Kegel exercises, counseling, psychotherapy, muscle relaxants and lubricants, vaginal dilators, cognitive-behavioral therapy, topical anesthetics, antianxiety medications, use of benzodiazepines, hypnotherapy, and Botox injections.[4,9,12] However, none of the treatment approaches are evaluated based on well-designed studies.

Botox injection effectively treats neuromuscular dysfunctions and has been widely used since the successful treatment of the first case in 1997.[21] Botulinum toxin is a protein neurotoxin produced by anaerobic sporulated bacteria of the *Clostridium* genus.[22] It induces peripheral muscle relaxation by degrading soluble N-ethylmaleimide-sensitive factor activating protein receptor (SNARE) proteins and blocking the release of acetylcholine responsible for neurotransmission of muscle contraction. Additionally, Botulinum A also decreases the substance P and glutamate levels as a part of central sensitization, thereby decreasing pain sensitivity.[23] The muscle inactivation lasts until the formation of new fibrils and reconnection of the neuromuscular junction.[24] The following factors must be considered during the delivery of Botox injections: The amount of Botox injected per muscle and the total amount and the number of sites injected.[24] To avoid antibody formation, the dose and frequency of Botox should be minimized. Although the extent of paralysis depends on the amount of toxin injected, the data on the minimum dosage required for vaginismus treatment are unclear. Botox doses ranging from 20 to 500 units per injection are deemed successful in treating vaginismus and pelvic pains.[12,23,25] In a comparative analysis, Ghazizadeh et al.[26] reported that a higher dose of Botox (500 U) is more effective than a lower dose (250 U) of Botox. Our study aimed to compare the efficacy of low-dose Botox (150 U) with higher-dose Botox (200 U) in vaginismus patients' treatment outcomes.

Pacik et al.[16] explained a direct relationship between muscular spasms and the severity of vaginismus. Spasms of increased muscle activity in levator ani, puborectalis, and bulbocavernosus muscles are common in severe vaginismus grades. Therefore, similar to Park and Paraiso,[27] in our study, Botox was injected explicitly into and around the bulbospongiosus muscle and the lateral submucosal areas of the introitus and additional injections into the levator ani muscle, wherever required. Successful paralysis or spasm of the bulbospongiosus muscle is indicative of improvement in vaginismus.[28] According to the manufacturer's instructions, we diluted 100 U of Botox with 2 mL of preservative-free saline. Reports also suggest replacing saline with anesthetic solutions for immediate antinociceptive effects. However, it must be used with caution.[25]

The ability to achieve satisfactory intercourse is considered the primary outcome in most studies.[8,9,24,29,30] Based on this, the success rate of botulinum injections in vaginismus ranges from 62% to 100%,[23] and patients achieved satisfactory intercourse on the same day of treatment.[9] In our study, Lamont criteria and psychosexual evaluation using a questionnaire by FSFI were used as indicators to check the efficacy of botulinum toxin in a broader perspective. Similar to Bertolasi et al.,[31] we observed significant improvement in finger penetration pain and anxiety scores, dilator anxiety and pain scores, and intercourse anxiety scores in individual treatment groups ($p < 0.05$). In intergroup comparisons of symptom improvements between 150 U and 200 U Botox, except for dilator pain scores ($p = 0.015$), the pain and anxiety scores of all other variables in both treatment groups were similar ($p > 0.05$).

Based on an Iranian study, factors including male partner involvement during treatment and cultural background not influencing the treatment outcome,[32] whereas marital and fertility-related anxiety, family and social pressure, and personal guilt negatively affect the treatment outcome.[33] According to Anğin et al.,[34] a positive history of vaginismus within a close family and environment negatively affects the treatment outcome. Additionally, sexual abuse decreases the prognosis. While the sexual health of the male partner does not influence the treatment outcome, it affects the duration of treatment. In our study, occupation, residency, type of vaginismus, and type of anesthesia did not significantly affect the overall study cohort's treatment outcome and individual groups.

Although botulinum toxin is generally safe, its use is contraindicated in patients with local infections, albumin hypersensitivity, neuromuscular and bleeding disorders, and the use of anticoagulants.[23] Adverse events are noted with higher doses that include pain, hematoma, and infection at the injection site, urinary and anal incontinence, transient blurred vision, and vaginal dryness.[14,25,35] However, urinary and fecal incontinence are seen in higher doses >100 U. Rarely, an ischiorectal fossa abscess may also occur.[36] To prevent injection-related adverse effects and complications, guidance techniques, such as electromyography, electrical stimulation, and ultrasound, can be used in an office setting to restrict injections to the muscles and vaginal soft tissue only. In our study, since the clinician was careful not to inject the solution anteriorly or posteriorly, side effects were seen in only 19.2% of patients (urinary incontinence versus anal incontinence; 17.2% vs. 2%). The frequency of side effects between the 150 U and 200 U Botox groups was comparable ($p = 0.997$).

In a country with strict social and religious norms where sexual problems are considered taboo, the present study is the first of its kind with the hope of saving families from breaking apart due to vaginismus-related consequences. The inclusion of a wide range of patients from within and outside the country was one of the strengths. Although the sample size was small, it seemed sufficient to identify differences in the study outcome. A short follow-up period is one of the study's major limitations, as previous studies have reported recurrences following Botox injections. According to previous research, a placebo had an equal or superior effect to Botox injections.[37,38] In their metanalysis, Weinberger et al.[39] conferred that the placebo effect accounts for 67.7% of outcomes in female sexual dysfunction treatment. The inclusion of a placebo arm will assist in assessing the accurate outcome of the test group. Hence, the inability to include a placebo arm in the study was another limitation. Therefore, further placebo-controlled, prospective randomized trials with controlled questionnaires are essential for vaginismus treatment.

In vaginismus patients, detailed discussions and history are mandatory to categorize a patient under an anatomical or psychological disorder, especially during the first gynecological visits. The botulinum injection is a simple, safe, cost-effective, and rapid treatment that can be performed in an inpatient or outpatient setting; clinicians widely appreciate it. However, the effect lasts for around 6 months. Based on the evidence, the frequency of patients discontinuing follow-up ranges from 1.2% to 47.8%.[34] Therefore, regular follow-ups may be required to check for recurrences. Severe vaginismus is one of the reasons for unconsummated marriages, and continuous failure to have intercourse secondarily leads to male impotence.[40] The fear and anxiety about sex could be due to a lack of sex education in women with no knowledge of sexual anatomy.[41] Therefore, it is of utmost importance to incorporate sex education into the school curriculum.

Moreover, some studies demonstrated no positive or inferior outcome of Botox in vaginismus as compared with other treatment modalities, including physiotherapy,[4] behavioral sex therapy,[42] and better outcomes with a multimodal approach, such as dilatators, physical therapy, psychotherapy, and sacral erector spinae block (ESB).[6] Therefore, pre- and postprocedure counseling and long-term follow-up are essential during vaginismus treatment. Along with satisfactory intercourse, domains of sexual function and FSFI must also be considered efficacy endpoints of vaginismus treatment.[4,42]

Along with Botox injections, it is paramount to incorporate psychotherapy and counseling in patients, especially those with severe anxiety, and fear of sex and gynecological examination. Further randomized controlled trials, including a placebo group, are warranted to evaluate the efficacy of low-dose Botox.

Several pathologies from the gynecological field for which BoNT treatment can be used. Most of these dysfunctions have been shown to be refractory to conventional treatments, but the results after single or repeated cycles of BoNT-A were favorable and the symptoms improved.

The dosage used ranged from 40 U to 400 U in a single administration. In some cases, repeated injection cycles were necessary, depending on the symptomatology and the scores obtained after the patients completed standardized questionnaires. The improvement of the symptomatology was objectively certified using standardized questionnaires before and after a certain period postinjection.

CONCLUSION

When compared to BoNT-B, we observed that BoNT-A is used more often with good results, especially because the paralysis resulting from BoNT-B is not as efficient as the one of BoNT-A. It is also desirable to carry out further studies to reach a consensus on the optimal BoNT-A dose and administration protocol to create a standardized treatment.

This review highlights that BoNT could be successfully used in treating symptoms of gynecological dysfunctions refractory to conventional treatments, having few side effects and high efficacy.

REFERENCES

1. Boyer SC, Goldfinger C, Thibault-Gagnon S, Pukall CF. Management of female sexual pain disorders. Adv Psychosom Med. 2011;31:83-104.
2. Ferreira JR, Souza RP. Botulinum toxin for vaginismus treatment. Pharmacology. 2012;89(5-6):256-9.
3. Velayati A, Sadatmahalleh SJ, Ziaei S, Kazemnejad A. The role of personal factors in quality of life among Iranian women with vaginismus: a path analysis. Health Qual Life Outcomes. 2021;19(1):166.
4. Yaraghi M, Ghazizadeh S, Mohammadi F, Ashtiani EM, Bakhtiyari M, Mareshi SM. Comparing the effectiveness of functional electrical stimulation via sexual cognitive/behavioral therapy of pelvic floor muscles versus local injection of botulinum toxin on the sexual functioning of patients with primary vaginismus: a randomized clinical trial. Int Urogynecol J Pelvic Floor Dysfunct. 2019;30(11):1821-8.
5. American Psychiatric Association. Diagnostic and Statistical Manual of Mental Disorders, 5th edition. Washington: American Psychiatric Association; 2013. pp. 1-7.
6. Yilmaz EPT, Ahiskalioglu EO, Ahiskalioglu A, Tulgar S, Aydin ME, Kumtepe Y. A novel multimodal treatment method and pilot feasibility study for vaginismus: initial experience with the combination of sacral erector spinae plane block and progressive dilatation. Cureus. 2020;12(10):e10846.
7. World Health Organization. (2021). International Classification of Diseases (ICD). [online] Available from: https://www.who.int/standards/classifications/classification-of-diseases. [Last assessed May, 2021].
8. Velayati A, Sadatmahalleh SJ, Ziaei S, Kazemnejad A. Can Botox offer help women with vaginismus? A systematic review and meta-analysis. Int J Sex Health. 2019;31(03):233-43.
9. Fageeh WM. Different treatment modalities for refractory vaginismus in western Saudi Arabia. J Sex Med. 2011;8(6):1735-9.
10. Michetti PM, Silvaggi M, Fabrizi A, Tartaglia N, Rossi R, Simonelli C. Unconsummated marriage: can it still be considered a consequence of vaginismus? Int J Impot Res. 2014;26(1):28-30.
11. Zheng Z, Yin J, Cheng B, Huang W. Materials selection for the injection into vaginal wall for treatment of vaginal atrophy. Aesthetic Plast Surg. 2021;45(3):1231-41.
12. Dick B, Natale C, Reddy A, Akula KP, Yousif A, Hellstrom WJG. Application of botulinum neurotoxin in female sexual and genitourinary dysfunction: a review of current practices. Sex Med Rev. 2021;9(1):57-63.
13. Yule MA. Female Sexual Function Index. Dordrecht: Springer; 2014. pp. 2244-6.
14. Achour R, Koch M, Zgueb Y, Ouali U, Hmid RB. Vaginismus and pregnancy: epidemiological profile and management difficulties. Psychol Res Behav Manag. 2019;12:137-43.
15. Anğın AD, Gün İ, Sakin Ö, Çıkman MS, Eserdağ S, Anğın P. Effects of predisposing factors on the success and treatment period in vaginismus. JBRA Assist Reprod. 2020;24(2):180-8.
16. Pacik PT, Babb CR, Polio A, Nelson CE, Goekeler CE, Holmes LN. Case series: redefining severe grade 5 vaginismus. Sex Med. 2019;7(4):489-97.
17. Rosen R, Brown C, Heiman J, Leiblum S, Meston C, Shabsigh R. The Female Sexual Function Index (FSFI): a multidimensional self-report instrument for the assessment of female sexual function. J Sex Marital Ther. 2000;26(2):191-208.
18. Maasoumi R, Lamyian M, Montazeri A, Azin SA, Aguilar-Vafaie ME, Hajizadeh E. The sexual quality of life-female (SQOL-F) questionnaire: translation and psychometric properties of the Iranian version. Reprod Health. 2013;10:25.
19. Potur DC, Satilmiş IG, Merih YD, Kakaşçi ÇG, Demirci N, Ersoy M. Does infertility affect the sexual function and sexual quality of life of women? A case control study. Int J Sex Health. 2020;32(1):22-32.
20. Fugl-Meyer KS, Bohm-Starke N, Petersen CD, Fugl-Meyer A, Parish S, Giraldi A. Standard operating procedures for female genital sexual pain. J Sex Med. 2013;10(1):83-93.
21. Foster L, Clapp L, Erickson M, Jabbari B. Botulinum toxin A and chronic low back pain: a randomized, double-blind study. Neurology. 2001;56(10):1290-3.
22. Chen CL, Meng E. Can botulinum toxin A play a role in treatment of chronic pelvic pain syndrome in female patients?—Clinical and animal evidence. Toxins (Basel). 2020;12(2):110.

23. Gari R, Alyafi M, Gadi RU, Gadi SU. Use of Botulinum Toxin (Botox®) in cases of refractory pelvic floor muscle dysfunction. Sex Med Rev. 2022;10(1):155-61.
24. Ghazizadeh S, Nikzad M. Botulinum toxin in the treatment of refractory vaginismus. Obstet Gynecol. 2004; 104(5 Pt 1):922-5.
25. Karp BI, Tandon H, Vigil D, Stratton P. Methodological approaches to botulinum toxin for the treatment of chronic pelvic pain, vaginismus, and vulvar pain disorders. Int Urogynecol J Pelvic Floor Dysfunct. 2019;30(7):1071-81.
26. Ghazizadeh S, Abedi J, Pourmatroud AJ, Raiisi F, Lesanpezeshki M. Comparison of 500 units vs 250 units of botulinum toxin (abobotulinumtoxinA) for the treatment of severe vaginismus. J Bacteriol Mycol (Monroe Township). 2016;3(3):1033-6.
27. Park AJ, Paraiso MFR. Successful use of botulinum toxin type a in the treatment of refractory postoperative dyspareunia. Obstet Gynecol. 2009;114(2 Pt 2):484-7.
28. Shafik A, El-Sibai O. Study of the pelvic floor muscles in vaginismus: a concept of pathogenesis. Eur J Obstet Gynecol Reprod Biol. 2002;105(1):67-70.
29. Moga MA, Dimienescu OG, Bălan A, Scârneciu I, Barabaş B, Pleş L. Therapeutic approaches of botulinum toxin in gynecology. Toxins (Basel). 2018;10(4):169.
30. Pacik PT. Understanding and treating vaginismus: a multimodal approach. Int Urogynecol J Pelvic Floor Dysfunct. 2014;25(12):1613-20.
31. Bertolasi L, Frasson E, Cappelletti JY, Vicentini S, Bordignon M, Graziottin A. Botulinum neurotoxin type A injections for vaginismus secondary to vulvar vestibulitis syndrome. Obstet Gynecol. 2009;114(5):1008-16.
32. Molaeinezhad M, Khoei EM, Salehi M, Yousfy A, Roudsari RL. Validation of the partner version of the multidimensional vaginal penetration disorder questionnaire: a tool for clinical assessment of lifelong vaginismus in a sample of Iranian population. J Educ Health Promot. 2014;3:114.
33. Rahman S. Female sexual dysfunction among Muslim women: increasing awareness to improve overall evaluation and treatment. Sex Med Rev. 2018;6(4):535-47.
34. Anğın AD, Gün İ, Sakin Ö, Çıkman MS, Eserdağ S, Anğın P. Effects of predisposing factors on the success and treatment period in vaginismus. JBRA Assist Reprod. 2020;24(2):180-8.
35. Butrick CW. Pelvic floor hypertonic disorders: identification and management. Obstet Gynecol Clin North Am. 2009;36(3):707-22.
36. Brueseke TJ, Lane FL. Ischiorectal fossa abscess after pelvic floor injection of botulinum toxin. Am J Obstet Gynecol. 2012;206(3):e7-e8.
37. Weinberger JM, Houman J, Caron AT, Anger J. Female sexual dysfunction: a systematic review of outcomes across various treatment modalities. Sex Med Rev. 2019;7(2):223-50.
38. Diomande I, Gabriel N, Kashiwagi M, Ghisu GP, Welter J, Fink D. Subcutaneous botulinum toxin type A injections for provoked vestibulodynia: a randomized placebo-controlled trial and exploratory subanalysis. Arch Gynecol Obstet. 2019;299(4):993-1000.
39. Weinberger JM, Houman J, Caron AT, Patel DN, Baskin AS, Ackerman AL. Female sexual dysfunction and the placebo effect: a meta-analysis. Obstet Gynecol. 2018;132(2):453-8.
40. Zargooshi J. Male sexual dysfunction in unconsummated marriage: long-term outcome in 417 patients. J Sex Med. 2008;5(12):2895-903.
41. Basson R, Wierman ME, van Lankveld J, Brotto L. Summary of the recommendations on sexual dysfunctions in women. J Sex Med. 2010;7(1 Pt 2):314-26.
42. Maseroli E, Scavello I, Rastrelli G, Limoncin E, Cipriani S, Corona G. Outcome of medical and psychosexual interventions for vaginismus: a systematic review and meta-analysis. J Sex Med. 2018;15(12):1752-64.

CHAPTER 15

Genitourinary Syndrome of Menopause: Novel Treatment Modalities

Ragini Agrawal

INTRODUCTION

With increasing years added to life, there are more chances for women to suffer from somatic and psychological symptoms due to aging and estrogen deficiency.[1] "Considering that women spend a third of their life in menopause, it is essential to recognize GSM in order to restore the vaginal and vulvar epithelium and ultimately improve quality of life."

The syndrome or its features manifest in approximately 15% of premenopausal women and 40–54% of postmenopausal women. Genitourinary syndrome of menopause (GSM) is often underdiagnosed due to sexual embarrassment or general disregard due to associating it as a liability of natural aging.

Genitourinary symptoms related to abrupt menopause tend to present in relatively younger women and cause greater sexual dysfunction and poorer quality of life (QOL) outcomes, the management of their menopausal symptoms has become an increasingly important issue.

The GSM is a term given in 2013 by "The International Society for Study of Women's Sexual Health and the North American Menopausal Society."[2] More and more women are suffering from it as their longevity of life is increasing. It is a complex of multiple symptoms such as vaginal dryness, the feeling of recurrent urinary burning, dyspareunia, stress and urge urinary incontinence, vulvodynia, and vulvovaginal atrophy (VVA) all linked to hypoestrogenism. It is an umbrella term to cover all urogenital and sexual problems occurring in females due to hypoestrogenism **(Flowchart 1)**.

Flowchart 1: Urogenital and sexual problems due to hypoestrogenism.

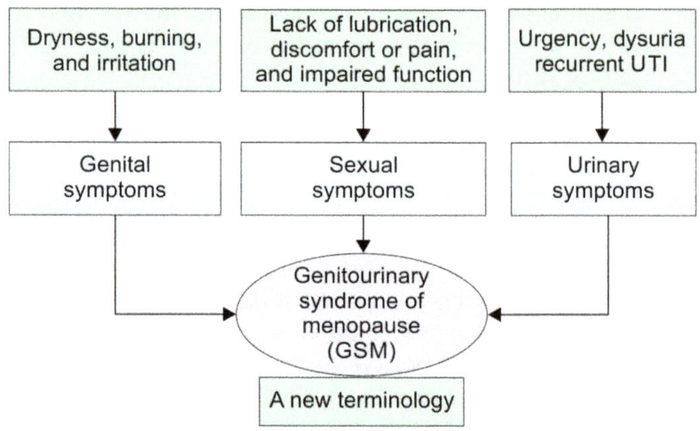

(UTI: urinary tract infection)

CAUSES

Hypoestrogenism in women may be linked to multiple causes, natural menopause being the most common. Surgical menopause is due to bilateral oophorectomy premenopausal, premature ovarian insufficiency, postpartum lactating state, and Iatrogenic due to hypothalamopituitary suffering drugs [such as gonadotropin-releasing hormone (GnRH) agonists], an aromatase inhibitor, methotrexate, oncology treatments, radiation, etc.

PATHOPHYSIOLOGY

Female genitalia and lower urinary tract have an embryologically common origin. Both have estrogen receptors. Postmenopause estrogen receptors decrease with age. It reduces collagen, elastin, and hyaluronic acid from epithelial layers. The flexible vaginal canal becomes rigid, dry, and atrophied. The nonkeratinized stratified squamous epithelium which is home to lactobacilli becomes thin. Lactobacillus helps in the conversion of glycogen to lactic acid and makes vaginal pH acidic (3.5–4.5). As the lactobacilli diminish, acidity also starts turning into alkalinity and leads to recurrent bacterial infections **(Fig. 1)**.[3]

Also, there is decreased secretion of other lubricants such as Bartholin gland secretions leading to dyspareunia and dryness. The bladder and urethra also become atrophic, causing urinary incontinence and frequency.[1]

According to an article in Acta, 50% of women postmenopause suffer stress urinary incontinence (SUI) (20% urge incontinence).[4,5]

Flowchart 2 explains the loss of estrogen leads to many anatomical changes which in turn is the reason for functional changes. These functional changes are the reason for VVA, urinary problems, and lack of lubrication leads to painful intercourse.

RISK FACTORS FOR GENITOURINARY SYNDROME OF MENOPAUSE

- Age
- Bilateral oophorectomy
- Premature ovarian failure

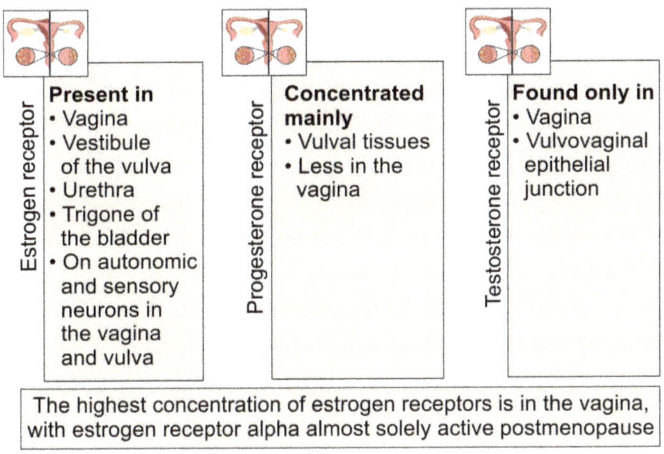

Fig. 1: Pathophysiology and anatomical changes.

- Smoking
- Alcohol abuse
- Decreased sexual frequency or abstinence
- Other causes of low estrogen (e.g., postpartum period and hypothalamic amenorrhea)
- Cancer treatments, including pelvic irradiation, chemotherapy, and endocrine therapy.

CLINICAL FEATURES

Table 1 explains the clinical features of GSM.

DIAGNOSIS AND TREATMENT

The aim of treatment is to improve the quality of life of women. Detailed history and local examination will help in reaching a diagnosis.

Repeated reports of sterile urine routine or culture despite severe symptoms of dysuria, urgency, and frequency clinch the diagnosis. Take the opportunity to do liquid-based cervical cytology, pelvic ultrasonography (USG), and mammography too. As per speculum, dry parched vulvovagina is seen with developing stenosis.

- Laboratory testing is not typically required, although cultures or biopsies could be indicated if appearance is nontypical or does not improve after therapy.
- The vaginal pH and the vaginal maturation index (VMI) are some tests to assess the efficacy of therapies.

Flowchart 2: Pathophysiology and anatomical changes.

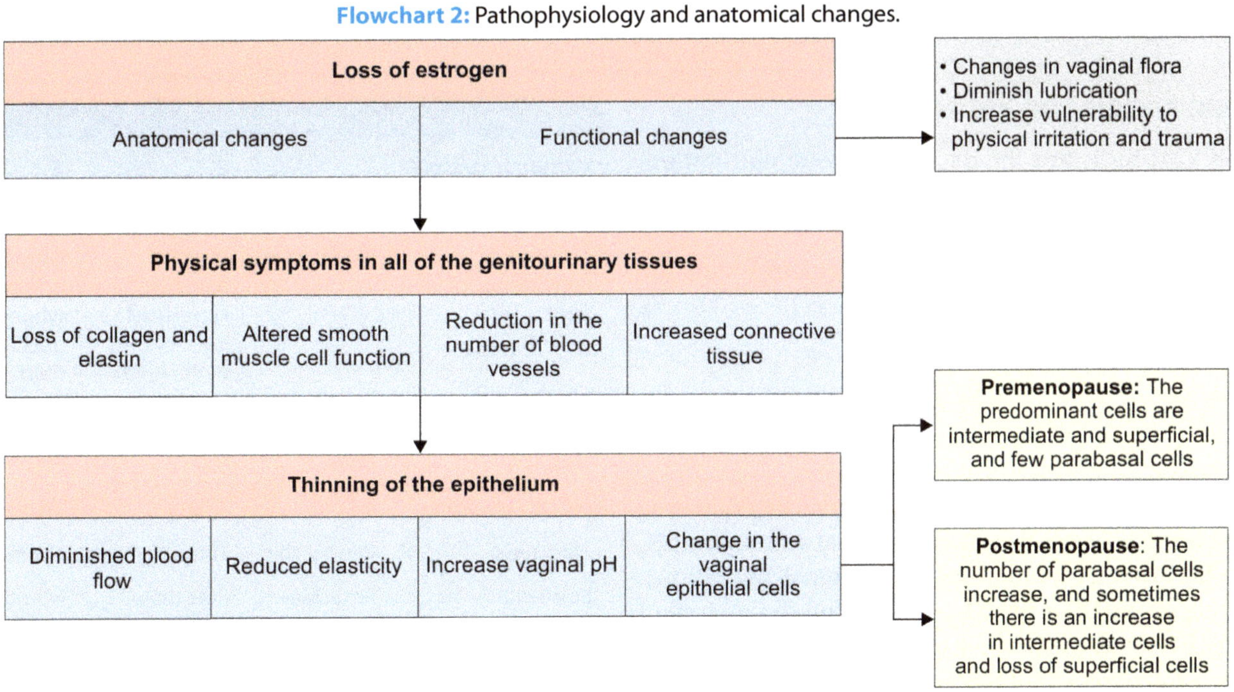

TABLE 1: External genital, urological, and sexual manifestations of genitourinary syndrome of menopause (GSM).

External genital		Urological		Sexual
Signs and symptoms	**Complications**	**Signs and symptoms**	**Complications**	**Signs and symptoms**
• Vaginal/pelvic pain and pressure • Dryness • Irritation/burning • Tenderness • Pruritus vulvae • Decreased turgor and elasticity • Suprapubic pain • Leukorrhea • Ecchymosis • Erythema • Thinning/graying pubic hair • Thinning/pallor of vaginal epithelium • Pale vaginal mucous membrane • Fusion of labia minora • Labial shrinking • Leukoplakic patches on vaginal mucosa • Presence of petechiae • Fewer vaginal rugae • Increased vaginal friability	• Labial atrophy • Vulvar atrophy and lesions • Atrophy of Bartholin glands • Intravaginal retraction of urethra • Alkaline pH (5–7) • Reduced vaginal and cervical secretions • Pelvic organ prolapse • Vaginal vault prolapse • Vaginal stenosis and shortening • Introital stenosis	• Frequency • Urgency • Postvoid dribbling • Nocturia • Stress/urgency incontinence • Dysuria • Hematuria • Recurrent urinary tract infection	• Ischemia of vesical trigone • Meatal stenosis • Cystocele and rectocele • Urethral prolapse • Urethral atrophy • Retraction of urethral meatus inside vagina associated with vaginal voiding • Uterine prolapse • Urethral polyp or caruncle	• Loss of libido • Loss of arousal • Lack of lubrication • Dyspareunia • Dysorgasmia • Pelvic pain • Bleeding or spotting during intercourse

Source: Gandhi J, Chen A, Dagur G, Suh Y, Smith N, Cali B, et al. Genitourinary syndrome of menopause: an overview of clinical manifestations, pathophysiology, etiology, evaluation, and management. Am J Obstet Gynecol. 2016;215(6):704-11.

Vaginal Maturation Index

- The VMI indicates the degree of tissue maturation, measuring the percentage of superficial, intermediate, and parabasal cells.
- The maturation value (MV) is calculated with the following formula: MV = % surface cells + (0.5 × % intermediate cells).

Vaginal Health Index Score and Genitourinary Syndrome of Menopause

The Vaginal Health Index Score is a tool that, by evaluating five parameters (vaginal elasticity, vaginal secretions, pH, epithelial mucous membrane, and vaginal hydration), allows us to obtain a final score defining the degree of atrophy in the genitourinary tract by assigning a single score to each parameter **(Table 2)**.

TABLE 2: Vaginal Health Index Score.

Parameters/score	*1*	*2*	*3*
pH	>6.5	5–6.5	<5
Moisture/consistency of fluid	No moisture	Minimal moisture/superficial layer of thin white fluid	Normal moisture/white flocculant fluid
Rugosity	None	Minimal	Good
Elasticity	Poor	Fair	Excellent
Length of vagina	<4 cm	4–6 cm	>6 cm
Thickness	Papery thin	Thin	Normal
Epithelial	Petechiae	Petechiae after scraping	Normal not friable
Vascularity	Minimal	Fair	Good

Differential Diagnosis

- Dermatological conditions of the vulva (e.g., lichen sclerosus or planus, eczema, dermatitis, and chronic vulvovaginitis)
- Vulvodynia
- Vaginismus
- Autoimmune disorders
- Malignancy
- Chronic pelvic pain
- Trauma and foreign bodies
- Diabetes
- Lupus

Treatment

Various treatment options are available:

- *Lubrication:* Moisturizing does help though
- *Hormones:* The last estrogen receptor can be replenished with exogenous administration of estrogen.[6] When genitourinary symptoms dominate, local therapy is sufficient.[7-9] This approach is not associated with systemic effects and requires no progestin for endometrial protection.

  In younger patients, especially in cases of primary ovarian insufficiency (POI), cancer patients, or surgical menopause, timely starting hormone replacement therapy (HRT), orally or locally, is the effective option until contraindicated.
- *Lifestyle modification:* Avoiding harsh chemicals, vaginal douching, and repeated washing help in restoring the moisture and biometrics of the area vaginal probiotics can also help.

Newer Treatments

Selective Estrogen Receptor Modulators (SERMs) (e.g., Ospemifene) for Vulvovaginal Atrophy and Dyspareunia

Ospemifene is the only SERM to be indicated for the treatment of VVA.

It has been approved by the US Food and Drug Administration (FDA) for the treatment of moderate to severe dyspareunia and by the European Medical Agency (EMA) for the treatment of moderate to severe VVA in women, with or without a uterus, who are not candidates for local estrogen therapy.

It is a tissue-specific estrogen complex (combination of SERM and estrogen), which is well-tolerated and effective for symptom relief.

It exerts a positive effect on the vaginal epithelium while having, at the same time, a neutral or minimal effect on the other estrogen-dependent organs.

Neutral effect on the endometrium and the cardiovascular system, and an antiestrogenic effect in preclinical studies on the breast.

Dose: 60 mg daily

The effects on the signs of VVA are visible after 4 weeks of treatment such as the increase of superficial cells, the reduction of basal cells, and the reduction of vaginal pH.[10,11]

A significant effect on symptoms such as dryness and dyspareunia has been demonstrated to occur after 12 weeks of treatment.[12,13]

The efficacy of ospemifene at a histological level in both vaginal and vulvar tissue has been demonstrated by observing increases in vaginal and vulvar epithelial thickness, glycogen content, proliferation index, and an increase in vaginal estrogen receptor alfa (ERα).

Ospemifene has also been shown to improve atrophy of the vulvar vestibule and to normalize vestibular sensitivity by increasing the perception threshold at a vulvar level.

In a short-term study, it has also been shown to increase the ratio of type I and type III collagen at the vaginal level, suggesting possible beneficial long-term effects on vaginal connective tissue.[14,15]

Contraindications

- A current or previous thromboembolic event
- Vaginal bleeding of unknown origin
- Presence of signs or symptoms of endometrial hyperplasia
- Malignant tumor-dependent on sex hormones
- Ongoing breast carcinoma

The EMA has also approved its administration in women with previous breast cancer after the completion of treatment including adjuvant therapy and after the performance of a control mammogram.[16]

Dehydroepiandrosterone (Androgens)

Dehydroepiandrosterone (DHEA) is used to increase epithelial thickness and secretions (local use).

It acts as a precursor of intracellular sex steroid androgens and estrogens.[17]

Since the conversion happens inside the cells, serum estradiol remains within the normal values for postmenopausal women, thereby probably avoiding the risk of systemic effects.

Dose: Daily intravaginal prasterone (6.5 mg).

The endometrium is not affected by DHEA, because the enzymes required to transform DHEA into estrogens are absent in the endometrium.[18]

Although no systemic increase in estrogen level has been reported, a history of breast cancer remains a contraindication.

Energy-based Devices

Laser, high-intensity focused ultrasound (HIFU), and radiofrequency (RF) have come as a boom to the treatment of these conditions.[19,20] In many studies the consequences of hypoestrogenism in the vulvovaginal area treated with physical energies, such as laser, RF, and USG are discussed.

Major benefits of energy-based device (EBD):

- Thickening of the nonkeratinized epithelium
- Increase in local angiogenesis
- Development of new collagen fibers and restoration of vaginal architecture.
- Improving elasticity
- Improvement in genitourinary symptoms
- Improvement in lubrification
- A decline in vaginal pH
- Normalization of the genital microbiome.

Mechanism of action: The EBDs add by the principal of thermal rejuvenation.

Laser or RF waves act by heating the connective tissue of the vaginal wall from 40°C to 42°C.

They induce collagen contraction, neocollagenesis, vascularization, and growth factor infiltration that ultimately revitalizes and restores the elasticity and moisture of the vaginal mucosa.

The proposed mechanism is the activation of heat shock proteins and tissue growth factors to stimulate new collagen synthesis and epithelial remodeling.

The added advantage of using EBD in postcancer-treated patients following radiotherapy, or for breast cancer survivors wherein hormone therapy is contra-indicated cannot be undermined.

- Minimally invasive, virtually painless procedure
- Gentle treatment for controlled safety and accuracy
- Maximum precision with carbon dioxide (CO_2) laser, the right wavelength, and perfect pulse
- Fast and efficient delivery of fractionated laser energy split into micro pixels
- No post-treatment downtime
- Excellent patient satisfaction and long-term success.

In 2020, the North American Menopause Society issued a norm regarding the use of EBDs. Although they have not yet been approved by the FDA for use in genitourinary system (GUS) and are still considered an experimental treatment, several clinical studies have shown them to be effective in the treatment of the syndrome.

In a recent meta-analysis, Pitsouni et al. reported improvements in both genitourinary symptoms and their repercussions of urinary incontinence, quality of life, the vaginal health index, and sexuality. In all parameters, analysis of the treatments showed that the laser was beneficial for women in the control group. They also reported low rates of nonsevere side effects. However, it should be noted that the number of participants was small, and follow-up was short; therefore, the long-term effects of such therapies cannot be assessed.

Platelet-rich Plasma Therapy

Autologous platelet-rich plasma (PRP) injected locally in the vaginal and vulval area helps in rejuvenating the troubled area and is found to be very effective.

CONCLUSION

Genitourinary symptoms are chronic, and rarely resolved spontaneously and often progress if left untreated. Symptoms are not life-threatening, but they are progressive and may have a profound impact on the QOL of postmenopausal women by negatively affecting self-esteem and intimacy with their partners. However, hormonal and nonhormonal treatments can provide patients with the solution to regain their previous level of function.

It is high time that clinicians especially gynecologists should take GSM seriously and offer help to women suffering from this problem. With adequate treatments, counseling, and tender long care, the women can lead a long life not only in quantity but also a quality.

REFERENCES

1. Barbo DM. The physiology of the menopause. Med Clin North Am. 1987;71:11-22.
2. Calleja-Agius J, Brincat M, Borg M. Skin connective tissue and ageing. Best Pract Res Clin Obstet Gynaecol. 2013;27:727-40.
3. Calleja-Agius J, Brincat MP. The urogenital system and the menopause. Climacteric. 2015;18(Suppl 1):18-22.
4. Nappi RE, Biglia N, Cagnacci A, Di Carlo C, Luisi S, Paoletti AM. Diagnosis and management of symptoms associated

with vulvovaginal atrophy: expert opinion on behalf of the Italian VVA study group. Gynecol Endocrinol. 2016;32(8): 602-6.
5. Bachmann G. Urogenital ageing: an old problem newly recognized. Maturitas. 1995;Suppl. 1:S1-5.
6. Huang AJ, Gregorich SE, Kuppermann M, Nakagawa S, Van Den Eeden SK, Brown JS, et al. Day-to-day Impact of vaginal aging questionnaire: a multidimensional measure of the impact of vaginal symptoms on functioning and well-being in postmenopausal women. Menopause. 2015;22(2): 144-54.
7. Kim H-K, Kang S-Y, Chung Y-J, Kim J-H, Kim M-R. The recent review of genito urinary syndrome of menopause. J Menopausal Med. 2015:21(2):65-71.
8. North American Menopause Society. The role of local vaginal estrogen for treatment of vaginal atrophy in post-menopausal women: 2007 position statement of the North American Menopausal Society. Menopause. 2007;14(3 Pt 1):355-69.
9. Jindal P, Kundal I, Kalra R, Sahdev S. Genitourinary syndrome of menopause. In: Jindal P, Malhotra N, Joshi S (Eds). Aesthetic and Regenerative Gynecology. Springer: Springer; 2022. pp. 265-71.
10. Jindal P, Madhu G, Isha K, Mittal M, Ridhi G, Cherry M, et al. Female urinary incontinence - A revisit on prevalence of this problem in today's society. Acta Scientific Women's Health. 2021;3(9):27-33.
11. Robinson D, Cardogio LD. The role of estrogen in female lower urinary tract dysfunction. Urol. 2003;62(syp):45-51.
12. Palecios S. Managing urogenital atrophy. Maturitas. 2009;63:315-8.
13. Robinson D, Cardozo LD. The role of estrogens in female lower urinary tract dysfunction. Urol. 2003;62:45-51.
14. https://www.menopause.org/for-women/sexual-health-menopause-online/changes-at-midlife/changes-in-the-vagina-and-vulva
15. Alvisi S, Gava G, Orsili I, Giacomelli G, Baldassarre M, Seracchioli R, et al. Vaginal health in menopausal women. Medicina (Kaunas). 2019;55(10):615.
16. The NAMS 2020 GSM Position Statement Editorial Panel. The 2020 genitourinary syndrome of menopause position statement of The North American Menopause Society. Menopause. 2020;27(9):976-92.
17. Ross EV, McKinlay JR, Anderson RR. Why does carbon dioxide resurfacing work? A review. Arch Dermatol. 1999; 135:444-54.
18. Eming SA, Wynn TA, Martin P. Inflammation and metabolism in tissue repair and regeneration. Science. 2017;356(6342):1026-30.
19. Soares-Júnior JM, Barbosa MTA, Aguiar LM, Seganfredo IB, de Pereyra EAG, de Melo NR, et al. Energy-based devices in gynecology: the new frontier for the treatment of genitourinary syndrome of post menopause? Clinics (Sao Paulo). 2021;76:e3066.
20. Pitsouni E, Grigoriadis T, Falagas ME, Salvatore S, Athanasiou S. Laser therapy for the genitourinary syndrome of menopause. A systematic review and meta-analysis. Maturitas. 2017;103:78-88.

CHAPTER 16

Labiaplasty and Clitoroplasty: A Comprehensive Review

Preeti Jindal, Pragati Tandon

LABIAPLASTY

Definition

Labiaplasty (labia reduction or labial reduction) is a surgical procedure for altering the labia minora (inner vulval lips) or labia majora, the folds of skin surrounding the vaginal introitus **(Figs. 1A to C)**.

Labiaplasty and clitoroplasty are two types of vulvo-vaginal surgery that can be performed to improve the appearance and function of the female genitalia. Labia-plasty involves reducing or reshaping the labia minora, while clitoroplasty involves surgery of the clitoris. The clitoral hood is an extension of labia minora folds over the clitoris and usually labiaplasty involves clitoral surgery also.

Introduction

The demand for genital cosmetic surgery has significantly increased due to patient knowledge. The American Society of Aesthetic Plastic Surgeons reported in 2017 that labiaplasty has increased by 217.2% between 2012 and 2017. Due to their differences, the labia majora and minora would be treated differently when it comes to aesthetic operations. Both procedures may be done for a number of reasons, including cosmetic surgery. Some women may choose these procedures to improve the appearance of the vulva. The cause can be enlarged or asymmetrical labia, or the clitoris is buried under the foreskin. Labiaplasty can also be done to improve the function of the vulva.[2] For example, enlarged labia may rub during exercise or intercourse, causing discomfort or pain.[3]

Clitoroplasty may be performed to improve sexual sensitivity and function.[4] Labiaplasty and clitoroplasty are sometimes performed as part of gender confirmation surgery for transgender people.[5]

Anatomy

Normal women vary widely in the size, shape, color, and thickness of their labia minora.[2] When a person is sexually aroused, they can sometimes grow two or three times their normal diameter and can either be visible or concealed by labia majora.[3] The glans clitoris is located immediately beneath the prepuce. As depicted in **Figures 2A and B**, the frenula are folds of skin that extend from the glans clitoris and combine with the extension of the clitoral hood to form the labia minora. The internal circumflex artery, external pudendal artery, and internal pudendal artery all have branches that give blood to the labia minora. The posterior labial nerve, a continuation of the pudendal nerve, innervates the labia minora.

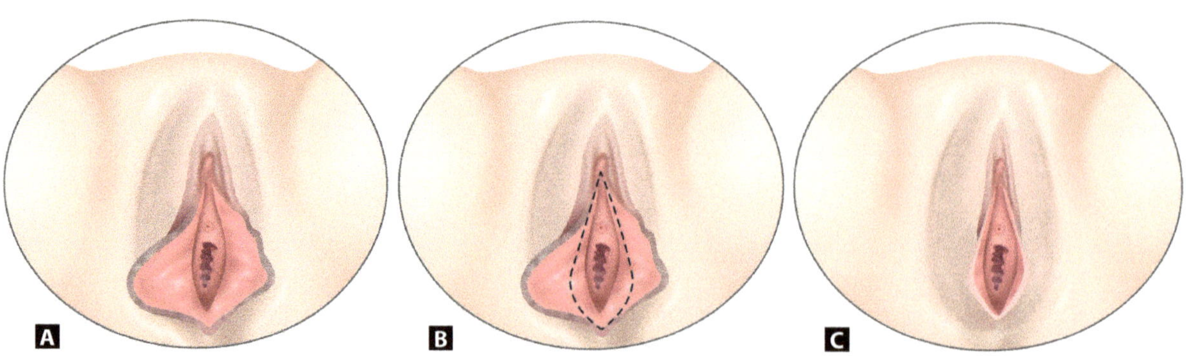

Figs. 1A to C: Labiaplasty.
Source: Jindal P et al.[1]

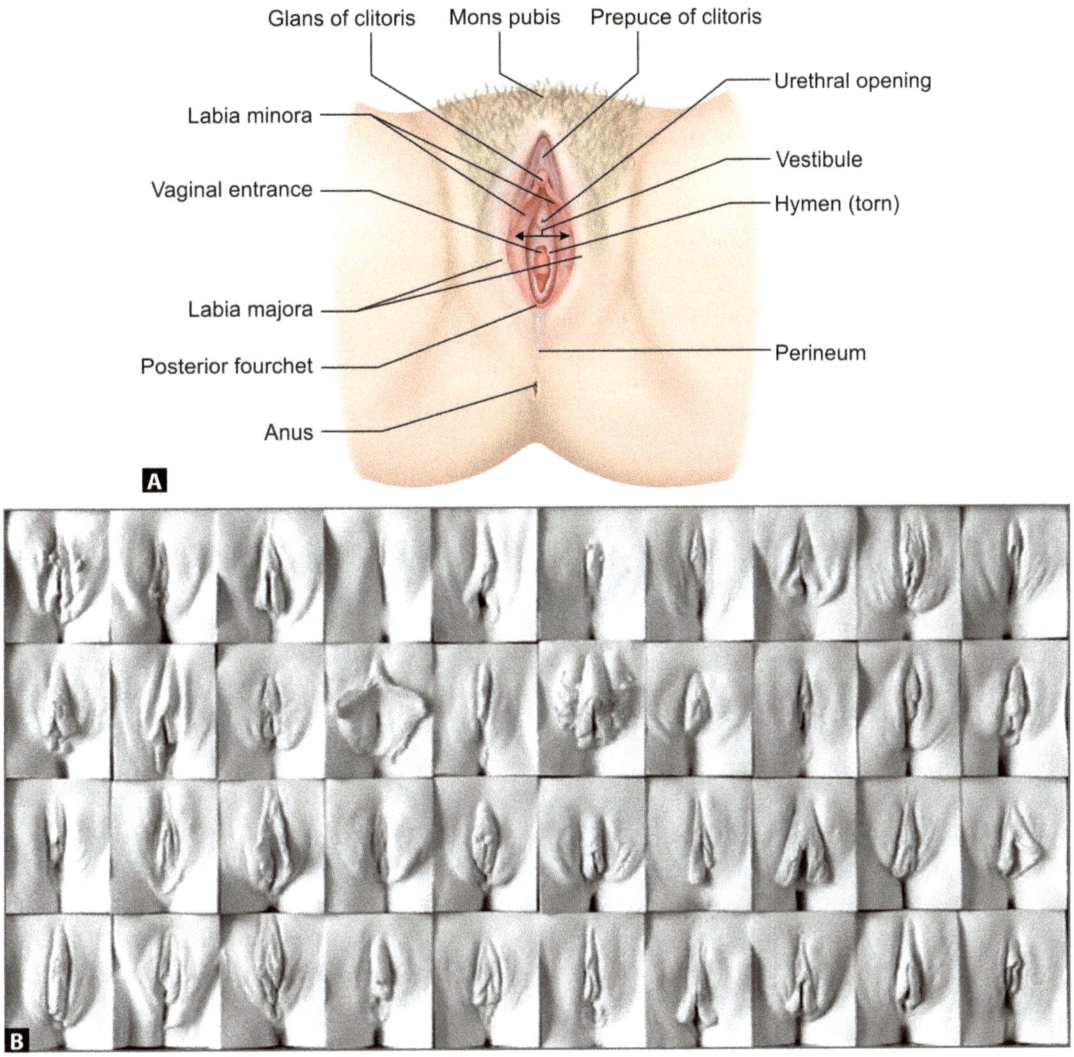

Figs. 2A and B: Vulval wall by British artist—Jamie McCartney.
Source: Jindal P, Kundal Isha. Introduction to the rising field of Aesthetic and Regenerative Gynecology: Aesthetic and Regenerative Gynecology. Singapore: Springer; 2022. pp. 3-4.

Desire for Labiaplasty (Labia Minora)

When the labia minora are enlarged, women seek labiaplasty. The enlargement of labia minora is primarily congenital, though some women do claim that enlargement occurred after:

- Childbirth
- Hormonal therapy
- With age
- Genital piercing can increase labial size and asymmetry because of the weight of the ornament.
- Hypertrophy of the labia minora can cause discomfort and lead to dyspareunia.
- Chronic urinary tract infection
- Local irritation
- Difficulty in maintaining hygiene
- Interference with tight clothes and sports such as horse riding.
- Aesthetically unpleasant although there is no standard.

All the mentioned are a reason for a patient to opt for labiaplasty. Cultural acceptance has further increased the incidence. Although there are no standard genital aesthetic ideals, basic guidelines for labia minora plasty include symmetrical labia minora that do not protrude past the labia majora, especially when standing.

Labia Minor Hypertrophy Classification

There is no universally accepted classification of labia minora as there are wide variations. An attempt has been made to classify labia minora hypertrophy in the following manner:

- Class I—Labia majora and minora are just about equal
- Class II—Protrusion of labia minora beyond the labia majora
- Class III—Includes an enlarged clitoral hood besides labia minora enlargement
- Class IV—Labia minora extends to the perineum

Indications

There are no widely accepted guidelines for labiaplasty, and it is carried out for a variety of reasons. Hypertrophy of the labia minora can cause:

- Dyspareunia
- Chronic urinary tract infections
- Irritation and hygienic difficulties and interference with sports

What constitutes labial hypertrophy is poorly defined in the literature. Others have advocated for surgery only in the presence of chronic symptoms.[3] The incidence has additionally increased due to cultural acceptance. Basic principles include symmetrical labia minora that do not extend past the labia majora, especially when standing, although there are no set standards for genital aesthetics.

Contraindications

Even though the desire to have labiaplasty is an individual choice, thorough medical and sexual history should be taken to rule out any contraindications such as:

- Active genital infections
- Sexually transmitted disease
- Gynecological malignancies
- Unrealistic aesthetic goals
- Body dysmorphic syndrome
- Smokers who are unwilling to quit either temporarily or permanently (as this will interfere with optimal wound healing).
- Pregnancy
- Severe coagulation disorder

Consenting and Consultation

Before labiaplasty or clitoroplasty, the patient undergoes a thorough surgical evaluation. This includes a physical examination, a discussion of the patient's medical history, and a review of the patient's goals for surgery. The surgeon also discusses the risks and benefits of the operation with the patient. During the consultation, the surgeon discusses the patient's expectations for the operation and assesses the patient's suitability for the procedure. The surgeon also provides information to the patient about the risks and benefits of the surgery and the recovery. It is important that patients have realistic expectations about the results of surgery. Labiaplasty and clitoroplasty can improve the appearance and function of the vulva, but they are not perfect procedures. Patients should be aware that there is a risk of complications and that the results of surgery may not be exactly what they expected.[1,5,6]

TECHNIQUES OF LABIOPLASTY

The techniques of labioplasty are as follows:

- Edge resection
- Wedge resection
- De-epithelialization
- Labiaplasty with ZIG-ZAG incision
- Labiaplasty is done with an extended W plasty incision.
- Laser labiaplasty
- Labiaplasty with clitoral hood resection

Edge Resection

It is a simple resection of tissue at the free edge of the labia minora. The clamp is placed across the area of labial tissue to the resected (clamp helps in hemostasis). The tissue to be removed is resected, and the cut labium is sutured as shown in **Figures 3A and B**.

Advantages

- It is easy to perform.
- Removes the hyperpigmented, irregular edge of the labia minora.

Disadvantages

- There is a loss of natural rugosity of the free edge of labia minora.
- Possibility of everting the inner lining of the labia
- Unable to excise the redundant tissue

Wedge Resection

It can be done either by central wedge resection or posterior wedge resection. It involves cutting and removing a partial thickness wedge of tissue from the thickest part of the labia minora.[4] Aesthetically it is superior to the edge resection,

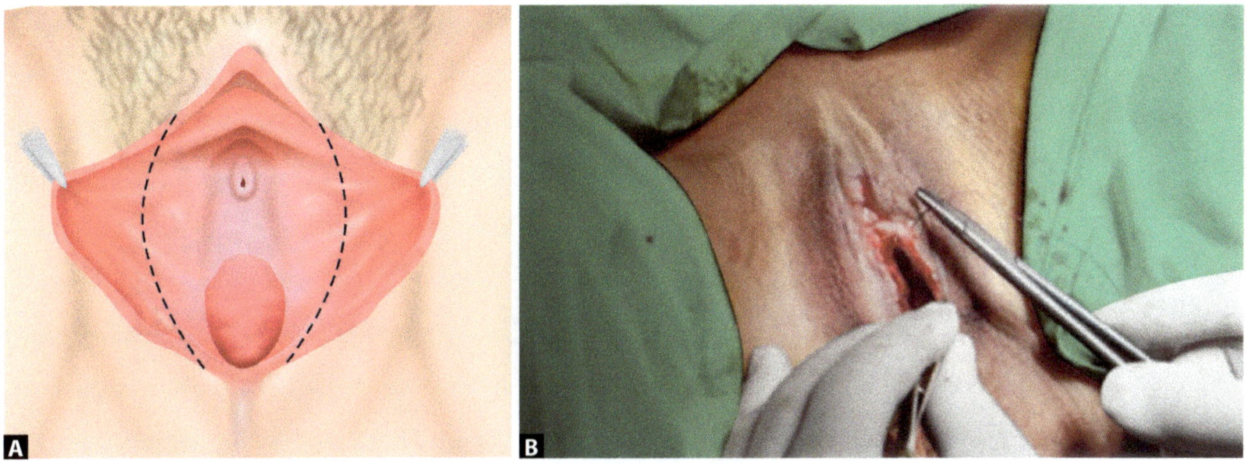

Figs. 3A and B: Edge resection.
Source: Jindal P et al.[1]

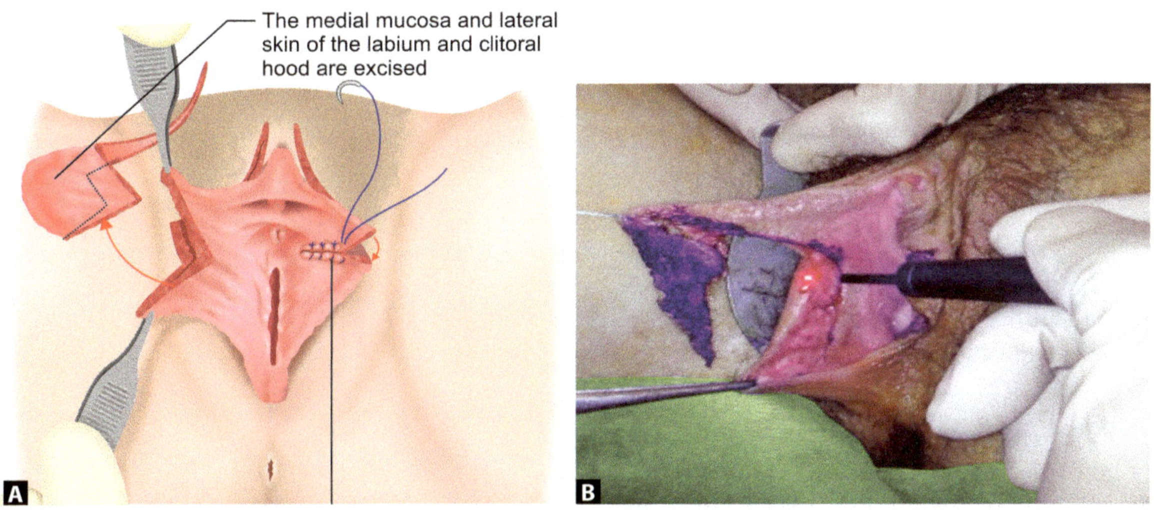

Figs. 4A and B: Wedge resection.

because it preserves the natural rugosity of the labia. Removal of the skin and mucosa should be done, leaving the submucosa intact. This decreases the risk of damaging pertinent labial nerves that can result in painful neuromas or numbness **(Figs. 4A and B)**.

F Geraldo improved the central wedge resection technique with an additional 90º Z plasty technique. This addition produces a redefined surgical edge that is less tethered and there is less livelihood of scalloped edge scars.[4,5]

Advantages

Central wedge can treat prominent clitoral without a separate incision (**Figs. 5A to D**).[1]

Disadvantages

- Very demanding surgical procedure
- Difficult to judge the correct amount of labial skin to resect. This can lead to either under or overcorrection.
- Increased probability of surgical wound dehiscence.

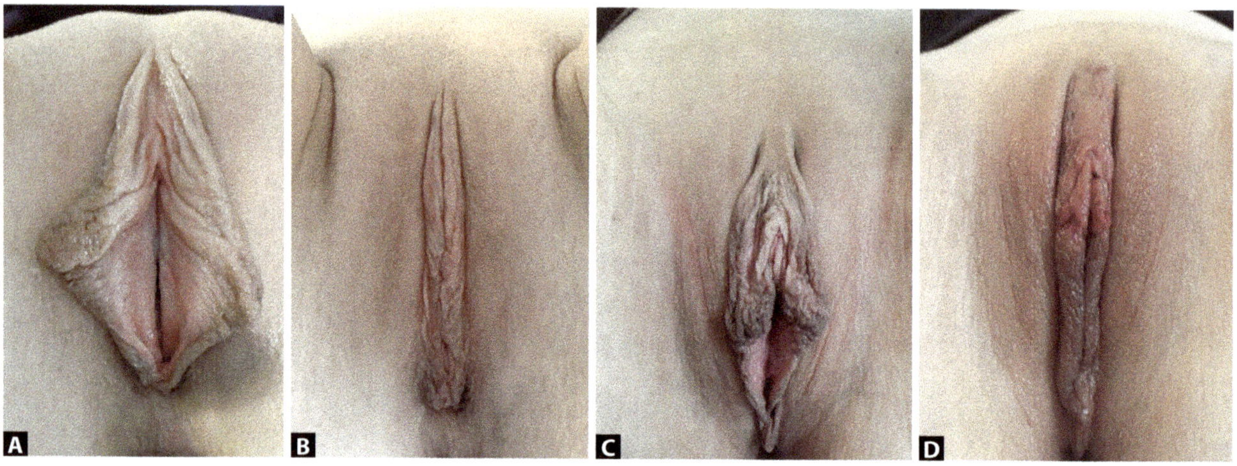

Figs. 5A to D: Patient 1 (A) Prelabiaplasty; (B) Postlabiaplasty and patient 2; (C) Prelabiaplasty; (D) Postlabiaplasty.
Source: Jindal P et al.[1]

De-epithelialization

This entails using a medical laser or a scalpel to cut the epithelium of the middle region of the medial and lateral portion of the labia minora **(Fig. 6)**.[6,7]

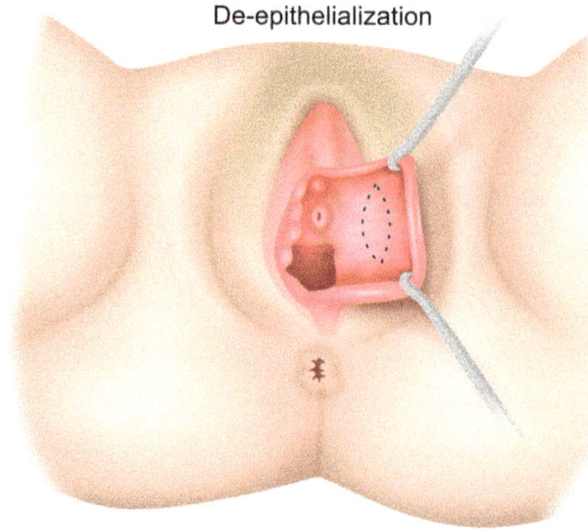

Fig. 6: De-epithelialization.

Advantages

- Lessens superfluous vertical tissue
- Keeps labia minora's inherent rugosity intact and retains the erectile and sensory qualities.

Disadvantages

To achieve labial reduction, a large region of labial tissue must be de-epithelialized, which is a technical drawback.

Zig-Zag Incision

In this type of labia, Z-shaped incisions are made and then stitched together in a new way **(Fig. 7)**.[8]

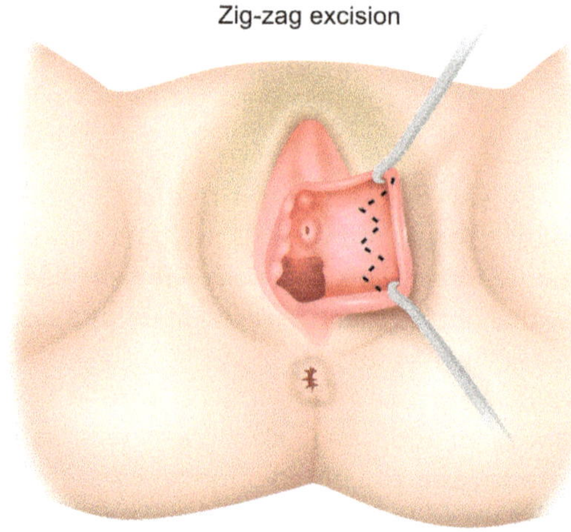

Fig. 7: Labia minora plasty with zig-zag incision.

Labiaplasty Done with an Extended W Plasty Incision

This incision is given by extending the W incision for labiaplasty **(Fig. 8)**.

Labiaplasty with Clitoral Hood Resection

This type of clitoroplasty involves removing the clitoral hood, which is the foreskin that covers the clitoris.[9] From each labium minus's most protuberant section, a central wedge, or V, is excised. In order to remove the extra lateral

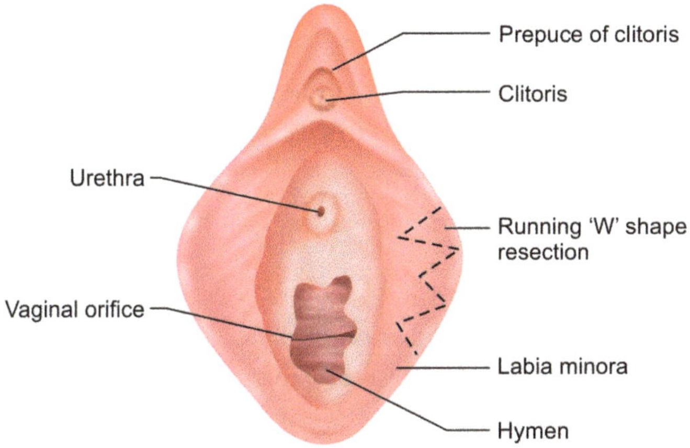

Fig. 8: Extended W plasty incision.

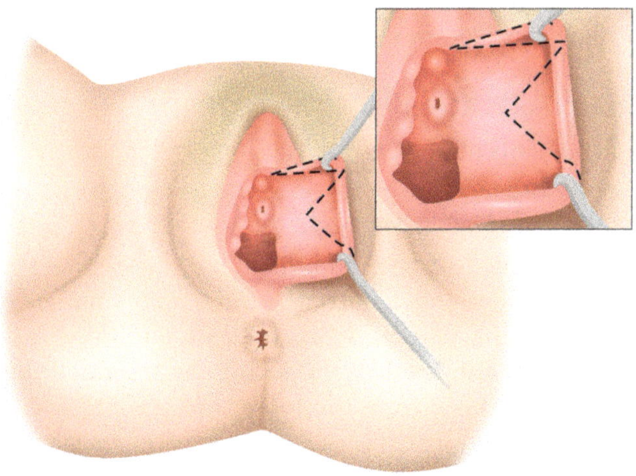
Fig. 9: Clitoral hood resection.

labium and lateral clitoral hood, the outer portion of the V excision is typically curved anteriorly and laterally **(Fig. 9)**.

Laser Labiaplasty

De-epithelialization of the labia occurs with laser excision of the minora. Rather than a surgical knife, a laser is employed.

Postoperative Care

- The patient can typically leave the hospital in a few hours.
- A vaginal pack is not necessary.
- Put on a sanitary pad for ease.
- Maintain the space dry and clean.
- Applying an antibiotic ointment locally two or three times per day for a few days.
- Making a follow-up visit.
- After 3 or 4 days following surgery, return to your regular, physically undemanding work.
- Do not use tampons
  - Avoid tight clothes
  - Avoid sexual intercourse for 4–6 weeks.

Postoperative Complications

Like all surgeries, there is a risk of complications associated with labiaplasty and clitoroplasty such as:

- Infection is a rare but serious complication of surgery.
- Bleeding may occur during or after surgery.
- Pain is normal after surgery but should be controlled with medication.
- Scarring is expected after surgery, but it usually fades over time.
- There is a small risk of loss of sensation in the vulva after surgery.
- Dyspareunia is a rare complication of vulvar and clitoroplasty.

LABIA MAJORA PLASTY

Definition

It is the procedure to improve the aesthetics of labia majora, giving permanent results.

Introduction

Less focus has been placed on labia majora plasty or surgical rejuvenation of the labia majora, but women are becoming more aware of labia minora plasty surgery, which entails shrinking and altering the labia minora.

This could also be a result of the labia majora's nonsurgical rejuvenation techniques. Nowadays, noninvasive rejuvenation is more appealing to women than surgical enhancement. For a variety of causes, the labia majora may lose their distinctive original appearance. These could be:

- Genetic reasons for supporting tissue or loosening
- Aging and childbirth
- Loss of weight

All the above leads to saggy, drooping labia, that is aesthetically unpleasing, sometimes sexually embarrassing, and yet another reminder of aging.

Anatomy

The outer lips of the vulva are the typical term used to describe the labia majora. The labia majora are two

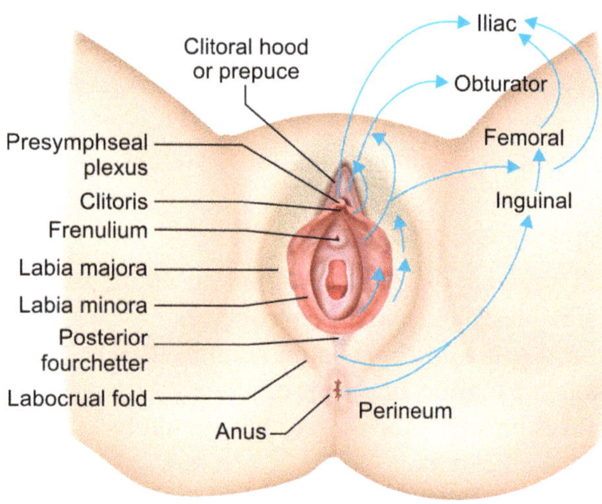

Fig.10: Anatomy of labia majora.

longitudinal, adipose tissues filled with cutaneous folds. They are made up of nerve endings, blood and lymphatic vessels, smooth muscle fibers, and the dermis, which contains the orifices of several glands, including sebaceous, sudoriferous, and apocrine ones. Each labia majora has two surfaces: A smooth inner surface covered in huge sebaceous glands and an outer surface that is pigmented and covered in long pubic hair. They join anteriorly to form the anterior labial commissure and posteriorly to form the posterior labial commissure. The vagina, clitoris, urethral orifice, and labia minora are situated between the labia majora as seen in **Figure 10**.

Desire for Labiaplasty

- Decreased sensation during sexual intercourse. Sometimes sexually embarrassing.
- Discomfort during exercising or while wearing tight clothes.
- Asymmetry
- Chronic urinary tract infection
- Aesthetically unpleasant look and loss of volume and firmness.

All these factors motivate the patients for labia majora rejuvenation.

Patients often opt for a nonsurgical procedure for labia majora rejuvenation, which could be done by injections and fillers such as:

- Fat fillers by fat harvested from another area
- Synthetic fillers
- Hyaluronic acid
- Platelet-rich plasma (PRP)
- Stem cells
- Use of carbon dioxide (CO_2) laser
- Use of radio frequency (RF) laser
- Amniotic fluid injection.

However, these noninvasive procedures have some limitations such as:

- They are expensive.
- Need to be repeated periodically.
- Irregular and slight bumps can occur if not uniformly injected.
- For this reason, some patients may opt for surgical correction.
- For performing surgical aesthetic procedures, knowledge of anatomy must be there.

Contraindications

Same as labia minora.

Labia Majora Plasty

A vertical line is drawn from the top of the clitoral hood to the labial crease, connecting the lateral labia majora and the medial clitoral hood and labia minora. The line is drawn to the level of the introitus. A semielliptical mark is produced from the top of the vertical line and extends laterally just over the top ridge of the labia majora before bending back down to the vertical line's lowest point.

This is repeated on the opposite side to achieve symmetry. To avoid the appearance of a gaping vaginal opening, only a moderate quantity of labia majora tissue should be excised. Excess, loose skin appears to be removed without causing injury to big vessels or nerves, nor does it impact skin sensitivity.

Bleeding is a significant risk when fat pad excision procedures are used and larger, deeper arteries are transected. Preliminary research indicates that high-frequency monopolar RF and ordinary electrocautery are effective surgical instruments for labia majora reduction surgery, as pain control becomes more problematic following fat pad removal. Labia minora plasty and labia majora plasty can be performed in stages on the same patient. When performed by surgeons with advanced expertise, a combined and unified approach to simultaneous labia minora plasty and labia majora plasty is both possible and safe in certain individuals.

REJUVENATION OF LABIA MAJORA BY NONSURGICAL PROCEDURES

Use of Hyaluronic Acid

Augmentation of labia majora involves increasing their fulness as a result of injecting. Suturing labia majora after removal of excess tissue cross-linked hyaluronic acid. The hyaluronic acid fillers moisturize the skin and mucous membrane and stimulate fibroblasts to produce collagen.

Carbon Dioxide Laser

Carbon dioxide fractional laser has a dermal rejuvenation effect, stimulated by gentle heating and subsequent selective induction of collagen regeneration and deposition in deeper layers. This results in the improvement of skin texture and wrinkles. CO_2 laser rejuvenates the skin tissue and promotes collagen production leading to tightening and shrinking of labia majora and minora **(Figs. 11A to C)**.

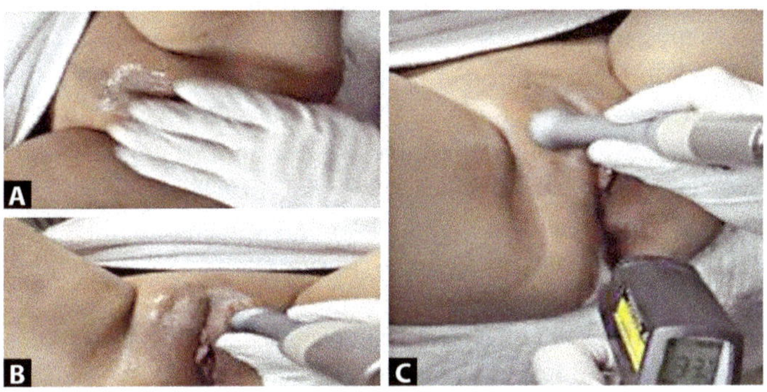

Figs. 11A to C: Carbon dioxide (CO_2) vulval laser demonstration.

Platelet-rich Plasma

Platelet-rich plasma is a portion of the plasma fraction of autologous blood, which has a platelet fraction above the baseline **(Fig. 12)**. PRP is an inexpensive and immunologically safe source of growth factors. PRP promotes tissue repair, influences angiogenesis, and reduces inflammation.[10]

Amniotic Fluid and Stem Cell Injection

These are the new methods that can be used for labial rejuvenation.

CLITORAL HOOD RESECTION

Clitoral hood resection, also termed clitoral hoodectomy, clitoral unhooding, clitoridotomy, or partial hoodectomy is a procedure for reducing the size and area of the clitoral hood (prepuce) in order to further expose the clitoral glans **(Fig. 13)**.

The upper part of labia minora diverges into two branches. The superior branch of labia minora is termed as clitoral prepuce and the inferior branch as clitoral frenulum. Clitoral hood reduction is rarely performed as an isolated procedure. It is most commonly performed in combination with labia minora reduction. The hood is prepuce of the glans clitoris. Clitoral hood redundancy, when present, may be in the horizontal or vertical plane or both. Clitoral hood folds may be unilateral or bilateral and result in a widened appearance. Vertical excess manifests as the ptotic, elongated clitoral hood. If this is

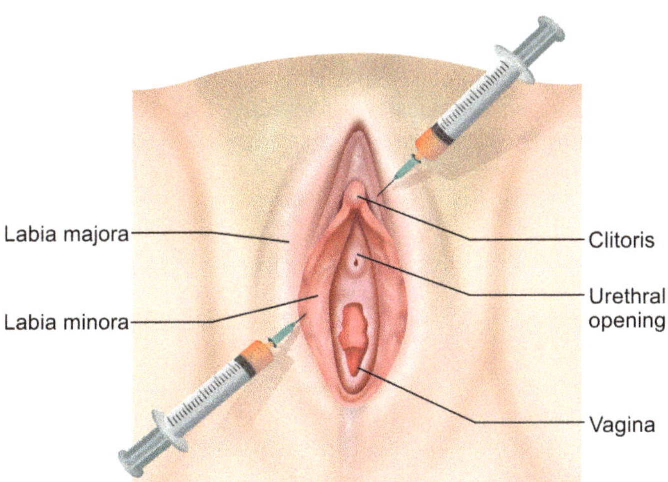

Fig. 12: Platelet-rich plasma (PRP) labial infiltration.

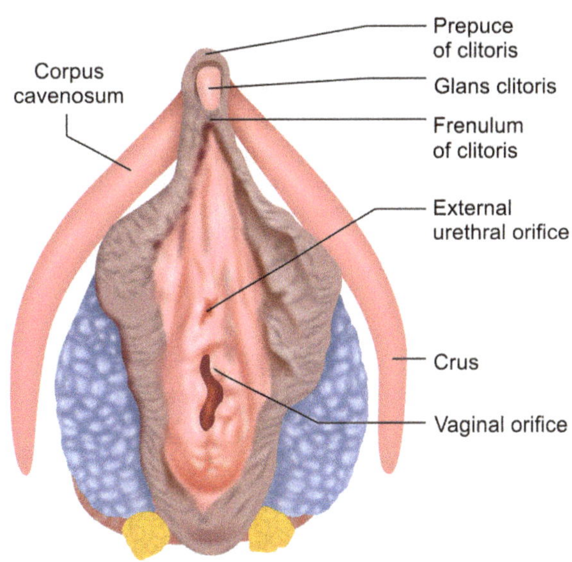

Fig. 13: Clitoral hood resection.

present, it should be dealt with during labiaplasty. Patients may opt for clitoral reduction in cases such as congenital or idiopathic enlargement, hormonal imbalance, hermaphroditism, and anabolic steroid intake.[11,12]

ETHICAL CONSIDERATIONS

Labiaplasty and clitoroplasty are two types of surgery that have been ethically debated. Some people argue that these procedures are unnecessary and can harm women's body image and self-esteem.

Others argue that these procedures are a form of female genital mutilation and should be banned. It is important to note that there is no consensus on the ethics of vulva and clitoroplasty. Ultimately, each patient must make an individual decision in consultation with their surgeon whether or not to perform any of these procedures.[13-18]

CONCLUSION

Labiaplasty and clitoroplasty are two types of vulvovaginal surgery that can be performed to improve the appearance and function of the female genitalia. Both procedures can be performed for a variety of reasons, including cosmetic, functional, and gender confirmation surgery. It is important for the patient to have realistic expectations about the outcome of the surgery and to discuss the risks and benefits with their surgeon. Labiaplasty and clitoroplasty can be life-changing surgeries for many patients, but they are not without risk.

REFERENCES

1. Joshi, S. Labiaplasty and clitoroplasty. In Jindal P, Malhotra N, Joshi S (Eds). Aesthetic and Regenerative Gynecology. Singapore: Springer; 2022. pp. 233-47.
2. Masters Z, William H, Johnson VE, Kolodny RC (Eds). Human Sexuality. New York: Harper Collins College Publishers; 1995. p. 47.
3. Sloane E. Biology of Women. Cengage Learning; 2002. p. 32.
4. Motakef S, Rodriguez-Feliz J, Chung MT, Ingargiola MJ, Wong VW, Patel A. Vaginal labiaplasty: current practices and a simplified classification system for labial protrusion. Plast Reconstr Surg. 2015;135(3):774-88.
5. Smith J. Labiaplasty and clitoroplasty: a comprehensive review. Int J Gynecol Obstet. 2023;160(2):209-18.
6. Jones M. Labiaplasty: Indications, techniques, and outcomes. Plast Reconstr Surg. 2022;150(1):289e-98e.
7. Brown K. Clitoroplasty: a systematic review of the literature. J Sex Med. 2022;19(10):623-33.
8. Alter GJ. A new technique for aesthetic labia minora reduction. Ann Plast Surg. 1998;40(3):287-90.
9. Williams L. Labiaplasty and clitoroplasty: a review of the literature. Female Pelvic Med Reconstr Surg. 2021;27(1): 10-9.
10. Eppeley BL, Pietrzak WS, Blauton M. Platelet-rich plasma: a review of biology and application in plastic surgery. Plast Reconstr Surg. 2006;118(6):147e-59e.
11. Purple I. Labiaplasty and clitoroplasty: a review of the literature and ethical considerations. J R Soc Med. 2015;108(3):121-7.
12. Hunter JG. Commentary on: postoperative clitoral hood deformity after labiaplasty. Aesthet Surg J. 2013;30(7):1037-8.
13. Hamori CA. Postoperative clitoral hood deformity after labiaplasty. Aesthet Surg J. 2013;33(7):1030-6.
14. Black F. Labiaplasty and clitoroplasty: a systematic review of the literature and ethical considerations. Ann Plast Surg. 2018;81(6):673-84.
15. Green D. Labiaplasty and clitoroplasty: Surgical techniques and outcomes. Clin Plast Surg. 2020;47(4):507-18.
16. White E. Labiaplasty and clitoroplasty: a review of the literature and ethical considerations. J Med Ethics. 2019; 45(12):788-92.
17. Grey G. Labiaplasty and clitoroplasty: a review of the literature and ethical considerations. J Am Med Assoc. 2017;317(1):76-7.
18. Pink H. Labiaplasty and clitoroplasty: a review of the literature and ethical considerations. Plast Reconstr Surg. 2016;137(5):1288e-96e.

CHAPTER 17

Female Orgasmic Disorder and Treatment

Kanika Singh

I really feel privileged to get this opportunity to pen down on such an important topic "female orgasmic disorders." It is nothing new which I am talking about...it was very much there in olden days, but was not talked and heard commonly. These days it is much heard...as today's woman is more empowered by all means...be it financially, emotionally, or by any other means.

She has her own choices and is very much vocal about it and has great clarity of all her rights to have complete physical, emotional, sexual, and mental health, whereas in olden days the women were suppressed, they did not have power to speak for their rights and if by chance some female did so was judged and tabooed, as a bad woman.

Before going in depth of "female orgasmic disorder" it would not be fair if I do not throw some light on "orgasm."

INTRODUCTION

It is an AHA moment.

The peak of sexual excitement, makes one feel lighter powerful feeling of sexual pleasure and sensation.

It can be mild or intense **(Fig. 1)**.

Orgasm can be "clitoral activated" versus "vaginally activated."

Jannini et al.[1] showed that orgasms resulting from direct clitoral stimulation have been reported to be sharp, bursting, short lasting, superficial and more localized, confined only to the pubic area.[2]

By contrast, vaginally activated orgasms have been described as more diffuse, whole body, radiating, psychologically more satisfying, and longer lasting.[1-2]

The most common orgasm (sometimes called a clitorally activated orgasm) also involves the vagina, because clitoral stimulation produces the contraction of the pubococcygeal muscle supporting the pelvic floor, which is where vaginal contractions are felt.

Orgasms that result from G-spot stimulation involves the vagina as well but causes contractions around the uterus, which is several inches above the pelvic floor, and may also involve the muscles of the lower part of the lower part of the anterior abdominal wall **(Fig. 2)**.

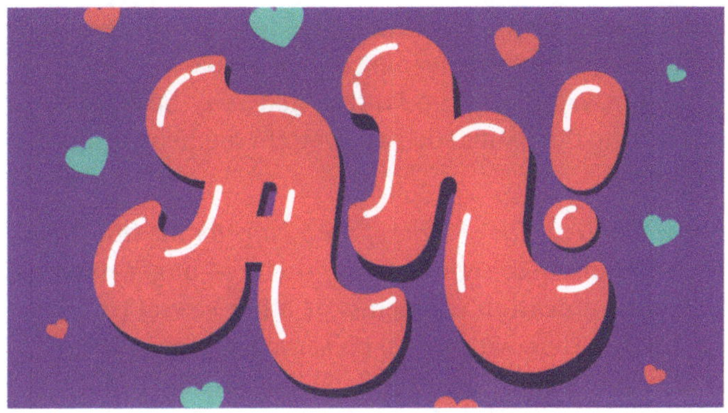

Fig. 1: Feelings expressed in words.

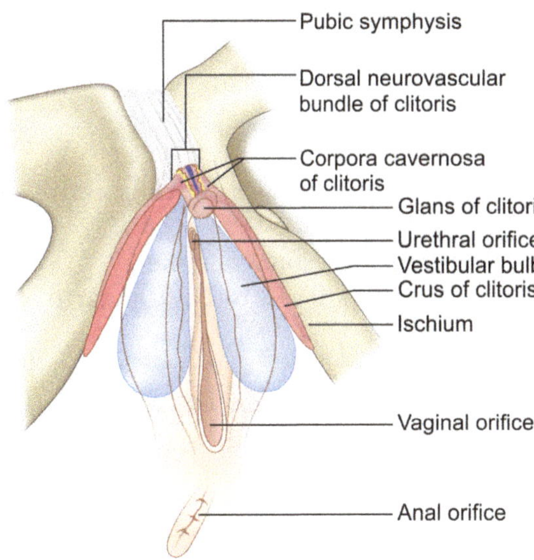

Fig. 2: External genitalia.

FEMALE SEXUAL DIFFICULTIES

These are more common than we think and impact couples inside and outside the bedroom. When sex is not even easy, how do you even begin this conversation with your partner or for those matters.

A subset of women with female sexual dysfunction (FSD) has female orgasmic disorders, there will be difficulty in achieving or complete inability to experience orgasm.[3]

These symptoms should last for 6 months or more.

Successful treatment of orgasmic disorders not only improves a woman's sexual pleasure but also can improve her emotional health and quality of life **(Fig. 3)**.

And the actual reason of problem is not known but could be related to problems with partner such as low moral, low self-esteem, or any medicines.

The desire of having sex can change in a women due to many reasons such as increasing age, any interpersonal relationship problems leading to divorce or pregnancy itself can be the cause leading to this problem.

There are many modalities that may be helpful in addressing the issues such as—certain medicines, lifestyle changes.

Following is the list of some of the factors for the disorders:

- Problems in the relationships such as—anger, mistrust, communication problems, or other sexual problems can interfere with sexual pleasure and orgasm.
- Bedridden and ill partners can have sexual problems.
- Previous emotional trauma such as assault or sexual abuse.
- Obesity and ugly looks
- Anxiety
- Cultural or religious beliefs
- Low academic level
- Having health problems
- Person on antipsychotic's, antihistamines, and antihypertensives
- Pelvic vascular congestion syndrome
- Genetics is also believed to be a factor in female orgasmic disorder
- Medical conditions such as nervous system disorder (multiple sclerosis, spinal cord lesions)
- Hormonal conditions such as thyroid disorders, hyperprolactinemia, asthma

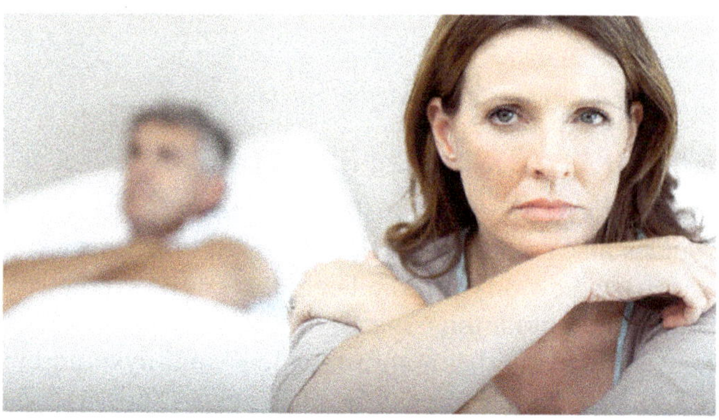

Fig. 3: Bad mood due to female orgasmic disorder.

But researchers have found that it is not medical condition alone, it is the stress of managing a chronic illness and pain, the effect of this on a woman's emotional well-being.

KINDS OF ANORGASMIA

- *Primary anorgasmia* when a person has never ever experienced an orgasm or complete absence of the perception of orgasm ever in life.
- *Secondary anorgasmia* when a person has experienced orgasm prior at some point of life but not able to perceive or feel now.
- *Situational anorgasmia* which is the type that women experience most frequently, an orgasm can be experienced in particular situation such as after having oral sex.
- *General anorgasmia* is where an orgasm is not attained in spite of maximum arousal.

MANAGEMENT OF FEMALE ORGASMIC DISORDERS

It is very important to correctly diagnose and treat these disorders, for that thorough history and physical examination is the key.

Besides this it is very important to know that whether that female has ever experienced orgasm in her life or not, her psychiatrist or psychological evaluation should be done.

Successful treatment of orgasmic disorders not only improves a woman's sexual pleasure but also can improve her emotional health.

There are multiple different treatments that are effective in FSD/female orgasmic disorder.

So, the treatment depends upon the cause like if it is hormonal deficiency then can be well treated by hormones.

If it is secondary to some drug then either change of drug or addition of some adjuvant to counter the side effect of that particular drug in the form of use of lubricants locally.

Various kinds of platelet-rich plasma shots such as O shots, k shots can be given to enhance the orgasm.

G-spot Augmentin can be done.

Use of sex toys or vibrators under supervision is taught regarding its usage so as to explore the G-spot or understand her erogenous zones.

Couple counseling for improvement of communication skills and address any conflicts that is affecting trust and intimacy **(Fig. 4)**.

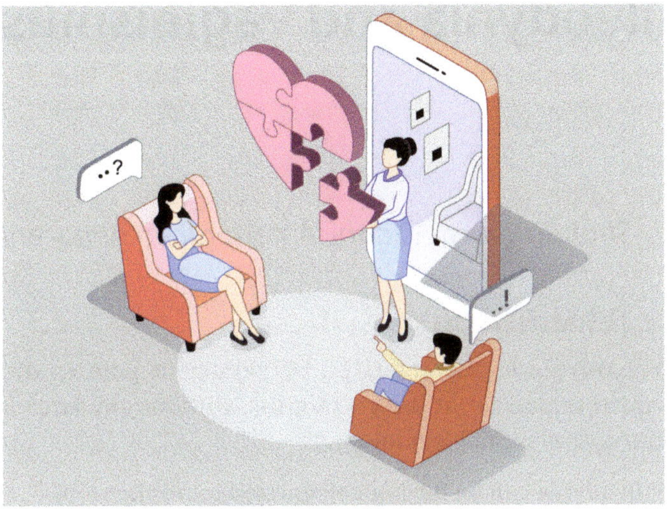

Fig. 4: Couple counseling.

Couples should be taught about the importance of foreplay, exploration of erogenous areas in each partner so as to have more satisfying sex life, like clitoral stimulation, use of different sexual techniques and let each other know which works best for whom.

Woman should be honest and open and should be vocal about her needs and should not feign orgasm. And should avoid discussing any sexual issue at the time of act as it affects the self-esteem of the other partner.

Avoidance of distractions and rather complete physical, emotional, and mental involvement should be there so as to have pleasure and orgasm as each is interrelated and absence of any one component can affect orgasm. Certain fantasies also work very well.

Instead of trying too hard for orgasm, try instead to enjoy the experience and closeness with the partner. Sometimes when trying to reach the goal, the stress people put on themselves cancels out finding enjoyment and reaching orgasm.

If you are able to discuss what you would like, when it comes to sex, inform your partner. While you may think he should know what you like that is not the case. By letting him know, he will be able to help fulfill your sexual desires.

Make sure to tell your partner when he is doing something you find enjoyable. He will know for future times that it gave you pleasure.

Ease up on yourself. If you do not reach orgasm or only do so sometimes, it does not mean you are a failure. It also does not help to beat yourself up, because it will not lead to better sex.

Just because your partner is finished does not mean you are, too let him know if you are fully aroused and would like to continue. If you feel like you are able to instruct him on what to do, especially if you feel you may have an orgasm.

CONCLUSION

"An orgasm is like a pleasurable, seductive music, played rhythmically in a right way, by a terrific musician".

REFERENCES

1. Jannini EA, Amati G, Lenzi A. Histology and immunohistochemical studies of female genital tissue. In: Goldstein I, Maston C, Davis S, Traish A, (Eds). Women's Sexual Function and Dysfunction Study, Diagnosis and Treatment. London: Taylor and Francis, 2006.
2. Komisaruk JB, Beyar-Flores C, Whipple B (Eds). The Science of Orgasm. Baltimore: John Hopkins University Press, 2006.
3. American College of Obstetricians and Gynecologists' Committee on Practice Bulletins—Gynecology. Female Sexual Dysfunction: ACOG Practice Bulletin Clinical Management Guidelines for Obstetrician-Gynecologists, Number 119. Obstet Gynecol. 2011;117:996.

CHAPTER 18

Vulvodynia and Vaginismus

Shahad Saeed Alzaabi, Amel Ibrahim Almaeeni

VULVODYNIA

INTRODUCTION

Vulvodynia is a condition characterized by persistent pain in the vulva area. About 18% of women have experienced vulvar pain that aligns with the symptoms of vulvodynia at some stage,[1] where women experience considerable distress due to chronic vulvar pain. Managing this condition can be difficult for healthcare professionals as the exact cause of the pain is unknown, and it persists for >3 months.[2]

The International Society for the Study of Vulvovaginal Disease (ISSVD) provides additional details about vulvodynia including its various descriptions. These descriptions include specifying the location of the pain (whether it is generalized or localized to specific areas like the vaginal entrance or clitoris), whether the pain is provoked by contact or unprovoked, the onset of the pain (primary if it started from the first genital contact or secondary if it occurred after a period of pain-free intercourse), and whether the pain is intermittent or persistent.[2,3]

Studies consistently indicate that vulvodynia is linked to a decline in overall quality of life, diminished sexual function, and impaired physical well-being.[3-5] Despite the significant burden and detrimental effects on women's lives, research suggests that <6% of women with vulvodynia receive an accurate diagnosis initially, resulting in prolonged pain that persists for several years.[6]

Addressing the various aspects of vulvodynia requires a multidisciplinary approach involving a team of healthcare professionals, such as a lead clinician, clinical psychologist, physiotherapist, psychosexual medicine clinician, and pain management specialist. Given the diverse causes of the condition, multimodal therapy is often recommended as the preferred approach in the majority of cases.[7]

TERMINOLOGY

Vulvodynia is characterized by persistent pain in the vulvar region for at least 3 months, without any known cause or identifiable etiology.

Vulvodynia can be further categorized into subgroups:[8]

- *Location:* The symptoms may manifest as localized (such as vestibulodynia or clitorodynia), generalized, or a combination of both (localized and generalized).
- *Provocation:* The pain can be triggered by specific factors, such as insertion or contact (provoked), occur spontaneously without any apparent cause (unprovoked), or a mix of both (provoked and spontaneous).
- *Onset:* The condition can be classified as primary, meaning the symptoms have been present since the beginning (e.g., discomfort during tampon insertion or sexual intercourse), or secondary, where symptoms develop after a period of normal function.
- *Temporal pattern:* The pain may occur intermittently, persistently, constantly, immediately after physical contact (immediate), or with a delay after contact (delayed).

EPIDEMIOLOGY

According to self-report studies, the prevalence of chronic vulvar pain, encompassing all types, varies between 3 and 15%.[9-12] Determining the prevalence of vulvar pain is difficult since many women experiencing this condition do not seek medical evaluation. Furthermore, when they do seek medical attention, vulvar pain is often misdiagnosed.[13]

Moreover, individuals who present with vestibular pain may exhibit diverse symptoms and also experience generalized pain in other areas of the pelvis. These symptoms can be exacerbated by various factors including vulvovaginal infections, hypoestrogenic states, and conditions associated with anxiety, depression, catastrophizing, and other psychosocial factors.[14,15]

PATHOGENESIS AND LIKELY CONTRIBUTORS

The exact cause of localized vulvar pain syndrome is not completely understood and is likely to involve multiple factors.[13,16] The prevailing theory suggests that a triggering event, such as an infection or trauma, initiates a localized inflammatory response.[8]

In women who are susceptible, the inflammatory response can result in the excessive growth of nerve fibers in the vestibular tissue and decreased pain thresholds. This, in turn, can lead to the central sensitization of pain.[17-20]

Inflammation

While the available data are inconclusive, an excessive or abnormal immune response has been suggested as a potential cause of vulvodynia. A systematic review encompassing 18 studies with 400 women revealed limited and conflicting evidence regarding the association between localized vulvodynia and inflammation, both locally and systemically.[21]

The heightened production of proinflammatory substances and/or impaired tissue clearance of inflammatory responses can sensitize neurons in the vulvar vestibule. This, in turn, can lead to the upregulation of neurons in the central nervous system.[13]

Research studies have documented an elevation in the levels of inflammatory markers such as interleukin-6, interleukin-1, and tumor necrosis factor-α. Conversely, a decrease has been observed in the levels of macrophage inhibitory protein 1β.[22,23] In women experiencing vestibular pain, there is an observed increase in the surface receptor dectin-1, which has a binding affinity for *Candida albicans*. This increase is not observed in women without vestibular pain (control group).[24]

As a result, women with vestibular pain syndromes may have a higher likelihood of binding *C. albicans* and triggering an inflammatory response compared to women without any symptoms.

Neurologic Proliferation and Sensitization

Studies have found that women diagnosed with localized vulvar pain syndrome exhibit a higher density of intraepithelial nerve fibers and increased levels of the vanilloid receptor 1 (VR1), which is activated by the inflammatory response.[25] Additionally, hyperesthesia, resulting from the sensitization of both the peripheral and central nervous systems, has been reported in these individuals.[26,27]

Furthermore, studies have indicated that patients diagnosed with localized vulvar pain syndrome exhibit lower sensory and pressure-pain thresholds.[24,28-30] The chronic inflammation of the vulvar vestibule may result in hyperinnervation and sensitization, causing even gentle touch to the vulva to elicit a significantly painful response, known as allodynia.

Infection

Research has documented a correlation between genital infections, specifically *C. albicans* and bacterial vaginosis, and the development of localized vulvar pain syndrome.[31,32] About 70% of women with vulvodynia report a history of recurrent or severe yeast infections.[4,33,34] Moreover, an increase in pelvic infections appears to elevate the risk of developing localized vulvar pain syndrome.[32]

Genetic Factors

Certain genetic polymorphisms have the potential to impact the immune system's response to trauma or infection, hinder the termination of inflammatory responses, or increase susceptibility to pain following exposure to infectious agents.[13,35] Studies have associated genetic polymorphisms related to interleukin-1β, tumor necrosis factor-α, interleukin-1 receptor antagonist, mannose-binding lectin, and melanocortin-1 receptor with vulvar pain.[35-39] In women diagnosed with localized vulvar pain syndrome, there is evidence to suggest heightened inflammatory reactions (e.g., increased interleukin-1β) and impaired ability to resolve inflammatory responses (e.g., impaired interleukin-1 receptor antagonist).[40,41] Studies have observed an increased number of cytosine-adenine-guanine (CAG) repeats in genes responsible for coding androgen receptors in adolescents who experience vulvar pain in response to combined hormonal contraceptives, in comparison to control subjects. This occurrence is hypothesized to be associated with reduced levels of free testosterone.[42,43]

Allergy

There is evidence linking allergic reactions to localized vulvar pain syndrome. In a study involving 220 women diagnosed with this condition, it was found that 20% of them had a vaginal allergy, characterized by elevated levels of immunoglobulin E. Furthermore, nearly half of these women experienced successful treatment with antihistamine medications.[31]

Hormonal

The impact of reproductive hormones on the development of vulvodynia remains uncertain. Some studies have indicated a decrease in estrogen receptor-α levels in women with localized vulvar pain syndrome compared to control women,[44] while others have reported an increase.[45] The effects of contraceptive hormone pills on vestibular pain are also conflicting. Women with weaker androgen receptors may be more vulnerable to vulvodynia when using hormonal contraceptives.[42] Additionally, hormonal changes could contribute to a lower likelihood of resolving localized vulvar pain syndrome in obese women [body mass index (BMI) ≥30 kg/m^2] compared to women of normal weight (BMI: 18.5–24.9 kg/m^2).[32]

Myofascial

Pelvic floor muscle dysfunction can worsen the symptoms of localized vulvar pain. Furthermore, patients with vulvodynia may develop pelvic myofascial disorders or pelvic floor hypertonus, as contact with the vulvar vestibule induces pain, triggering a reflex contraction and subsequently increasing tension in the levator ani and other pelvic floor muscles.[46,47]

Psychological Dysfunction

The correlation between psychological dysfunction and localized vulvar pain syndrome is a topic of ongoing debate. Women with this condition often display lower pain thresholds, heightened systemic pain perception, increased levels of anxiety, depression, hypervigilance, and somatization compared to women without vulvodynia.[44,48-50] However, there is no evidence suggesting that psychological factors are the primary cause of localized vulvar pain syndrome. The mental health stigma surrounding vulvar pain can have various negative consequences including dismissive experiences within the healthcare system, feelings of shame and guilt, low self-esteem, social isolation, and negative societal views regarding sexuality and femininity.[51]

DIAGNOSTIC CRITERIA

The characteristics defining localized vulvar pain syndrome are as follows:[13]

- Pain specifically in the vulvar vestibule, with or without involving the clitoris
- No identifiable cause for the pain
- Duration of at least 3 months
- Pain triggered by pressure-point testing.

Furthermore, the appearance of symptoms can be classified as primary, occurring from the initial contact with the vestibule, or secondary, developing after a period of normal function. The symptoms may exhibit different temporal patterns, such as intermittent, persistent (without remission), or continuous. Additionally, the timing of symptoms after vestibular contact can vary, ranging from immediate to delayed. The most prevalent form of the disorder is characterized by pain provoked by genital contact in an otherwise asymptomatic woman. However, there are other variations including women experiencing spontaneous pain or a combination of provoked and spontaneous symptoms.[13]

It is possible for women to experience both vulvar pain with a known cause (such as lichen sclerosus, herpes, or candida) and localized vulvar pain syndrome simultaneously. These cases are usually identified when the symptoms of vulvodynia persist even after treating all identified causes of vulvar pain.[13]

DIAGNOSTIC EVALUATION

The diagnostic assessment for localized vulvar pain syndrome involves a comprehensive examination and a thorough review of the patient's medical history including targeted pressure-point testing of the vulvar vestibule. One of the aims of this evaluation is to identify any potential underlying causes of the woman's pain, such as infections or genitourinary syndrome of menopause. It is important to note that localized vulvar pain syndrome is a diagnosis made by excluding other identifiable causes of symptoms. Women who have a specific cause for their pain, such as an infection, do not meet the criteria for localized vulvar pain syndrome. However, it can be challenging to differentiate between vulvar pain caused by a specific condition and localized vulvar pain syndrome, as they can coexist.[2]

History

During the evaluation process, the patient's history is carefully examined, which involves a thorough review of various systems, a detailed gynecologic history, and an exploration of the patient's specific experiences with vulvar pain. This helps to characterize the nature of the pain and identify any potential underlying causes of vulvar pain.[2]

The International Pelvic Pain Society has created a comprehensive form for assessing women with chronic pelvic pain, regardless of its cause. Within the review of systems, specific inquiries are made about prior skin conditions (regardless of location), allergies, and dietary/nutritional factors, as these factors can contribute to specific vulvar pain. While excessive urinary oxalate excretion has been suggested as a potential irritant for vulvodynia patients, it has not been identified as a cause of localized vulvar pain syndrome.[3] Some individuals with localized vulvar pain syndrome may find that acidic or sugary foods worsen their symptoms. By eliminating certain foods and monitoring pain levels, it can help determine if there is any correlation between diet and localized vulvar pain.[2]

The gynecologic history plays a crucial role in identifying potential causes of the woman's symptoms and assessing the risk factors associated with localized vulvar pain syndrome. Specific inquiries are made regarding prior genital infections, the use of topical treatments, and exposure to hormones. Women diagnosed with localized vulvar pain syndrome often have a history of multiple genital infections. It is important to note that topical treatments, such as antifungal creams, can either cause or exacerbate dermatitis, which is a known cause of vulvar pain. Some studies have suggested a possible association between hormone use, particularly oral contraceptive pills, and localized vulvar pain syndrome. Additionally, a detailed sexual history is obtained to assess for female sexual dysfunction including issues related to desire, arousal, orgasm, and pain. Screening for intimate partner violence is also conducted. Furthermore, inquiries are made regarding pelvic floor dysfunction (such as urinary or fecal incontinence and prolapse), obstetric injuries, and prior abdominal/pelvic surgeries. It is worth noting that in rare cases, renal stones can cause pain in the corresponding vulva.[2]

Psychological factors and anatomical trauma can both contribute to the development or worsening of vulvodynia and other specific types of vulvar pain, such as vaginismus. In order to diagnose localized vulvar pain syndrome, it is necessary to ensure that any identifiable specific causes of pelvic and vulvar pain have been treated effectively (for example, using antifungal medications for candida and undergoing pelvic floor physiotherapy for vaginismus), address any associated psychological issues, and confirm that the vestibular pain persists despite these interventions.

During the assessment of vulvar vestibular symptoms, we specifically focus on gathering information about the following aspects of the patient's history.

Pain Characteristics

Characteristics of pain: Women diagnosed with localized vulvar pain syndrome are often able to consistently describe, pinpoint the location, and rate the intensity of their pain. Approximately 90% of women with this condition describe their symptoms as a burning sensation specifically localized to the vulvar vestibule.[52] Other descriptors used to convey the nature of the pain include sharp, cutting, hot, knife-like, "like razor blades," and throbbing. The pain can be classified as primary, occurring with initial contact, such as during sexual activity or tampon use, or secondary, developing after a period of normal function.[13]

Location: Utilizing an anatomical diagram that allows the woman to pinpoint the specific areas of pain can be beneficial. In the case of localized vulvar pain syndrome, the pain is confined to the vestibule or clitoris.[13]

Intensity: Patients are also asked to rate the intensity of their symptoms over time using a numerical 10-point pain scale. This information helps in understanding the duration and severity of the pain, as well as its impact on the woman's daily activities.[13]

Pain timeline: A record is created to track the occurrence and length of pain, along with any events that may have triggered it (such as a genital infection, tampon use, or intercourse), and the treatment received. Symptoms may appear suddenly or with a delay, and they can be constant or sporadic. To be classified as localized vulvar pain syndrome, symptoms must persist for at least 3 months.

Associated Symptoms

Dyspareunia: We assess if the woman experiences introital dyspareunia, which is a key symptom of vestibulodynia.[42] Women who report general dyspareunia or pain during deep penetration undergo additional evaluation to rule out other potential causes, such as vaginismus or endometriosis.

Tampon usage: Women diagnosed with localized vulvar pain syndrome often experience intense pain when attempting to insert tampons, rendering them unable to use them. According to a study involving a questionnaire administered to 30 women with vulvar vestibular pain, nearly half of them reported pain during tampon insertion.[33] If a woman is capable of regularly using tampons without pain, it is less likely that she has localized vulvar pain syndrome, and we proceed to investigate other potential causes for her symptoms.

Myofascial pain: There is evidence to suggest that myofascial pain syndromes increase the likelihood of developing localized vulvar pain syndrome, and women diagnosed with localized vulvar pain syndrome may experience secondary myofascial pain due to escalating tension in the pelvic floor muscles. To screen for myofascial pain, we inquire if women experience deep burning pain, pelvic heaviness, or pain that radiates to other areas.[33]

Menstruation: Typically, localized vulvar pain syndrome is not exacerbated by menstrual periods. However, if a woman experiences worsened symptoms during her menstrual cycle, further evaluation is conducted to explore potential hormonally dependent causes of pelvic pain, such as endometriosis or pelvic congestion syndrome.

Symptoms related to semen exposure: The clinical presentations of women with both localized vulvar pain syndrome and seminal plasma allergy can be similar. However, there is a key distinction between the two conditions. Women diagnosed with localized vulvar pain syndrome experience symptoms even when using a condom, whereas women with seminal plasma allergy do not.

Psychosocial Impact

Women diagnosed with localized vulvar pain syndrome often experience various negative effects including impaired sexual function, diminished psychological well-being, and strained interpersonal relationships. Furthermore, their ability to engage in routine activities may be compromised. To assess the impact, we inquire whether women avoid or cease certain activities due to their symptoms and how these symptoms influence their relationships.

Physical Examination

In cases of generalized vulvodynia (GVD), the vulva typically appears normal during examination. To differentiate localized vulvodynia from other causes of vulval pain, a pelvic examination is performed, specifically focusing on localizing the symptoms and signs to the vestibule area.

- During vulval inspection, it is valuable to look for signs such as erythema, fissures, excoriations, ulceration, hypopigmentation, or architectural changes in the vulva, as it helps rule out vulvovaginal infection and vulval dermatosis. In localized vulvodynia, the presence of vulvar erythema on visual inspection at the vestibule can be a significant finding, although it can also be observed in women without any underlying condition.[53]
- To assess for vulvodynia, a moistened cotton swab test, also known as the Q-tip test, is conducted. Gentle pressure is applied to various areas, including the inner thigh, labia majora, interlabial sulcus, clitoris, perineum, and specific positions along the vestibule (2, 4, 6, 8, and 10 o'clock). Women with vulvodynia typically experience discomfort during this test, particularly in the posterior introitus and hymenal remnants.[54]
- The presence of allodynia and hyperesthesia throughout the vestibule indicates intrinsic pathology likely caused by neuronal proliferation, particularly if these sensations are perceived in the posterior vestibule, which may suggest hypertonicity of the levator ani muscles.
- To rule out peripheral neuropathy, the bulbocavernosus reflex (elicited by gently stroking the labia majora) and the anal wink tests are performed.[55]
- During the vaginal examination, minimal pressure is applied to any painful area, and a narrow speculum is used to examine the vaginal wall (epithelium). This helps identify signs of atrophy, erosions, or synechiae that may suggest erosive lichen planus.
- Digital examination is conducted using one finger to internally palpate the pelvic floor musculature, allowing for the identification of vaginismus and tenderness in the pelvic floor muscles. The uterus and adnexa are also palpated to check for evidence of pelvic masses or endometriosis.[56]

Investigations

Screening for infections: To rule out vulvovaginal infections as a potential cause of vulval pain, infection screening includes various tests, such as wet smears, vaginal pH measurement, and fungal and bacterial cultures. These screenings help identify infections, such as bacterial vaginosis, trichomoniasis, and candidiasis. A study conducted in Norway highlighted bacterial vaginosis as a notable risk factor for localized vulvodynia and recommended the inclusion of wet smears as a routine evaluation for patients.[57]

Colposcopy: Colposcopy is performed to rule out subclinical human papillomavirus (HPV) infection and localized fungal infections. However, a recent review suggests that colposcopy and the use of acetic acid provide little or no additional benefit compared to a visual examination of the vulva without any aids.[58]

Human papillomavirus testing: The available evidence does not strongly support HPV as a cause of vulvodynia, therefore testing for HPV infection is not recommended.[6]

Vulval biopsy: The routine practice of conducting vulval biopsies is not widely supported. A study involving Danish women with vulvodynia found that only 12.5% of those with vulval erythema showed histopathological signs of vulval dermatosis. This raises doubts about the usefulness of routine vulval biopsies in these cases. However, vulval biopsies are warranted in situations where there are indications of vulvar dermatoses, intraepithelial neoplasia, or when vulvodynia becomes refractory to other treatments.[59]

Imaging: In general, localized vulvar pain syndrome does not typically exhibit specific imaging findings. However, imaging techniques can be valuable in identifying alternative causes of pain, such as uterine fibroids or ovarian cysts. Patients who present with symptoms or have risk factors for kidney stones may also benefit from imaging to rule out this condition. Routine magnetic romance imaging (MRI) is not typically indicated for unprovoked pain, as sacral cysts causing referred pain to the vulva are extremely rare.[60]

MANAGEMENT

The management approach for women with vulvodynia encompasses the following:

- Patient education and psychological support
- Vulval care measures
- Medical treatment
- Surgical therapy

Adopting a multidisciplinary team approach is recommended, where the lead clinician triages patients based on their specific needs to other healthcare professionals, such as clinical psychologists, physiotherapists, psychosexual medicine specialists, and pain management teams.[61]

Patient Education and Psychological Support

To ensure that the patient is well-informed about vulvodynia and its treatment, it is important to provide them with realistic information about the condition. It is crucial to acknowledge the patient's pain as genuine and explain that there is no single treatment that is universally effective. Instead, a combination of therapies may be necessary, and it may take several weeks to months to see an improvement in symptoms. The approach to treatment should be personalized and patient-centered, taking into account the patient's preferences, the involvement of their partner, local healthcare guidelines, and any associated costs. Additionally, healthcare providers should offer information on support groups and patient resources to help the patient navigate their condition.[62] Research has shown that educational seminars conducted by gynecologists who specialize in managing vulvodynia, in a group setting, have had a significant positive impact on the psychological well-being and sexual function of women affected by the condition.[62]

Vulval Care

The primary focus of initial management is to implement gentle vulval care measures in order to minimize irritation. A recent study examining the effectiveness of vulval care has shown a statistically significant improvement in symptoms, such as dyspareunia, burning, itching, and pain.

The recommended vulval care measures include the following:[63,64]

- Avoiding the direct application of perfumes, dyes, chemicals, and soaps to the vulva or on clothing that comes into contact with the vulva
- Avoiding tight and synthetic clothing, with a preference for 100% cotton
- Using sufficient lubrication prior to intercourse when experiencing dyspareunia
- Utilizing a sitz bath and applying a preservative-free emollient, such as petroleum jelly, to seal moisture in the skin and improve the skin's protective barrier
- Applying cold gel packs to the vulval area.

Medical Treatment

Medical treatment includes topical, intralesional, and oral drugs are summarized based on recent systematic reviews on the pharmacotherapy of vulvodynia.

Topical Therapy

Research supports the use of lidocaine ointment at 2% or 5% concentration, which has been shown to improve symptoms when applied overnight or before intercourse, resulting in a 50% reduction in dyspareunia (painful intercourse).[65] Another study found that topical gabapentin at 2–6% concentration led to a 50% reduction in pain and improved sexual relationships. However, caution should be exercised when prescribing topical agents to avoid allergic contact dermatitis. Other topical medications like nifedipine, capsaicin, amitriptyline, baclofen, nitroglycerine, and sodium cromoglycate have not been proven to provide significant benefits.[66]

Intralesional Therapy

In the first controlled trial comparing botulinum toxin type A injection in the vestibular epithelium to a placebo, positive outcomes were observed in terms of pain reduction, sexual function, and quality of life. However, the long-term effects may require further investigation.[57] Additionally, there have been reports of successful treatment for stubborn vulvodynia using submucosal infiltration with a combination of betamethasone and lidocaine.[67]

Systemic Therapy

Tricyclic antidepressants (TCAs), such as amitriptyline, imipramine, nortriptyline, and desipramine, as well as selective serotonin reuptake inhibitors (SSRIs) and serotonin and noradrenaline reuptake inhibitors (SNRIs), are commonly used medications for managing unprovoked pain at lower doses than those used for depression. Amitriptyline, in particular, has been extensively studied and is typically prescribed at a nightly dose of 5–25 mg. The dosage can be gradually increased by 10–25 mg/week until adequate pain control is achieved, up to a maximum daily dose of 150 mg. It is important to note that it may take at least 4 weeks before the full pain-relieving effects become evident.[3] In a prospective nonrandomized study, it was found that women who were prescribed TCAs experienced a 47% reduction in pain scores.[68]

In a recent systematic review investigating the effectiveness of antidepressants in vulvodynia, the authors emphasized the need for additional well-controlled trials to identify the specific characteristics that would help predict which women would benefit from antidepressant treatment.[69] Should TCAs not be well-tolerated or fail to produce the desired response, anticonvulsants like gabapentin and pregabalin may be considered as alternative options.[70]

Side effects, such as sedation, dry mouth, dizziness (specifically associated with TCAs), and cognitive impairment are common concerns with the use of systemic medications. Achieving optimal pain control may often require a multimodal approach, and it is crucial to exercise caution and check for potential drug interactions. When prescribing these medications to individuals of reproductive age, it is important to provide sufficient contraceptive counseling.[71]

To summarize, the use of 2–5% lidocaine in topical therapy has been shown to be effective and can be recommended for treating provoked localized vulvodynia. For unprovoked vulvodynia, TCAs, gabapentin, or pregabalin are viable treatment options. However, the optimal drug therapy for vulvodynia remains uncertain due to a lack of well-controlled trials providing sufficient evidence.[72]

Surgical Treatment

Modified vestibulectomy is currently recommended for women with localized provoked vulvodynia when other treatment options have been exhausted.[61] This procedure involves removing a U-shaped section of the vestibular mucosa up to Hart's line (the edges of the vulvar vestibule) and advancing the posterior vaginal mucosa to cover the resulting defect. Modified vestibulectomy has shown high patient satisfaction rates and low complication rates.[73] Interestingly, a critical review of various treatment strategies for provoked localized vulvodynia suggests that vestibulectomy is the most effective treatment option thus far. However, more robust data is needed to further support its efficacy.[74,75]

Laser ablation of the vulvar epithelium, using either the potassium titanyl phosphate (KTP)-neodymium-doped yttrium aluminum garnet (Nd:YAG) laser or the CO_2 laser, has been proposed as an alternative to the more invasive vestibulectomy procedure. The laser treatment disrupts angiogenesis, increases nerve density, and promotes collagen remodeling while preserving the macroscopic anatomy. The effectiveness of laser therapy for vulvodynia was found to be comparable to that of vestibulectomy. A recent study with a 2-year follow-up on the use of KTP-Nd:YAG laser for vulvodynia reported that 68% of patients experienced reduced pain during sexual intercourse and improved sexual satisfaction.[76]

VAGINISMUS

INTRODUCTION

Historically, vaginismus has been described as involuntary muscle spasms that occur during vaginal penetration. However, the definition and criteria for diagnosing vaginismus have evolved to encompass a broader range of symptoms. When no identifiable cause is found, patients with vaginismus often require a multimodal approach to treatment.

DEFINITIONS AND CRITERIA

The terminology and diagnostic criteria for vaginismus are often encompassed within the broader category of female sexual pain (FSP). While the terminology may overlap, individual patients may resonate more with one description than the other.

Diagnostic and Statistical Manual of Mental Disorders, Fifth Edition (DSM-5)

The DSM-5 categorizes "vaginismus" as a symptom under the broader classification of "genito-pelvic pain/penetration disorder" (GPPPD).[77] This represents a shift from previous definitions of vaginismus, which focused on "involuntary (pelvic) muscle spasm,"[78] "pain and fear of vaginal penetration,"[78] and "recurrent or persistent involuntary spasm of the musculature of the outer third of the vagina that interferes with sexual intercourse."[79] In the DSM-5, GPPPD is characterized by significant difficulty with at least one of the following: (1) vaginal intercourse/penetration, (2) genito-pelvic pain, (3) fear of vaginal intercourse/penetration/pain, or (4) heightened pelvic floor muscle tension during attempted penetration.[77]

International Consultation on Sexual Medicine

In 2016, the fourth International Consultation on Sexual Medicine (ICSM) provided further clarification on the components of specific disorders and grouped them together as "female genital-pelvic pain dysfunction". According to the ICSM, this term encompasses persistent or recurring difficulties associated with at least one of the following actions or symptoms:[1]

- Experience of pain during vaginal penetration during intercourse
- Significant vulvovaginal pain during genital contact
- Intense fear or anxiety about vulvovaginal or pelvic pain before, during, or as a result of genital contact
- Excessive tension or overactivity of pelvic floor muscles, with or without genital contact.

EVALUATION

Patients undergo evaluation to identify the causes of their symptoms, and once diagnosed, specific etiologies are treated accordingly. For instance, if the symptoms are related to genitourinary syndrome of menopause (GSM), appropriate treatment is provided to address the pain. However, even if a direct cause is not identified, patients may still require additional therapy to manage symptoms of fear or anxiety that arises from either anticipated pain or relationship difficulties.[1]

TREATMENT

Vaginismus does not have a one-size-fits-all treatment approach, and patients with this condition often find relief through a multimodal strategy. This approach typically includes myofascial pelvic physical therapy, medications, other interventions, such as trigger point injections, and mental health support like pain psychiatry or cognitive behavioral therapy.[80,81]

CONCLUSION

In conclusion, vulvodynia and vaginismus are complex conditions that significantly impact the quality of life and well-being of those affected. Both disorders, though distinct in their presentation, share common challenges related to diagnosis, treatment, and the emotional toll they exert on patients. Understanding the multifaceted nature of these conditions is crucial for developing effective treatment plans. Advances in medical research, coupled with a holistic approach that includes psychological support, physical therapy, and patient education, offer hope for better way of management and improved outcomes. It is imperative for healthcare providers to foster a compassionate and informed approach to make sure that patients feel validated and supported throughout their journey to recovery.

REFERENCES

1. McCabe MP, Sharlip ID, Atalla E, Balon R, Fisher AD, Laumann E, et al. Definitions of Sexual Dysfunctions in Women and Men: A Consensus Statement From the Fourth International Consultation on Sexual Medicine 2015. J Sex Med. 2016;13(2):135-43.
2. Bornstein J, Goldstein AT, Stockdale CK, Bergeron S, Pukall C, Zolnoun D, et al. 2015 ISSVD, ISSWSH and IPPS Consensus Terminology and Classification of Persistent Vulvar Pain and Vulvodynia. Obstet Gynecol. 2016;127(4):745-51.
3. Haefner HK, Collins ME, Davis GD, Edwards L, Foster DC, Hartmann ED, et al. The vulvodynia guideline. J Low Genit Tract Dis. 2005;9(1):40-51.
4. Arnold LD, Bachmann GA, Rosen R, Kelly S, Rhoads GG. Vulvodynia: characteristics and associations with comorbidities and quality of life. Obstet Gynecol. 2006; 107(3):617-24.
5. Arnold LD, Bachmann GA, Rosen R, Rhoads GG. Assessment of vulvodynia symptoms in a sample of US women: a prevalence survey with a nested case control study. Am J Obstet Gynecol. 2007;196(2):128.e1-6.
6. Reid R. The management of genital condylomas, intraepithelial neoplasia, and vulvodynia. Obstet Gynecol Clin North Am. 1996;23(4):917-91.
7. Ben-Aroya Z, Edwards L. Vulvodynia. Semin Cutan Med Surg. 2015;34(4):192-8.
8. Bonham A. Vulvar vestibulodynia: strategies to meet the challenge. Obstet Gynecol Surv. 2015;70(4):274-8.
9. Harlow BL, Stewart EG. A population-based assessment of chronic unexplained vulvar pain: have we underestimated the prevalence of vulvodynia? J Am Med Womens Assoc (1972). 2003;58(2):82-8.
10. Metts JF. Vulvodynia and vulvar vestibulitis: challenges in diagnosis and management. Am Fam Physician. 1999;59(6):1547-56, 1561-2.
11. Reed BD, Crawford S, Couper M, Cave C, Haefner HK. Pain at the vulvar vestibule: a web-based survey. J Low Genit Tract Dis. 2004;8(1):48-57.
12. Reed BD, Haefner HK, Harlow SD, Gorenflo DW, Sen A. Reliability and validity of self-reported symptoms for predicting vulvodynia. Obstet Gynecol. 2006;108(4): 906-13.
13. Akopians AL, Rapkin AJ. Vulvodynia: The Role of Inflammation in the Etiology of Localized Provoked Pain of the Vulvar Vestibule (Vestibulodynia). Semin Reprod Med. 2015;33(4):239-45.
14. Barnabei VM. Vulvodynia. Clin Obstet Gynecol. 2020; 63(4):752-69.
15. Chisari C, Monajemi MB, Scott W, Moss-Morris R, McCracken LM. Psychosocial factors associated with pain and sexual function in women with Vulvodynia: A systematic review. Eur J Pain. 2021;25(1):39-50.
16. De Andres J, Sanchis-Lopez N, Asensio-Samper JM, Fabregat-Cid G, Villanueva-Perez VL, Monsalve Dolz V, et al. Vulvodynia—An evidence-based literature review and proposed treatment algorithm. Pain Pract. 2016;16(2):204-36.
17. Bohm-Starke N, Hilliges M, Falconer C, Rylander E. Increased intraepithelial innervation in women with vulvar vestibulitis syndrome. Gynecol Obstet Invest. 1998; 46(4):256-60.
18. Clare CA, Yeh J. Vulvodynia in adolescence: childhood vulvar pain syndromes. J Pediatr Adolesc Gynecol. 2011; 24(3):110-5.
19. Wesselmann U, Bonham A, Foster D. Vulvodynia: Current state of the biological science. Pain. 2014;155(9):1696-701.
20. Weström LV, Willén R. Vestibular nerve fiber proliferation in vulvar vestibulitis syndrome. Obstet Gynecol. 1998; 91(4):572-6.
21. Chalmers KJ, Madden VJ, Hutchinson MR, Moseley GL. Local and systemic inflammation in localized, provoked vestibulodynia: a systematic review. Obstet Gynecol. 2016;128(2):337-47.
22. Foster DC, Hasday JD. Elevated tissue levels of interleukin-1 beta and tumor necrosis factor-alpha in vulvar vestibulitis. Obstet Gynecol. 1997;89(2):291-6.
23. Ventolini G, Gygax SE, Adelson ME, Cool DR. Vulvodynia and fungal association: a preliminary report. Med Hypotheses. 2013;81(2):228-30.
24. Foster DC, Falsetta ML, Woeller CF, Pollock SJ, Song K, Bonham A, et al. Site-specific mesenchymal control of inflammatory pain to yeast challenge in vulvodynia-afflicted and pain-free women. Pain. 2015;156(3):386-96.
25. Tympanidis P, Casula MA, Yiangou Y, Terenghi G, Dowd P, Anand P. Increased vanilloid receptor VR1 innervation in vulvodynia. Eur J Pain. 2004;8(2):129-33.
26. Fenton BW. Limbic associated pelvic pain: a hypothesis to explain the diagnostic relationships and features of patients with chronic pelvic pain. Med Hypotheses. 2007; 69(2):282-6.
27. Hampson JP, Reed BD, Clauw DJ, Bhavsar R, Gracely RH, Haefner HK, et al. Augmented central pain processing in vulvodynia. J Pain. 2013;14(6):579-89.
28. Pukall CF, Binik YM, Khalifé S, Amsel R, Abbott FV. Vestibular tactile and pain thresholds in women with vulvar vestibulitis syndrome. Pain. 2002;96(1-2):163-75.
29. Zhang Z, Zolnoun DA, Francisco EM, Holden JK, Dennis RG, Tommerdahl M. Altered central sensitization in subgroups of women with vulvodynia. Clin J Pain. 2011; 27(9):755-63.
30. Zolnoun D, Bair E, Essick G, Gracely R, Goyal V, Maixner W. Reliability and reproducibility of novel methodology for assessment of pressure pain sensitivity in pelvis. J Pain. 2012;13(9):910-20.

31. Ledger WJ, Kessler A, Leonard GH, Witkin SS. Vulvar vestibulitis-a complex clinical entity. Infect Dis Obstet Gynecol. 1996;4(5):269-75.
32. Nguyen RH, Swanson D, Harlow BL. Urogenital infections in relation to the occurrence of vulvodynia. J Reprod Med. 2009;54(6):385-92.
33. Donders G, Bellen G. Characteristics of the pain observed in the focal vulvodynia syndrome (VVS). Med Hypotheses. 2012;78(1):11-4.
34. Friedrich EG Jr. Vulvar vestibulitis syndrome. J Reprod Med. 1987;32(2):110-4.
35. Jeremias J, Ledger WJ, Witkin SS. Interleukin 1 receptor antagonist gene polymorphism in women with vulvar vestibulitis. Am J Obstet Gynecol. 2000;182(2):283-5.
36. Babula O, Danielsson I, Sjoberg I, Ledger WJ, Witkin SS. Altered distribution of mannose-binding lectin alleles at exon I codon 54 in women with vulvar vestibulitis syndrome. Am J Obstet Gynecol. 2004;191(3):762-6.
37. Babula O, Linhares IM, Bongiovanni AM, Ledger WJ, Witkin SS. Association between primary vulvar vestibulitis syndrome, defective induction of tumor necrosis factor-alpha, and carriage of the mannose-binding lectin codon 54 gene polymorphism. Am J Obstet Gynecol. 2008;198(1):101.e1-4.
38. Gerber S, Bongiovanni AM, Ledger WJ, Witkin SS. Interleukin-1beta gene polymorphism in women with vulvar vestibulitis syndrome. Eur J Obstet Gynecol Reprod Biol. 2003;107(1):74-7.
39. Gerber S, Witkin SS, Stucki D. Immunological and genetic characterization of women with vulvodynia. J Med Life. 2008;1(4):432-8.
40. Gerber S, Bongiovanni AM, Ledger WJ, Witkin SS. Defective regulation of the proinflammatory immune response in women with vulvar vestibulitis syndrome. Am J Obstet Gynecol. 2002;186(4):696-700.
41. Pociot F, Mølvig J, Wogensen L, Worsaae H, Nerup J. A TaqI polymorphism in the human interleukin-1 beta (IL-1 beta) gene correlates with IL-1 beta secretion in vitro. Eur J Clin Invest. 1992;22(6):396-402.
42. Goldstein AT, Belkin ZR, Krapf JM, Song W, Khera M, Jutrzonka SL, et al. Polymorphisms of the androgen receptor gene and hormonal contraceptive induced provoked vestibulodynia. J Sex Med. 2014;11(11):2764-71.
43. Hersh JE. Vulvodynia in adolescents: presentation, diagnosis and treatment options. Curr Opin Obstet Gynecol. 2018;30(5):293-9.
44. Eva LJ, MacLean AB, Reid WM, Rolfe KJ, Perrett CW. Estrogen receptor expression in vulvar vestibulitis syndrome. Am J Obstet Gynecol. 2003;189(2):458-61.
45. Johannesson U, Sahlin L, Masironi B, Hilliges M, Blomgren B, Rylander E, et al. Steroid receptor expression and morphology in provoked vestibulodynia. Am J Obstet Gynecol. 2008;198(3):311.e1-6.
46. Butrick CW. Pelvic floor hypertonic disorders: identification and management. Obstet Gynecol Clin North Am. 2009;36(3):707-22.
47. Gentilcore-Saulnier E, McLean L, Goldfinger C, Pukall CF, Chamberlain S. Pelvic floor muscle assessment outcomes in women with and without provoked vestibulodynia and the impact of a physical therapy program. J Sex Med. 2010;7(2 Pt 2):1003-22.
48. Alappattu MJ, Bishop MD. Psychological factors in chronic pelvic pain in women: relevance and application of the fear-avoidance model of pain. Phys Ther. 2011;91(10):1542-50.
49. Bohm-Starke N, Hilliges M, Blomgren B, Falconer C, Rylander E. Increased blood flow and erythema in the posterior vestibular mucosa in vulvar vestibulitis(1). Obstet Gynecol. 2001;98(6):1067-74.
50. Granot M, Lavee Y. Psychological factors associated with perception of experimental pain in vulvar vestibulitis syndrome. J Sex Marital Ther. 2005;31(4):285-302.
51. Shallcross R, Dickson JM, Nunns D, Mackenzie C, Kiemle G. Women's subjective experiences of living with vulvodynia: a systematic review and meta-ethnography. Arch Sex Behav. 2018;47(3):577-95.
52. Bergeron S, Binik YM, Khalifé S, Pagidas K, Glazer HI. Vulvar vestibulitis syndrome: reliability of diagnosis and evaluation of current diagnostic criteria. Obstet Gynecol. 2001;98(1):45-51.
53. Masheb RM, Lozano-Blanco C, Kohorn EI, Minkin MJ, Kerns RD. Assessing sexual function and dyspareunia with the Female Sexual Function Index (FSFI) in women with vulvodynia. J Sex Marital Ther. 2004;30(5):315-24.
54. Winters U, Hart F, Al-Quragooli K. Vulvodynia. Obstet Gynaecol Reprod Med. 2018;28(4):116-9.
55. Previnaire JG. The importance of the bulbocavernosus reflex. Spinal Cord Ser Cases. 2018;4:2.
56. Goldstein AT, Pukall CF, Brown C, Bergeron S, Stein A, Kellogg-Spadt S. Vulvodynia: assessment and treatment. J Sex Med. 2016;13(4):572-90.
57. Petersen CD, Kristensen E, Lundvall L, Giraldi A. A retrospective study of relevant diagnostic procedures in vulvodynia. J Reprod Med. 2009;54(5):281-7.
58. Mascherpa F, Bogliatto F, Lynch PJ, Micheletti L, Benedetto C. Vulvodynia as a possible somatization disorder. More than just an opinion. J Reprod Med. 2007;52(2):107-10.
59. Edgardh K, Abdelnoor M. Vulvar vestibulitis and risk factors: a population-based case-control study in Oslo. Acta Derm Venereol. 2007;87(4):350-4.
60. Lewis FM, Harrington CI. Use of magnetic resonance imaging in vulvodynia. J Reprod Med. 1997;42(3):169.
61. Nunns D, Murphy R. Assessment and management of vulval pain. BMJ. 2012;344:e1723.
62. Brotto LA, Sadownik L, Thomson S. Impact of educational seminars on women with provoked vestibulodynia. J Obstet Gynaecol Can. 2010;32(2):132-8.
63. Goldstein AT, Burrows L. Vulvodynia. J Sex Med. 2008;5(1):5-14; quiz 15.

64. Lifits-Podorozhansky YM, Podorozhansky Y, Hoffstetter S, Gavard JA. Role of vulvar care guidelines in the initial management of vulvar complaints. J Low Genit Tract Dis. 2012;16(2):88-91.
65. Zolnoun DA, Hartmann KE, Steege JF. Overnight 5% lidocaine ointment for treatment of vulvar vestibulitis. Obstet Gynecol. 2003;102(1):84-7.
66. Itza F, Zarza D, Gómez-Sancha F, Salinas J, Bautrant E. Puesta al día en el diagnóstico y tratamiento de la vulvodinia [Update on the diagnosis and treatment of vulvodynia]. Actas Urol Esp. 2012;36(7):431-8.
67. Dede M, Yenen MC, Yilmaz A, Baser I. Successful treatment of persistent vulvodynia with submucous infiltration of betamethasone and lidocaine. Eur J Obstet Gynecol Reprod Biol. 2006;124(2):258-9.
68. Munday PE. Response to treatment in dysaesthetic vulvodynia. J Obstet Gynaecol. 2001;21(6):610-3.
69. Leo RJ, Dewani S. A systematic review of the utility of antidepressant pharmacotherapy in the treatment of vulvodynia pain. J Sex Med. 2013;10(10):2497-505.
70. Ben-David B, Friedman M. Gabapentin therapy for vulvodynia. Anesth Analg. 1999;89(6):1459-60.
71. Schwarz EB, Maselli J, Gonzales R. Contraceptive counseling of diabetic women of reproductive age. Obstet Gynecol. 2006;107(5):1070-4.
72. Nagandla K, Sivalingam N. Vulvodynia: Integrating current knowledge into clinical practice. Obstet Gynaecol. 2014;16(4):259-67.
73. Lavy Y, Lev-Sagie A, Hamani Y, Zacut D, Ben-Chetrit A. Modified vulvar vestibulectomy: simple and effective surgery for the treatment of vulvar vestibulitis. Eur J Obstet Gynecol Reprod Biol. 2005;120(1):91-5.
74. Eva LJ, Narain S, Orakwue CO, Luesley DM. Is modified vestibulectomy for localized provoked vulvodynia an effective long-term treatment? A follow-up study. J Reprod Med. 2008;53(6):435-40.
75. Landry T, Bergeron S, Dupuis MJ, Desrochers G. The treatment of provoked vestibulodynia: a critical review. Clin J Pain. 2008;24(2):155-71.
76. Leclair CM, Goetsch MF, Lee KK, Jensen JT. KTP-Nd:YAG laser therapy for the treatment of vestibulodynia: a follow-up study. J Reprod Med. 2007;52(1):53-8.
77. Berenguer-Soler M, Navarro-Sánchez A, Compañ-Rosique A, Luri-Prieto P, Navarro-Ortiz R, Gómez-Pérez L, et al. Genito Pelvic Pain/Penetration Disorder (GPPPD) in Spanish Women-Clinical Approach in Primary Health Care: Review and Meta-Analysis. J Clin Med. 2022; 11(9):2340.
78. Binik YM. The DSM diagnostic criteria for vaginismus. Arch Sex Behav. 2010;39(2):278-91.
79. Guze SB. (1995). Diagnostic and Statistical Manual of Mental Disorders, 4th ed. (DSM-IV). [online] Available from https://ajp.psychiatryonline.org/doi/abs/10.1176/ajp.152.8.1228 [Last accessed May, 2024].
80. Damagum FM, Garko AA. Successful management of penetration disorder: a holistic approach to an age-old problem. Niger J Clin Pract. 2023;26(1):125-7.
81. Eserdag S, Ezberci Akgün M, Şükrü Gürbüz F. Outcomes of vaginismus therapy assessed by penetrative intercourse, psychiatric symptoms, and marital satisfaction. J Sex Marital Ther. 2023;49(4):412-9.

CHAPTER 19

Cosmetic Breast Surgery in Gynecology

Mohan Thomas, James Dsilva

INTRODUCTION

Breasts have played a central part in feminine beauty and have been prominently displayed as art and paintings which is integral to a beautiful form. Perfectly symmetrical breasts are rare and a difference in breast size of about 20% between the two breasts is considered normal.

Breasts undergo significant changes over a woman's lifetime. At some stage in their lives, many women have noticed a change in their breast that is different to their usual cyclical changes. Most of these changes are not cause for concern but some changes in the breast may make a woman feel less confident or incomplete.

Young women usually have dense breasts because of the predominance of glandular tissue needed for breastfeeding. Sometimes this thickness is felt as a lump or a mass of tissue. Young ladies may also be concerned about the inadequate size of their breasts which now can be safely enhanced to an appropriate size. As women age, the glandular tissue shrinks and are replaced by fat. By menopause, most women's breasts are completely soft. This can make normal lumps more palpable.

Sometimes women find that their breasts feel different when they lose or gain weight and sometimes breasts change due to presence of genetic factors. Deflation of breasts due to weight loss and postbreastfeeding is akin to having loose clothes. This is part of the "deflation syndrome". Women who are well endowed have to fight the vagaries of gravity which causes continuous strain and pain on the neck and shoulders.

The female breast is one of the rare anatomical organs that have no bony or cartilaginous supports to keep it in place while gravity is continuously acting on it. It is suspended to the chest wall by its soft fibrous structures and its shape is substantially influenced during growth by the genetic predisposition and the bone, cartilage and muscle elements that surround the breast's base. A "perfect breast" for an adult woman involves the right match of glandular tissue, fat, skin, and connective tissue that hold everything in place on a chest which is proportionate to her height, weight, and lower body.[1]

Aesthetically breast surgery may include enlargement, reduction, or need for a breast lift.

Breast augmentations: Breast augmentation using a prosthesis is one of the most common surgical procedure undertaken as part of body enhancement surgery for people having small breasts, asymmetric breasts, as part of gender reassignment as well as for reconstruction after mastectomy. Two types of breast prostheses are currently available: silicone gel implants and saline implants. These are further classified into smooth, textured, and silk textured based on the implant surface and round and anatomic based on their shape. Silicone implants, consisting of a silicone polymer shell filled with silicone gel, are preferred for augmentation because they provide a more natural appearance and feel and there are no chances of sudden deflation. Saline implants on the other hand offer the advantage of a smaller incision, can be placed remotely as well as have no risk of silicone leak because they are inserted as empty silicone shells and inflated using sterile saline.

Breast implants as part of aesthetic surgery can be placed through an inframammary, periareolar, axillary or a remote umbilical incision. Pockets for breast implant are dissected through these incisions so that the implant can be placed in the subglandular or submuscular plane. When implants are used for breast reconstruction, they are usually placed in the submuscular plane so as to have sufficient tissue for implant coverage. Sometimes an expander may be required to enlarge the surrounding tissue (postmastectomy or congenital amastia) followed by the implant placement. An acellular dermal matrix, composed of extracellular matrix structures of bovine, porcine, or human cadaveric origin, or synthetic mesh can be used as an adjuncts to tissue expanders for shaping the reconstructive breast and anchoring the implant to the chest wall. Breast enhancement procedures are an important part of cosmetic surgery. Both the mental and physical well-being from chest wall enhancement are equally an important component of the transformation. Fat transfer to the breast is an option for those who want additional volume with no incisions and less down time. Fat transfer with additional platelet-rich plasma (PRP) can offer additional benefits by making the skin healthier from the inside out.

Breast reductions and breast uplifts (also known as a mastopexy) are different types in the same procedure spectrum. The principal aim of both these procedures is to reposition the droopy breast having a low nipple and a large areola into a well-positioned, uplifted, and perky breast with nipple pointing forward and outward. Breast lift surgery involves repositioning the nipple on a pedicle which is the supply of the nipple along with reshaping the breast tissue and tailoring the excess skin without reducing the breast volume. It may be combined with an implant to add volume, firmness, and enlarge the breast which is called an augmentation mastopexy. A breast reduction on the other hand includes moving the nipple on its vascular pedicle which includes the residual breast tissue left behind after adequate excision of the breast tissue has been undertaken.

Excess of the breast tissue, fat deposits and skin either naturally or due to pathologies can lead to breast enlargement and drooping, or what we call breast ptosis. Age, gravity, and smoking also affect the breast and induce glandular and skin stretching, especially in the periareolar area and in the lower pole where weight is maximal.

SURGICAL ANATOMY OF THE BREAST

A woman's breast extends from the 2nd rib superiorly to the level of the 6th rib inferiorly with the base lying over the pectoralis major muscle sliding easily on the pectoral fascia and covers a large part of the chest wall **(Fig. 1)**. Medially it extends from the middle of the sternum to continue laterally into the axilla (usually to the anterior axillary line) and may reach as far as the latissimus dorsi on the lateral chest wall. The nipple-areola complex (NAC) is usually in the center of the mound when the person lies down flat while in the standing position it is usually situated in the midclavicular axis at the level of the inframammary crease (4th or 5th intercostal space). The nipple-areolar complex contains the Montgomery glands that are embryologically transitional between sweat glands and mammary glands and are capable of secreting milk. The Montgomery glands

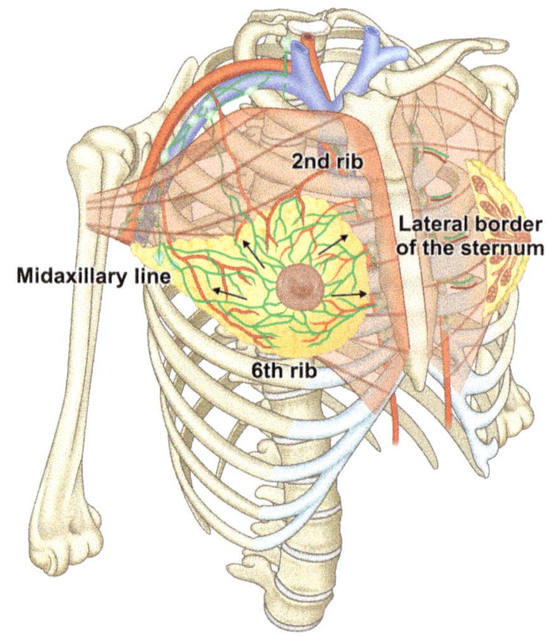

Fig. 1: Anatomical extent of the breast.

open at the Morgagni tubercles, which are small (1–2-mm diameter) raised papules on the areola. The nipple-areolar complex also contains many sensory nerve endings, smooth muscle, and an abundant lymphatic system called the subareolar or Sappey plexus.[2]

The breast is not a homogeneous structure and contains different tissue layers **(Fig. 2)**; however, the two predominant types of tissue within the breast are fat (becomes predominant during weight gain) and glandular tissue (which supports lactation). Each breast has 15–20 sections, or lobes, that surround the nipple in a radial manner, which are further divided into smaller sections, called lobules. At the end of each lobule are tiny "bulbs" that produce milk. These structures are linked together by small tubes called ducts, which carry milk to the nipples. Each nipple has up to 20 ducts draining milk to the surface. Fat fills the spaces between the lobes and ducts.

The size and weight of the breast varies substantially in individuals and can be 500 g or less in a small to moderate breast and about 750–1,000 g in a large heavy breast. The ratio of fat to connective tissue content determines the firmness of the breast and this ratio varies genetically as well as depends on the age of the person as well as the hormonal levels. The size and shape also varies over time in the same woman because of the changes during menstrual cycle, pregnancy, after weaning, and during menopause.[3] The mammary gland forms a cone with its base at the chest wall and its apex at the nipple **(Fig. 2)**.

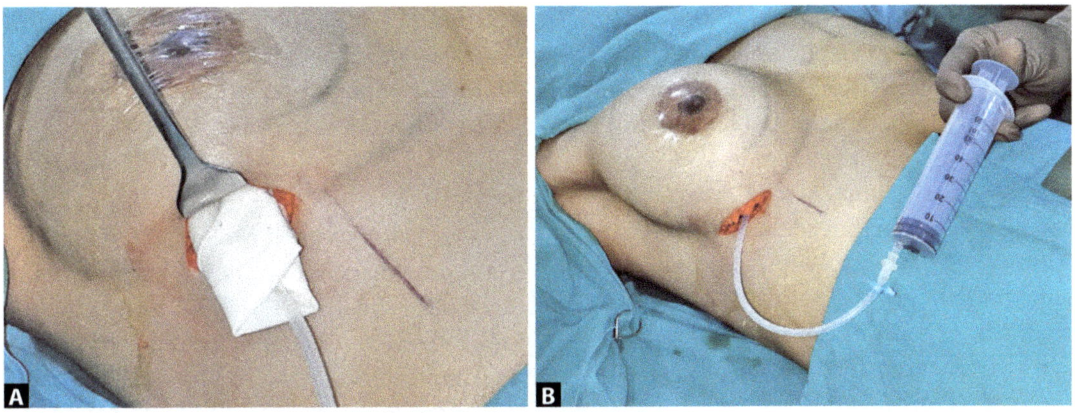

Figs. 2A and B: (A) Saline implant being rolled and placed in the pocket; (B) The implant inflated to the adequate size using sterile saline.

BREAST AUGMENTATION

Breast augmentation can be undertaken using either a breast implant or using autologous fat which is natural. Breast implant surgery is a safe and reversible procedure which gives the patient an option of choosing the size and type of implant. The only limiting factor being the skin envelope. Fat grafting to the breasts on the other hand requires at least two surgical procedures and more than one session. The procedure includes liposuction to harvest fat from the abdomen and/or thighs which is then processed to separate live adipocytes along with stem cells. These are then injected in very small aliquots in various layers of the breast so as to achieve adequate vascularity of the grafted fat for a permanent result.

Breast augmentation using an implant can be undertaken through the inframammary approach which is a standard against which all other techniques for breast augmentation are compared. The critical part of the breast augmentation operation is the accuracy and symmetry of the pocket creation, and anatomically the most critical aspect of this dissection lies at the inframammary fold. The inframammary approach unquestionably offers the greatest visualization of this area and results in the least damage to normal tissue. The transaxillary and periareolar approaches create trauma to tissue that is undisturbed using the inframammary approach, and does so at the price of less visualization of the critical aspects of the surgery.

Today, there are two types of breast implants commonly used:

1. Saline implant filled with sterile saline
2. Silicone implant filled with viscous silicone gel.

Saline breast implants are filled with sterile saline during the augmentation procedure. Should the implant shell leak, a saline implant will collapse, and the saline will be absorbed and naturally expelled by the body. The technical goal of saline-implant technology is a physically less invasive surgical technique for emplacing an empty breast implant device through a smaller surgical incision **(Fig. 2)**.

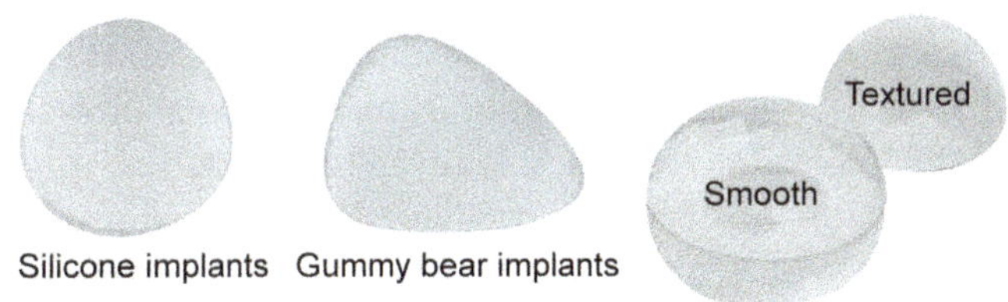

Fig. 3: Fifth-generation implants in various shapes and textures.

Silicone breast implants are prefilled implants which have standard volumes and sizes. They have a solid silicon elastomer shell filled with cohesive silicone gel. The shell can be smooth or textured. These implants are placed in the subglandular or submuscular plane and they feel like normal breast tissue **(Fig. 3)**.

Operative Technique

To place the breast implant in the appropriate location, the surgeon will make a single cut (incision) in one of these three places:

1. The crease under your breast (inframammary line)
2. Under your arm (axillary)—scar is hidden in the shadow.
3. Around your nipple (periareolar)—injury to the breast gland ducts is a possibility.

After making an incision, the surgeon will separate the breast tissue from the muscles and connective tissue of your chest. This creates a pocket either behind or in front of the outermost muscle of the chest wall (pectoral muscle). A sizer is placed in the pocket to check for the adequacy of the enlargement. Once the size is confirmed, the implant will then be placed into this pocket and it is centered behind the nipple.

Once the appropriate size implant is placed, hemostasis is achieved and closure of the pocket is completed using sutures and appropriate dressing material. Rest is advised for a few days and patients are prevented from lifting heavy weight, driving a car, or exercise for 6 weeks. Exercise is taught so as to prevent tightness in the breast and to achieve a normal feel **(Fig. 4)**.

Possible Complications

- Common complications which are possible in any surgery include bruising, swelling, pain, numbness, and blood clots. Pigmentation or increased scar thickness is always a possibility in Indian skin.
- Infection—skin related or atypical—managed usually with antibiotics
- Breast capsule contracture
- Breast implant illness
- Rare implant associated anaplastic large cell lymphoma (ALCL) arising from the capsule

BREAST REDUCTION

Patients with very large breast usually present with the following complaints which may include neck and back pain, headaches, shoulder grooving with painful indentations in the skin secondary to support garments and traction on the spinal ligaments, fungal infection in the inframammary area due to presence of moisture and sweat and numbness in the hands and fingers due to traction on the brachial plexus. More often than not, there is a general discomfort about the upper torso related to years of excess weight dragging down from the shoulders.

Breast reduction surgery usually combines reduction of skin and breast tissue with a pedicle to maintain blood supply to the NAC which allows movement of the NAC to the right level.

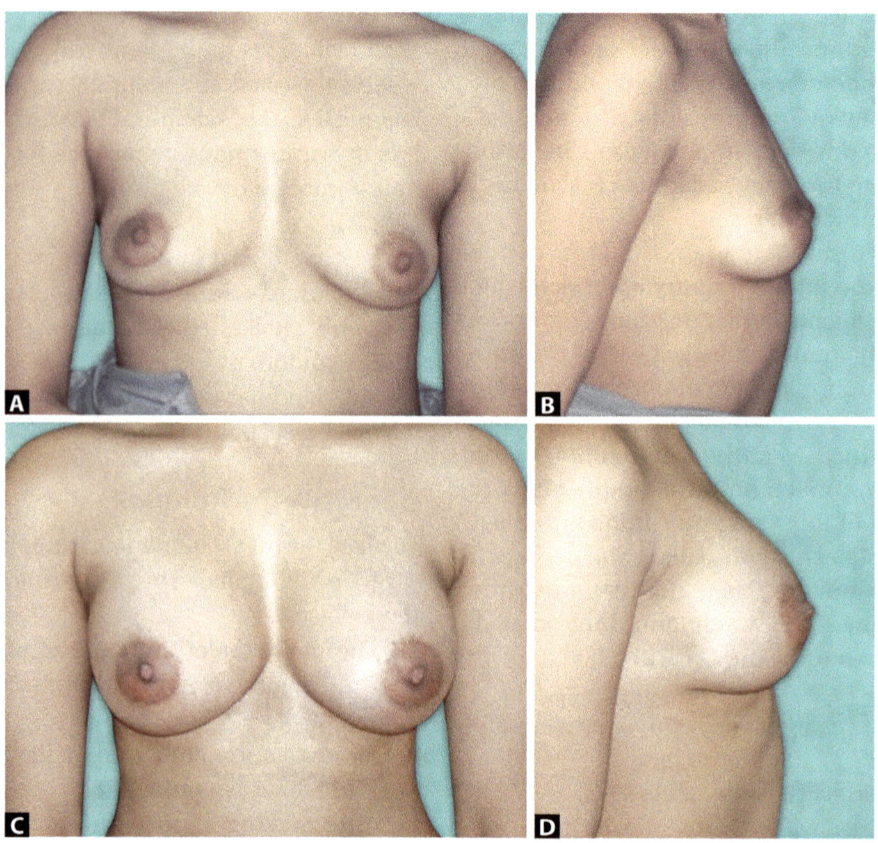

Figs. 4A to D: Preoperative (A and B) and postoperative (C and D) are photographs of a young lady who underwent enlargement of her breast using silicone cohesive gel implants of 290 gms.

Examination of the patient: The patient is examined in the standing position and the following measurements are taken:

- Distance between the nipple and the sternal notch is taken to check for symmetry on both sides.
- The breast diameter is measured along with its foot print.
- The extent of breast ptosis along with the distance of the NAC to inframammary crease is taken on both sides. Patient is checked for fungal infections and venous congestion in the lower pole.

Operative Technique

The surgical technique varies from surgeon to surgeon. Some surgeons use a modification of the same technique for all sizes and shapes of breast while others choose the technique based on the amount of reduction, the drooping of the breast as well as the extent of skin excess.

Since the various techniques described for breast reduction are primarily based on two variables namely the technique of glandular resection which is different from the skin incision and excision. Although the "one technique" approach has served many surgeons well over the years, familiarity with other techniques allows the surgeon to customize based on evidence for better outcomes with minimal or no complications.

- *NAC and its blood supply:* All breast reduction procedures require movement of NAC to a higher level as they are at a lower level.

  Each pedicle choice has certain advantages and disadvantages associated with it, depending on what the other elements of the operative plan may include.
- *Excision of breast parenchyma:* Once the pedicle along with the NAC has been created and the vascularity of NAC has been found to be safe, the remaining breast parenchyma is excised keeping the skin flap sufficiently thick.
- *Addressing the excess skin:* The ptotic redundant skin envelope must be reduced in a manner that it creates a conical shape of the breast and at the same time minimizes and hides the suture line.
- *Management of shape:* Once all resections have been completed and the adequate breast volume has been achieved, it becomes important to hold the remaining tissue together so that the breast is not only smaller but also looks shapely. Here again, different techniques have been described to provide "shape" which ranges from simply relying on the skin envelope to support the breast, to the use of internal suturing techniques, and even internally based chest wall flaps **(Fig. 5).**[4]

BREAST PTOSIS

Ptosis of the breast in lay man terms means "drooping of the breasts" which were at one time situated at a higher level. The treatment of breast ptosis involves reducing the discrepancy between the skin envelope and breast parenchyma which can be undertaken from the "outside-in" through tailoring and reducing the excess skin envelope, from the "inside-out" by increasing the breast volume, or a combination of the two procedures. "Mastopexy" procedure is primarily aimed to create a beautiful, perky breast by primarily addressing shape, and differs from breast augmentation where the so-called lift is achieved by altering the breast volume.

For an adult woman, the "perfect" balance of a glandular tissue, fat, skin, and connective tissue that hold everything in place may theoretically give rise to a "perfect breast". Time and gravity affect the breast and induce glandular and skin stretching, especially in the periareolar area and in the lower pole where weight is maximal **(Fig. 6)**.

Regnault[5] as shown in **Figure 7** proposed one of the most common classifications to date, using a combination of position of the NAC, the inframammary fold (IMF) and the lowest point on the breast as landmarks to define various grades as well as the "normal breast", "pseudoptosis" and "parenchymal maldistribution". This classification has been accepted worldwide.

Operative Technique

- *Periareolar mastopexy:* This technique is usually used in patients with Grade I or II breast ptosis and can raise the nipple by 2–2.5 cm. The markings for this procedure are drawn as an eccentric oval around the entire circumference of the areola with preferential height difference superiorly to elevate the nipple. The benefit of this technique is that the scar is hidden. Use of a "cartwheel permanent suture" prevents widening of the NAC posthealing but flattening of the breast has to be expected.
- *Crescent mastopexy:* This is a variant of the periareolar mastopexy where the incision is made superior to the areola in a crescent manner and is indicated in patients

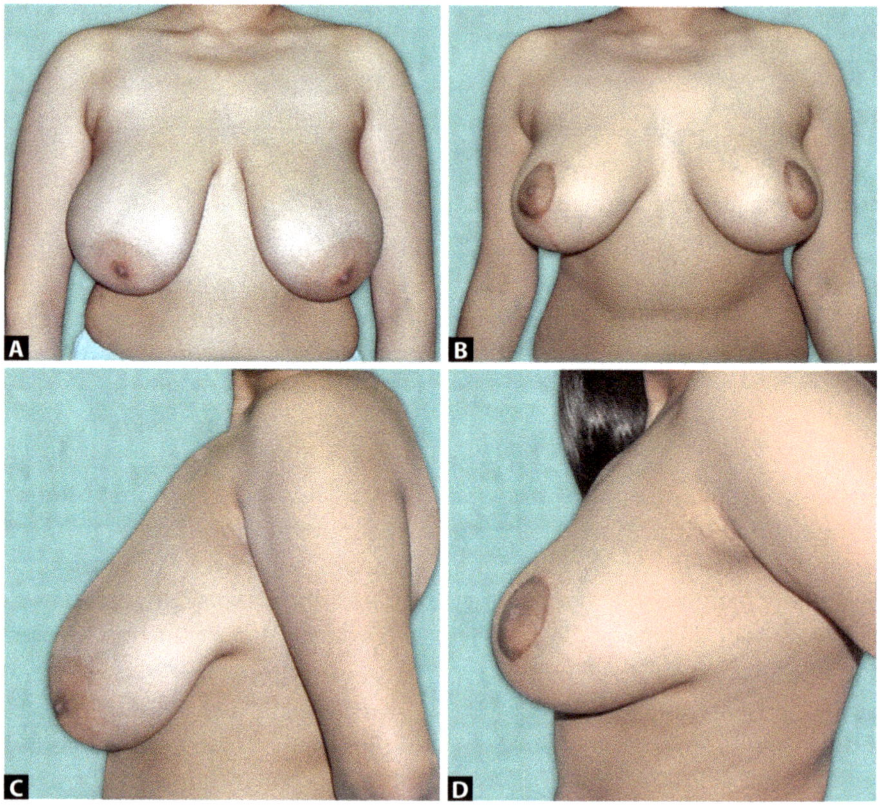

Figs. 5A and D: (A and C) Preoperative photographs of a 25-year-old unmarried female who had neck and back pain. She underwent resection of 550 g of breast tissue from the right and 625 g from left breast using a medial pedicle breast reduction with a vertical scar (lollipop) skin excision; (B and D) Postoperative images 2 months after surgery.

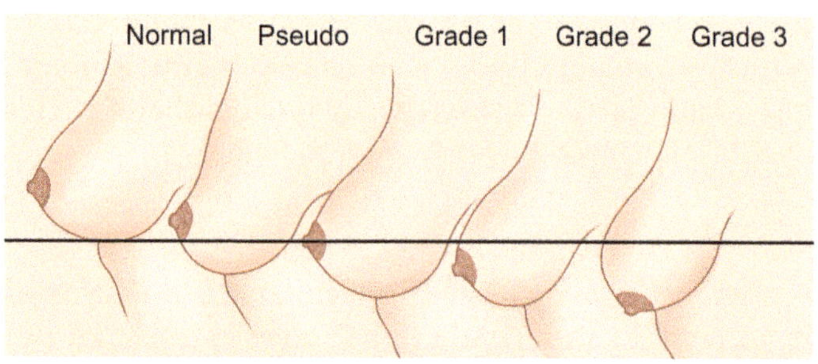

Fig. 6: Normal breast has the lower pole at the level of the inframammary fold (IMF). Pseudoptosis has the nipple-areola complex (NAC) above the IMF but the lower pole is below the level of the IMF. Grade I breast ptosis with areola at the IMF but above the contour of the gland, Grade II breast ptosis is NAC below the level of the IMF but above the contour of the gland, Grade III breast ptosis is NAC is below the level of IMF and contour of the gland.

where the breast tissue is at the normal level but the NAC is lower.

- *Vertical mastopexy:* Vertical mastopexies use suspension sutures to pick the breast tissue superiorly and tightening of the remaining glandular tissue is achieved by the use of sutures inferiorly. Skin is then tailor-tacked and excised with closure in a vertical orientation. This glandular tightening provides support to the repositioned NAC and also narrows the breast. This is the most suitable technique for simultaneous breast augmentation with an implant in the submuscular or subfascial/subglandular plane.
- *Inverted T or Wise-pattern mastopexy:* This type of mastopexy has been used in patients with severe excess of skin relative to breast parenchyma in a patient with Grade III ptosis. The marked area is de-epithelized and then the medial and lateral skin flaps are dissected up to the edge of the breast. The NAC is then repositioned and the gland in plicated to tighten as well as lift it. The medial and lateral skin flaps are then sutured to get an inverted T scar. This technique has the greatest frequency of bottoming out which is most likely due to the inferior pedicle rather than the skin excision

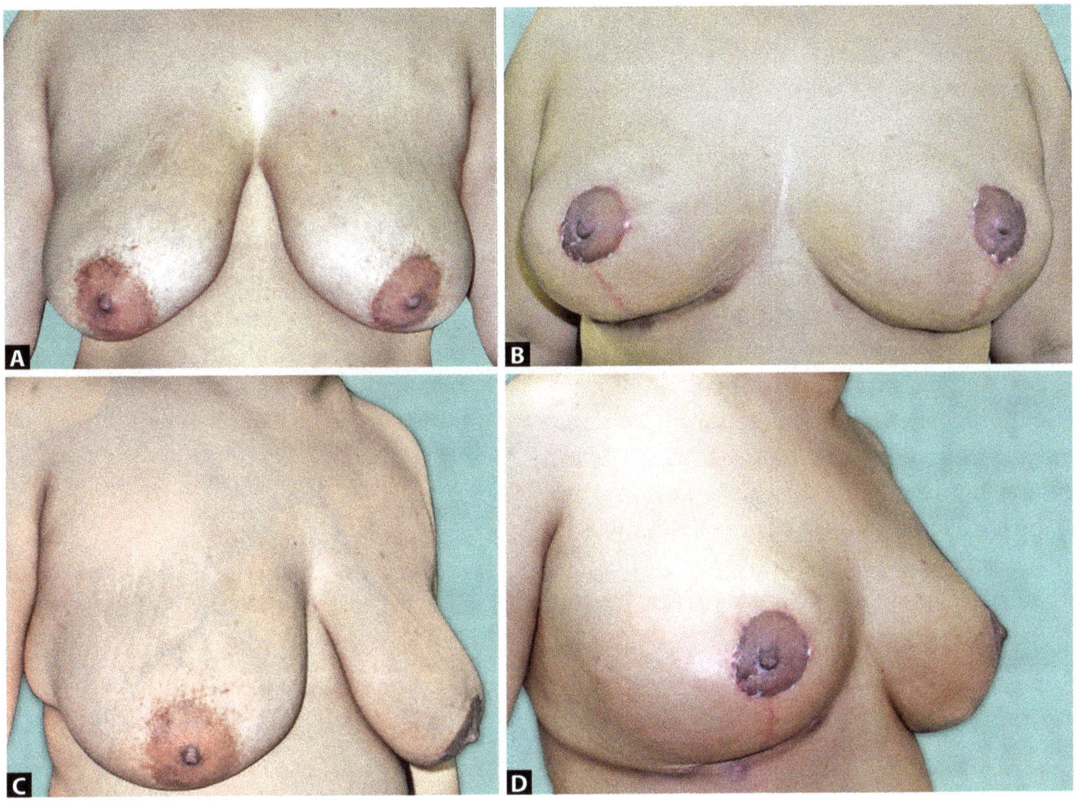

Figs. 7A to D: A 52-year-old postmenopausal lady wanted a mastopexy procedure. She had Grade III ptosis with significantly excess skin envelope as seen in A and C. She underwent a "Wise pattern" mastopexy with outstanding results. Postoperative images (B and D) taken after 4 weeks.

pattern, also the risk of breakdown at the T-junction is highest, especially when an implant is added.[6]

Postoperative Advice

- Supportive surgical bra at the end of the case to support the operated breast. This acts like a splint to offload the effects of gravity as the healing process begins. The supportive bra is used for 4–6 weeks before the underwire bra is advised.
- Drains are not used routinely.
- Broad-spectrum antibiotics may be advised at the surgeon's discretion. Rarely, it is advised beyond hospital stay.
- Pain medication or muscle relaxants, particularly if an augmentation is also performed in the subpectoral plane will be required.
- Physical activity is advised only after 4–6 weeks depending on the nature of the mastopexy and reduction procedure.

COMPLICATIONS[4]

Early

- *Hematoma and seroma:* Not very common and tend to get absorbed spontaneously over a period of time. Large hematomas may have to be evacuated.
- *Flap necrosis:* More common with inverted T technique, especially in smokers. Secondary procedures may be required.
- *Infection:* Usually seen due to underlying tissue necrosis

Late

- Asymmetry is possible. Preoperative asymmetry has to be assessed and resection planned accordingly.
- *Under-resection:* Not very common with the inverted T resections but more likely with vertical resections. May need correction by liposuction or direct resection.
- *Over-resection:* Not a common problem. Need to understand patient's requirements before and counsel her accordingly.

- *Unsightly scars:* Usually scars settle down over a period of time but in some "scar formers" the scar can be a problem and have to be dealt with in the usual manner.

CONCLUSION

A number of women who are unsatisfied with their breasts prefer to undergo breast surgeries and therefore it is growing in popularity. The size, shape, or asymmetry of the breasts can affect a person's self-confidence and may lead them to consider cosmetic breast surgery. The types of cosmetic breast surgery typically can be divided into three general categories, such as augmentation, reduction, and lifts. Usually, the aim of cosmetic breast surgery is to correct a problem that is causing dissatisfaction for the patient. For many individuals, breast shape or volume is a very important aspect of body image and so by correcting any areas perceived as unsightly by the patient, we can often make a significant improvement in the way they perceive themselves.

REFERENCES

1. Kotti B. A simple classification and a simplified treatment's algorithm for ptotic breasts. Plast Aesthet Res. 2018;5:16.
2. Kopans D. Breast anatomy and basic histology, physiology, and pathology. In: Kopans D, (Ed). Breast Imaging, 3rd edition. Philadelphia, Pa: Lippincott Williams & Wilkins; 2007. pp. 7-43.
3. Dufourmentel C, Mouly R. Chirurgie plastique. Paris: Flammarion; 1959. pp. 327-70.
4. Purohit S. Reduction mammoplasty. Indian J Plast Surg. 2008;41(Suppl):S64-S79.
5. Regnault P. Breast ptosis. Definition and treatment. Clin Plast Surg. 1976;3:193-203.
6. Rohrich RJ, Gosman AA, Brown SA, Reisch J. Mastopexy preferences: a survey of board-certified plastic surgeons. Plast Reconstr Surg. 2006;118(7):1631-8.

CHAPTER 20

Overactive Bladder Syndrome

Indranil Banerjee, Ami Shukla

INTRODUCTION

Overactive bladder (OAB) disorder is a persistent ailment which colossally affects the personal satisfaction in all kinds of people.[1] OAB influences execution of day-to-day activities and social and sexual capability. The meaning of OAB as refreshed in 2018 by International Continence Society Standardised Subcommittee definition is as follows—*"Urinary urgency, usually with urinary frequency and nocturia with or without urinary incontinence."*[2]

Determination of OAB is viewed as involuntary urinary leakage without urinary tract infection, metabolic problems (influencing urination), or urinary stress incontinence (created by exertion or overexertion). OAB can be both wet and dry. Just 33% of OAB patients demonstrate urge incontinence likewise called wet OAB.

This is in difference to stress incontinence because of inability of urethra and pelvic floor to endure increased intra-abdominal pressure that is typically unassociated with "urgency." A few patients might have both the symptoms and are analyzed as having mixed urinary symptoms. This condition was demonstrated to be common in a few European and American population 12–17%.[1,3,4]

In the United States alone, the prevalence of OAB was estimated to be 7% in 2013 with a projected increase to 48% by 2027.[5]

Despite the fact that OAB can influence all age groups, this situation is most normal in patients >40 years of age.[6] Since the socioeconomic and long-term impact is most profound in this age group, the investigations and treatment options are mostly directed to this group. This chapter will mainly focus on the pathophysiology, physical examination, and treatment options for this syndrome **(Table 1)**.

PATHOPHYSIOLOGY

The control of bladder is achieved by the interaction between sympathetic and parasympathetic nervous system. The storage function is mostly mediated by the sympathetic nervous system by relaxation of the detrusor muscles. Once the volume of urine crosses 250 mL, the bladder walls are stimulated via receptors on the detrusor muscle and a signal is send to two different sets of neurons. Parasympathetic neurons contract the detrusor muscle and relax the internal urethral sphincters. The somatic motor neurons supplying the external urethral sphincter via the pudendal nerve is also stimulated resulting in opening of the external urethral sphincter. The second action is however voluntary.

Different variables might be engaged with OAB and the main cause be different in different individuals. The etiology of OAB is still being scrutinized and is not surely known. However, the most up to date explanation of pathophysiology was provided by Malone-Lee et al. in his article published in 2018. In this landmark study, it was hypothesized the role of recurrent microbial invasion as a predecessor for developing OAB in later stage of life.[7]

TABLE 1: Different terminology and definitions related to overactive bladder.[2]

Terminology	*Definition*
Detrusor overactivity	An urodynamic observation characterized by involuntary spontaneous or provoked detrusor contractions during the filling phase
Nocturnal polyuria	An excess (>20–30%) proportion of urine excretion at night
Polyuria	>40 mL urine/kg body weight during 24 hours
Postvoid residual volume	The volume of fluid remaining in the bladder at the end of micturition
Urgency	A sudden compelling desire to void which is difficult to defer
Urinary frequency	>8 micturition in 24 hours
Urge urinary incontinence	Involuntary loss of urine associated with urgency

There are four other speculations other than this speculation which can be the possible mechanism to describe the pathophysiology of OAB:

1. The neurogenic hypothesis[8]
2. The myogenic hypothesis[9]
3. The independent bladder hypothesis[10]
4. The afferent flagging hypothesis[11]

The end point of all the possible underlying mechanism essentially involves the rise of intravesical pressure as a result of premature excitation of the detrusor muscles. It also involves simultaneous relaxation of the internal urethral sphincter to facilitate leakage if present.[12]

CLINICAL ASSESSMENT OF OVERACTIVE BLADDER

History Taking

Detailed history taking is important to differentiate between different types of urinary incontinence. The history taking should include basic questions about the main issue and its impact on quality of life.

The specific questions should be targeted to:

- Most bothersome symptom (along with the duration and progression)
- Urgency
- Nocturia
- Leakage with exertion (along with the type of exertion)
- Symptoms of urinary tract infection (along with any past history of urinary tract infection)
- Strain during passage of urine
- Fluid intake and types of fluid taken
- Any lump in the vagina
- Any discomfort in the vagina
- Any discharge from the vagina
- Any painful sexual intercourse (also the site of pain)
- Bowel habits
- Leakage or soiling of stool
- Leakage of wind

There should be information obtained regarding past obstetric history and gynecological history as well. History regarding intake of any hormone replacement therapy (HRT) should also be elicited at this point.

Current medications ongoing with the patient and her perceptions concerning what exacerbates the side effects ought to likewise be considered. Certain medications might add to urinary incontinence through the accompanying systems.[13]

For example:

- Diminished urethral pressure (neuroleptics, benzodiazepines, and α-adrenergic blockers)
- Increased urine output (diuretics)
- Lithium (increased fluid intake)

Beta-adrenergic blockers and antiparkinsonian medications however might prevent from further administration of anticholinergic medication at the time of treatment.

History taking is of immense importance as targeted questions will be of help to determine the pattern and type of incontinence. It has been proven beyond doubt that following a Proforma will be of good help to include every point necessary in the history taking.

This ensures that no piece of information is missed during the procedure **(Appendix 1)**.

PHYSICAL EXAMINATION

The actual assessment ought to start with general assessment of the patient followed by systematic examination focused on the systems related to urinary incontinence. These surveys include an abdominal examination including palpation to rule out any abdominal mass and also to find out any abdominal scar related to past surgeries. Also, any fullness of the urinary bladder suggestive of retention needs to be ruled out as well.

Inspection of vulva and vagina is important as there might be signs of vulval and vaginal atrophy. Inspection should also include examination under Valsalva maneuver and inspection in Sims positions. A vaginal examination is mandatory as it will reveal the presence of both cystocele and rectocele which can interfere with bladder performance. Mobility of the urethra and tone of the pelvic muscles also needs to be assessed in this step.

A digital rectal assessment is also necessary to the determine the rectal tone. It can help to determine fecal loading in the sigmoid colon as overstretching of the sigmoid colon can cause improper detrusor activity **(Box 1)**.[14]

INVESTIGATIONS

A bladder diary is an essential tool to determine the incontinence pattern in day-to-day life. It gives a vivid idea about the frequency, volume, and activity associated with any event of leakage.[15] The patients are usually instructed to fill up the bladder diary for 3 days and this gives the physician a cross-sectional idea about the current situation related to incontinence.[16,17]

BOX 1: Targeted physical examination in overactive bladder.

Abdominal examination			
Inspection/palpation		Yes	No
Percussion/auscultation		Yes	No
Inspection/per speculum examination/per speculum examination of vagina			
Observation			
Effect of cough			
Hypermobile urethra		Yes	No
Leakage of urine (Valsalva induced)		Yes	No
Urine loss without provocation		Yes	No
Perineum and vaginal atrophy			
Vaginal examination			
Atrophy		Yes	No
Cystocele	Rectocele	Vault prolapse	Uterine prolapse
Sensation left	Sensation right	Pain left	Pain right
Aware of pelvic floor contraction		Yes	No
Bimanual examination			
Uterus size/adnexa/pouch of Douglas (POD)			

The essential point of care test includes a urine dipstick to rule out infections, blood in urine, and presence of glucose in urine. Urine to be send for culture and sensitivity if the result is positive in nitrates or the patient is symptomatic of urinary tract infection. Further blood investigations which might add extra information include urea and electrolytes, creatinine, and glomerular filtration rate (eGFR).

Postvoid residual urine is measured using bladder scanner. The patient should be instructed to empty her bladder immediately before the test provided, she has not emptied her bladder in last 30 minutes (residual volume measured should be <150 mL). Urodynamics is a specific investigation which is directed to determine the pattern of urinary leakage which will determine the future course of treatment of that particular patient. It essentially consists of two components: (1) Uroflowmetry and (2) cystometry. Uroflowmetry determines the flow rate of urine and cystometry determines the capacity of urinary bladder

BOX 2: Investigations related to overactive bladder.[18]

Primary investigation

- Urinalysis to exclude infection, hematuria, and glycosuria
- Measurement of postresidual volume
- Frequency/volume chart (3 days)
- Bladder diary (3 days)

Secondary investigation

- Urodynamics—performed only if patient does not respond to initial medical treatment

along with an idea and elasticity and leakage pattern **(Box 2)**.

TREATMENT

The European Association of Urology has described both primary and secondary treatments for OAB.[19,20]

Primary Management

Aim of primary management is to inform ladies about OAB and assist them with creating services to control the symptoms. It is vital to convey to the lady that this mode will require long-term attachment and dedication from the patient to achieve success in this regard.

Lifestyle modifications like stoppage of smoking, weight reduction, dietary restriction, restriction of fluid intake to 1.5 L, reduction of caffeine, acidic foods, and alcohol, bowel regulation, and exercise can be very effective in this regard.[21,22]

Bladder retraining includes passing urine regular intervals irrespective of the usual urge to void. To begin with, the voiding intervals can be as small as half an hour which can be gradually increased until the patient can hold urine for up to 3–4 hours. This process will lead to a gradual increment of bladder capacity. Along with this, pelvic floor physiotherapy is another mode which is highly effective in reducing the natural progress of the syndrome.[23] During the training, patients are advised to contract and relax the pelvic floor in a series of 10 sequences, the entire set to be repeated for three times **(Boxes 3 and 4) (Figs. 1 and 2)**.[24]

Secondary Management

The cutting-edge drug treatment for OAB is the utilization of anticholinergic medications and β-adrenergic agonists. The expected outcome of these medications is to accomplish relaxation of the detrusor muscle to provide

BOX 3: Behavioral training as first-line therapy.

Target

To enrich the holding capacity by educating the ladies about the methods to stop bladder muscle contraction

The patients are educated about the practice of reinforcement of the pressure of urethra, vaginal muscles, and stoppage of detrusor contractions to prevent any event of leakage

- The initial appointment should be in the clinic to facilitate communication
- A verbal communication of legitimate compression of the pelvic floor muscles is to advise the fact to compress out pelvic floor which they will do to prevent any leakage of flatus
- A viable activity solution for more seasoned grown-ups is to contract and loosen up their pelvic floor muscles for 2 seconds with 15 sets, three times each day. The subjects ought to continuously build the span of press/relaxations by around 1 second out of each week, until they accomplish 10 seconds withdrawals. Right now, the patients can start an upkeep remedy of 10 seconds constrictions and relaxations with 10 sets one time per day
- *Freeze and squeeze:* At the point when a need to keep moving happens, rather than racing to the restroom, remain still and contract the pelvic floor muscle until the urge is not there anymore

Needs to be continued for 3 months

BOX 4: Bladder training as first-line therapy.

Target

To enhance the performance of bladder musculature and enhance the bladder volume by instructing the patient to void regularly rather than voiding on demand

- First step is to identify the lengthiest intervoid break is selected
- Patients are told to void in the morning and afterward at regular intervals, and again prior to retrieving back to bed
- In the event that the patient wants to void before the interval, patients are told to utilize concealment methods, like interruption or unwinding strategies, to make them reach the planned voiding time
- Following 14 days, target is increment of the time span by 15 minutes, continuously expanding intervoid interval

Patients are likewise requested to consider to settle down and take five full breaths, focusing on other activities rather than the voiding issues

The initial block should be for 6 weeks

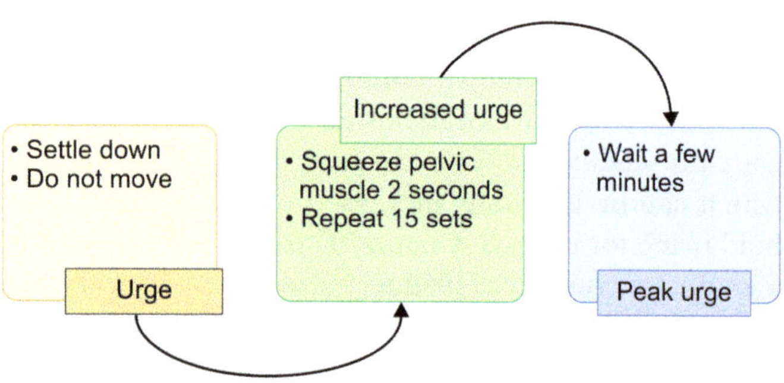

Fig. 1: Graphical representation of behavioral training.

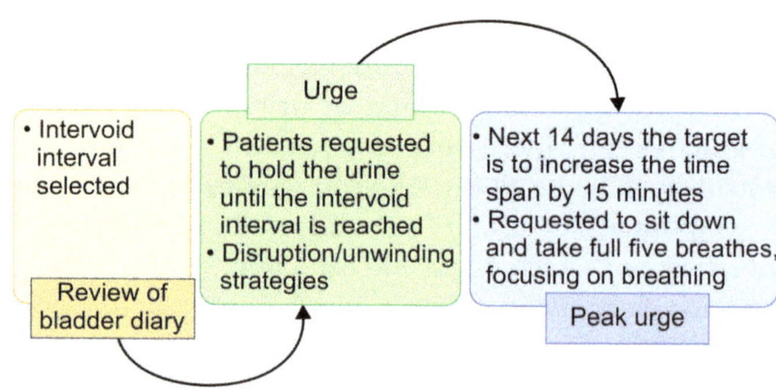

Fig. 2: Graphical representation of bladder retraining.

symptomatic improvement. This medication treats OAB symptoms by two pathways. The main system of activity works at the level of the neuromuscular junction on cholinergic-muscarinic receptors creating an inhibition of the mechanism through which parasympathetic excitement prompts detrusor muscle relaxation. Another way of activity might deal with urothelial receptors depressing afferent nerve activity.[25]

Side effect of anticholinergic drugs might restrict their actions. Dry mouth and constipation are the most common side effects leading to discontinuation of antimuscarinic medications in >50% of cases.[26] If constipations are predominant then early use fiber and stool softeners is recommended. This is the cause for discontinuation of the medication in >50% of cases. Patients should be notified that these medications cause gradual improvement of symptom over 2–3 months. Anticholinergic side effects also include blurred vision and dizziness.[27] Other adverse effects include deranged mental state, ill effect on the heart, typically, prolongation of the QT interval. These are usually more evident in elder population[26] who might suffer from neurological side effects from cerebrovascular disease.[26] The prescription of medicines with less blood-brain barrier penetrance (such as trospium and darifenacin) may alter the vagolytic effect on the cardiovascular system that may lead to change in heart and neurological systems.[28] Hence, an M3 selective muscarinic receptor agent like solifenacin may be first line in women with cardiovascular compromise. Elderly patients who receive multidrug therapy have renal and hepatic impairment should have anticholinergics prescribed with caution as these agents can cause interaction with other drugs which act through the cytochrome p450 pathway.[29]

Contraindications for the use of antimuscarinic drugs are patients with closed-angle glaucoma, myasthenia gravis, severe ulcerative colitis, a toxic megacolon, or intestinal obstruction.

Any medical treatment should be started with the lowest possible dose.

Oxybutynin has a transdermal preparation (patch and gel). Patients should be made aware about potential side effects. In general, initial regimen should be planned with lowest dose possible of antimuscarinic medications. Few studies suggested that extended-release formulation may have better effect to the immediate release preparations and increased compliance. In addition, solifenacin is similar in achieving results as extended-release tolterodine and fesoterodine is better than it. However, adverse effects are dose dependent.[30]

Beta-adrenergic agonist mirabegron 50 mg has comparable viability to most antimuscarinics with a lower rate of dry mouth, the most well-known unfavorable side effect detailed with antimuscarinics and one of the primary drivers of suspension of treatment **(Table 2)**.

TABLE 2: Different drug regimen and their adverse effects.[25]

Drug	Adverse effects	Notes
Oxybutynin CR	• Dry mouth • Constipation	• Dose-dependent effect • To be taken 1 hour before food intake
Oxybutynin transdermal	• Itchiness • Erythema • Dry mouth • Constipation	Transdermal delivery reduces anticholinergic side effect
Tolterodine	• Dry mouth • Constipations • Dry eyes	Dose-dependent effect with immediate release
Solifenacin	• Dry mouth • Constipation • Blurred vision	Steady state at 10 days with longer half-life
Darifenacin	• Dry mouth • Constipation	Steady state in 4–5 hours
Vaginal estrogen	• Increased risk of breast cancer • Breast discomfort • Local reactions	For postmenopausal women with vaginal atrophy
Duloxetine	• Nausea • Dry mouth • Constipation • Insomnia • Fatigue	Can be used if anticholinergics are contraindicated in OAB

Second-line Treatment

If the symptoms still persist even after using the first-line medication or patient noncompliance needs urodynamic assessment and multidisciplinary discussion. These secondary methods should be carefully planned after discussion with specialist urogynecologist.

The most common minimally invasive second-line treatment options include botulinum toxin injections, posterior tibial nerve neuromodulation, and sacral neuromodulation.

Botulin toxin is injected into detrusor muscles with the help of cystoscopy. This blocks presynaptic release of acetylcholine from nerve endings and as a result decreases contractility, and muscular atrophy is obtained at the site of infiltration. This form of management can be provided as an outpatient form of treatment as well.

There is option of peripheral tibial nerve stimulation, transcutaneous tibial nerve stimulation, and sacral neuromodulation. An external electrical signal is sent through the tibial nerve to the sacral plexus, through a needle embedded close to the ankle. This management modality has got a success rate of >50%.[31] This method continued for 30 consecutive sessions for 3 months was found to have no serious unfavorable impacts. This technique can be utilized for fecal incontinence too.

In more severe cases, S3 nerve root stimulation by an implanted electrical pulse generator is highly effective in providing benefit to patients in case of severe OAB not responding to medications and Botox.[32] Continuous

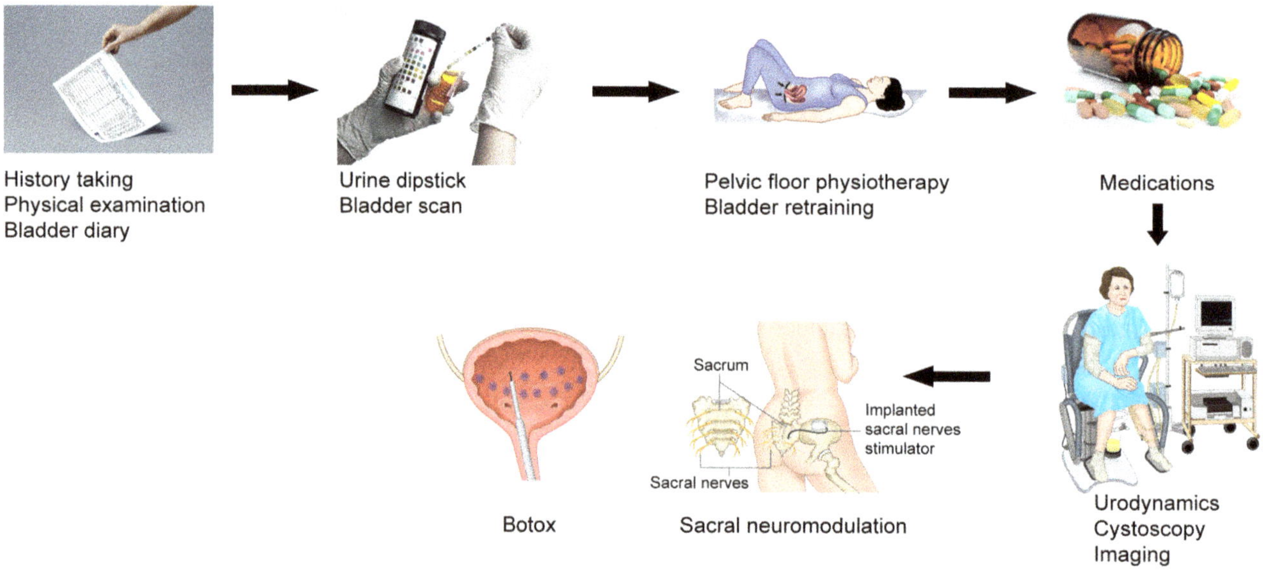

Fig. 3: Diagrammatic depiction of management strategies.
Source: Pictures collected from various sources via internet.

impulse is provided by an impulse generator lying close to the nerve roots. The most common therapy-related event was new onset pain. The implanted patients, if successful at 1 year, continued to have a successful outcome at a 5-year follow-up.

The final step is augmentation cystoplasty.[33] However, these procedures are performed rarely and is associated with prolonged period of recovery might need intermittent self-catheterization at the end. It can be used in a small subset of patients.[34] Bowels problems cannot be resolved in this route however.

For some patients, however, the only management option available can be long-term indwelling catheterization for refractory OAB.

Among other investigational therapies, neurokinin receptor antagonists, α-adrenoceptor antagonists, nerve growth factor inhibitors, gene therapy, and stem cell-based therapies are of considerable interest. The future development of new modalities in OAB treatment appears promising **(Fig. 3)**.[35-38]

CONCLUSION

The reasons for OAB are not totally perceived, and side effects might contrast among patients and might confound. A total fix is interesting and the treatment of an OAB can be a difficult issue for the doctor, with the need to tailor the choices as per the patient's situations. Patient satisfaction and improvement of symptoms are the ultimate goals to be achieved. There is a huge impact of OAB on well-being-related personal satisfaction. The significance of appropriate treatment cannot be overemphasized, particularly in old patients.

REFERENCES

1. Stewart WF, Van Rooyen JB, Cundiff GW, Abrams P, Herzog AR, Corey R, et al. Prevalence and burden of overactive bladder in the United States. World J Urol. 2003;20:327-36.
2. Wein AJ, Rovner ES. Definition and epidemiology of overactive bladder. Urology. 2002;60(5 Suppl 1):7-12; discussion 12.
3. Onukwugha E, Zuckerman IH, McNally D, Coyne KS, Vats V, Mullins CD. The total economic burden of overactive bladder in the United States: a disease-specific approach. Am J Manag Care. 2009;15(suppl 4):S90-97.
4. Marinkovic SP, Rovner ES, Moldwin RM, Stanton SL, Gillen LM, Marinkovic CM. The management of overactive bladder syndrome. BMJ. 2012;344:e2365.
5. Puckrein G, Walker D, Xu L, Congdon P, Gooch K. The Prevalence and Forecast Prevalence of Overactive Bladder in the Medicare Population. Clin Med Insights Urol. 2019;12.
6. Milsom I, Abrams P, Cardozo L, Roberts RG, Thuroff J, Wein AJ. How widespread are the symptoms of an overactive bladder and how are they managed? A population-based prevalence study. BJU Int. 2001;87:760-6.
7. Gill K, Kang R, Sathiananthamoorthy S, Khasriya R, Malone-Lee J. A blinded observational cohort study of the microbiological ecology associated with pyuria and overactive bladder symptoms. Int Urogynecol J. 2018;29(10):1493-500.

8. de Groat WC. A neurologic basis for the overactive bladder. Urology. 1997;50(6A suppl):36-52.
9. Brading AF. Spontaneous activity of lower urinary tract smooth muscles: correlation between ion channels and tissue function. J Physiol. 2006;570:13-22.
10. Drake MJ, Mills IW, Gillespie JI. Model of peripheral autonomous modules and a myovesical plexus in normal and overactive bladder function. Lancet. 2001;358:401-3.
11. Andersson KE. Detrusor myocyte activity and afferent signaling. Neurourol Urodyn. 2010;29:97-106.
12. Wein AJ, Rackley RR. Overactive bladder: a better understanding of pathophysiology, diagnosis and management. J Urol. 2006;175:S5-10.
13. Steele AC, Kohli N, Mallipeddi P, Karram M. Pharmacologic causes of female incontinence. Int Urogynecol J Pelvic Floor Dysfunct. 1999;10:106-10.
14. Borrie MJ, Campbell K, Arcese ZA, Bray J, Hart P, Labate T, et al. Urinary retention in patients in a geriatric rehabilitation unit: prevalence, risk factors, and validity of bladder scan evaluation. Rehabil Nurs. 2001;26:187-91.
15. Locher JL, Goode PS, Roth DL, Worrell RL, Burgio KL. Reliability assessment of the bladder diary for urinary incontinence in older women. J Gerontol A Biol Sci Med Sci. 2001;56:M32-35.
16. Abrams P, Cardozo L, Fall M, Griffiths D, Rosier P, Ulmsten U, et al. The standardisation of terminology in lower urinary tract function: report from the standardisation sub-committee of the International Continence Society. Urology. 2003;61:37-49.
17. Gormley EA, Lightner DJ, Burgio KL, Chai TC, Clemens JQ, Culkin DJ, et al. Diagnosis and treatment of overactive bladder (non-neurogenic) in adults: AUA/SUFU guideline. J Urol. 2012;188(6 suppl):2455-63.
18. Bottiggi KA, Salazar JC, Yu L, Caban-Holt AM, Ryan M, Mendiondo MS, et al. Long-term cognitive impact of anticholinergic medications in older adults. Am J Geriatr Psychiatry. 2006;14(11):980-4.
19. Thüroff JW, Abrams P, Andersson KE, Artibani W, Chapple CR, Drake MJ, et al. Guías EAU sobre incontinencia urinaria [EAU Guidelines on Urinary Incontinence]. Actas Urol Esp. 2011;35(7):373-88.
20. Yamaguchi O, Nishizawa O, Takeda M, Yokoyama O, Homma Y, Kakizaki H, et al. Clinical guidelines for overactive bladder. Int J Urol. 2009;16:126-42.
21. Hashim H, Abrams P. How should patients with an overactive bladder manipulate their fluid intake? BJU Int. 2008;102:62-6.
22. Lohsiriwat S, Hirunsai M, Chaiyaprasithi B. Effect of caffeine on bladder function in patients with overactive bladder symptoms. Urol Ann. 2011;3:14-8.
23. Shafik A, Shafik IA. Overactive bladder inhibition in response to pelvic floor muscle exercises. World J Urol. 2003;20:374-7.
24. Burgio KL, Locher JL, Goode PS. Combined behavioral and drug therapy for urge incontinence in older women. J Am Geriatr Soc. 2000;48:370-4.
25. Robinson D, Cardozo L. Antimuscarinic drugs to treat overactive bladder. BMJ. 2012;344:e2130.
26. Peeker R, Samsioe G, Kowalski J, Andersson AS, Bergqvist A. A prospective observational study of the effects of treatment with extended-release tolterodine on health-related quality of life of patients suffering overactive bladder syndrome in Sweden. Scand J Urol Nephrol. 2010;44:138-46.
27. Rosenberg MT, Newman DK, Tallman CT, Page SA. Overactive bladder: recognition requires vigilance for symptoms. Cleve Clin J Med. 2007;74(Suppl 3):S21-29.
28. Olshansky B, Ebinger U, Brum J, Egermark M, Viegas A, Rekeda L. Differential pharmacological effects of antimuscarinic drugs on heart rate: a randomized, placebo-controlled, double-blind, crossover study with tolterodine and darifenacin in healthy participants > or = 50 years. J Cardiovasc Pharmacol Ther. 2008;13:241-51.
29. Chapple CR, Martinez-Garcia R, Selvaggi L, Toozs-Hobson P, Warnack W, Drogendijk T, et al. A comparison of the efficacy and tolerability of solifenacin succinate and extended release tolterodine at treating overactive bladder syndrome: results of the STAR trial. Eur Urol. 2005;48:464-70.
30. Arnold J, McLeod N, Thani-Gasalam R, Rashid P. Overactive bladder syndrome—management and treatment options. Aust Fam Physician. 2012;41(11):878-83.
31. Ridout AE, Yoong W. Tibial nerve stimulation for overactive bladder syndrome unresponsive to medical therapy. J Obstet Gynaecol. 2010;30:111-4.
32. Schmidt RA, Jonas U, Oleson KA, Janknegt RA, Hassouna MM, Siegel SW, et al. Sacral nerve stimulation for treatment of refractory urinary urge incontinence. Sacral Nerve Stimulation Study Group. J Urol. 1999;162:352-7.
33. Mast P, Hoebeke P, Wyndaele JJ, Oosterlinck W, Everaert K. Experience with augmentation cystoplasty. A review. Paraplegia. 1995;33:560-4.
34. Holm J, Struckmann JR, Frimodt-Moller C. Augmentation ileo-cystoplasty in women with disabling urge incontinence. Ugeskr Laeger. 1995;157:1528-30.
35. Andersson KE. New pharmacologic targets for the treatment of the overactive bladder: an update. Urology. 2004; 63(3 suppl 1):32-41.
36. Chancellor MB. New frontiers in the treatment of overactive bladder and incontinence. Rev Urol. 2002;4(Suppl 4): S50-6.
37. Epstein BJ, Gums JG, Molina E. Newer agents for the management of overactive bladder. Am Fam Physician. 2006;74:2061-8.
38. Ng CK, Gonzalez RR, Te AE. Refractory overactive bladder in men: update on novel therapies. Curr Urol Rep. 2006;7:456-61.

APPENDIX 1

New Patient Questionnaire

a. *Personal details*

1. How old are you?
2. What is your occupation?
3. What is your best telephone contact number?

b. *Your presenting complaint*

Patient Answer

1. Please describe the symptoms that bother you the most.
2. How long have you had these problems for?
3. Are these problems getting worse? Yes ☐ No ☐

Office Use

c. *Questions about your bladder symptoms*

Patient Answer

1. How often do you have to visit the toilet to urinate in the day time?
2. How often do you have to wake up at night to urinate?
3. Do you have to rush to go to the toilet? (urgency)
   a. Is the feeling: Yes ☐ No ☐
   Mild ☐ Moderate ☐ Severe ☐
   (Please tick)
4. Do you get urgency to urinate if you are washing dishes or put a key in the door? Yes ☐ No ☐
   (Please tick)
5. Do you leak with exertion? Yes ☐ No ☐
   (Please tick)
6. If you do leak with exertion what causes the leakage? Cough ☐ Walk ☐ Bending down ☐
   Sneeze ☐ Jump ☐ Exercising ☐ Laugh ☐ Lifting a heavy object ☐
   (Please tick all appropriate activities)
7. Do you leak at the time of intercourse? Yes ☐ No ☐
   (Please tick)
8. If you do leak with intercourse is it: On penetration ☐ On orgasm ☐
   (Please tick)
9. Is there anything else that can make you leak?
10. Do your urinary symptoms stop you doing anything?
11. Have you ever experienced stinging or burning when passing urine? Yes ☐ No ☐
    (Please tick)
12. Have you ever noticed blood in your urine? Yes ☐ No ☐
    (Please tick)
13. Have you ever wet the bed? Yes ☐ No ☐
    (Please tick)
14. When you go to the loo do you have to: Strain to pass urine? ☐ Hover or lean forward to pass urine? ☐
    (Please tick)
15. Once you have finished urinating do you get a small dribble? Yes ☐ No ☐
    (Please tick)

16. Do you feel that you always empty your bladder completely? Yes ☐ No ☐
    (Please tick)
17. Do you think you have to get up and go back again? Yes ☐ No ☐
    (Please tick)
18. Does your leakage happen:
    On a daily basis? ☐
    More than once a week? ☐
    Less than once a week? ☐
    About once a month? ☐
    (Please tick)
19. If you do leak how severe is your leakage?
    A few drops? ☐
    You wet your underwear? ☐
    You wet your outer clothing? ☐
    You wet the floor? ☐
    (Please tick)
20. What is your total fluid intake during the day?
21. What drinks do you take during the course of the day?
22. How many pads do you have to use in the day?
    (Please mention the thickness of the pads also)
23. In the last 6 months have you had several urine infections? Yes ☐ No ☐
    (Please tick)
    If so, how many?
24. Were you given antibiotics for this? Yes ☐ No ☐
    (Please tick)

Office Use

d. *Questions regarding your vaginal symptoms*

Patient Answer

1. Are you aware of a lump in your vagina? Yes ☐ No ☐
   (Please tick)
2. Do you have any discomfort in the vaginal area? Yes ☐ No ☐
   (Please tick)
3. Do you have any pain in the vaginal area? Yes ☐ No ☐
   (Please tick)
4. Do you suffer with regular discharge from the vagina? Yes ☐ No ☐
   (Please tick)
5. Do you experience any pain at the time of intercourse? Yes ☐ No ☐
   (Please tick)
6. If so, is it on the outer side or on deep penetration? Outer side ☐ Deep penetration? ☐
   (Please tick)

Office Use

e. *Questions regarding your bowel symptoms*

Patient Answer

1. Do you open your bowels daily? Yes ☐ No ☐
   (Please tick)
2. How frequently do you open your bowels if not daily?

3. What is the consistency of your stool?
   Type 1: □
   Type 2: □
   Type 3: □
   Type 4: □
   Type 5: □
   Type 6: □
   Type 7: □
   (Please tick one)
4. Do you ever suffer with leakage or stool soiling? Yes □ No □
   (Please tick)
   If so, how often in a week?
5. Have you ever experienced inappropriate loss of wind which you find difficult to control? Yes □ No □
   (Please tick)
6. Do you suffer with stool urgency? Yes □ No □
   (Please tick)
7. Do you suffer with increased frequency of bowels? Yes □ No □
   (Please tick)
8. Do you find it difficult to empty the bowels? Yes□ No □
   (Please tick)
   If so, do you have to support:
   Perineum? □
   (area between the vagina and anus)
   Vagina? □
   Rectum? □
   (Please tick)

Office Use

f. *Questions regarding your gynecological history*

Patient Answer

1. How many children have you had?
2. Did you have a vaginal birth or caesarean section?
3. Have you ever had any gynecological operations in the past?
   Yes □ No □
   (Please tick)
4. If you did have any gynecological operations, what were they and roughly when were they performed?
5. Do you still have your periods?
   Yes □ No □
   (Please tick)
6. If you are having your periods are they: Regular?
   Yes □ No □
   Heavy/Moderate/Light (Please circle)
7. Is your cycle regular?
   Yes □ No □
   (Please tick)
8. Do you get any bleeding in between periods?
   Yes □ No □
   (Please tick)

9. Do you get any bleeding after intercourse?
   Yes ☐ No ☐
   (Please tick)
10. Are you up to date with your smear tests?
   Yes ☐ No ☐
   (Please tick)
11. Have you ever had any issues with smears in the past?
   Yes ☐ No ☐
   (Please tick)
12. If you have stopped having periods, how long ago was your last period?
13. Have you ever been on HRT?
   Yes ☐ No ☐
   (Please tick)
   If yes, when did you stop HRT?
14. Do you have any plans of pregnancy in the future?
   Yes ☐ No ☐ N/A ☐
   (Please tick)
15. Are you on any hormone/contraception? Yes ☐ No ☐
   (Please tick)

Office Use

g. *Questions regarding your past medical history*

Patient Answer

1. Have you ever had any other operations, other than your gynecological operations?
   Yes ☐ No ☐
   (Please tick)
   If so, what were they, and when?
2. Do you suffer with any medical issues?
   Yes ☐ No ☐
   (Please tick)
   Medical Issues - Please tick as appropriate

Raised blood pressure:	Yes ☐	No ☐	Asthma:	Yes ☐	No ☐
Epilepsy:	Yes ☐	No ☐	Diabetes:	Yes ☐	No ☐
Hypermobility:	Yes ☐	No ☐	Renal disease:	Yes ☐	No ☐
Liver disease:	Yes ☐	No ☐	Cancer:	Yes ☐	No ☐
Cardiac disease:	Yes ☐	No ☐	Allergies:	Yes ☐	No ☐

Please list:

Smoker: Yes ☐ No ☐ No/day/years Alcohol: Yes ☐ No ☐ Units/week

Give details.. Give details..

Additional health problems:

Office Use

h. *Questions regarding your current medications*

Patient Answer

1. Please list all medications that you are on. Please refer to your latest prescription given to you by your Doctor: (GP can assist with this)
2. Please list all medications that you are allergic to:

Office Use

FOR DOCTORS USE ONLY – do not complete

Colorectal questionnaire completed Yes No Not applicable

Quality of life questionnaire

- ICIQ – OAB OAB Score .... Bother score.......................................
- ICIQ – LUTSqol LUTs Score .... Bother score.......................................
- ICIQ – VS Vaginal symptoms score .... Sex matters score .... QOL score...................

MSU: BMI: Height

Leuc Nit PH Blood PVR: Weight

FOR DOCTORS USE ONLY – do not complete

Date:

Effect of cough: Hypermobile urethra Yes No Leakage of urine Yes No Urine loss without provocation Yes No

Perineum and vaginal introitus: ....

Vaginal examination

Atrophy Yes No

Cystocele: Rectocele: Vault prolapse: Uterine prolapse: Sensation (left) and (right):

Pain (left) and (right): Aware of pelvic floor contraction? Yes No

Bimanual examination: POP-Q:

Ultrasound scan:

Pelvic floor exercise offered Yes No Referred to Physiotherapy Yes No

Urodynamics organized Yes No

Indication:

Management plan:

Clinician signature: PRINT name:

Abbreviations: MSU: midstream specimen of urine, BMI: body mass index, gms: grams, mLs: milliliters, POP-Q: Pelvic Organ Prolapse Quantification

FOR DOCTORS USE ONLY – do not complete

Date: Follow up duration:

Surgical procedure: Date of procedure:

Reason

Return to theatre for procedure related event within 72 hours? Yes ☐ No ☐................

Catheterization required for more than 10 days postoperative? Yes ☐ No ☐................

Return to hospital within 30 days for procedure related event? Yes ☐ No ☐................

Long term problem identified? Yes ☐ No ☐................

Visit to GP within 6 weeks? Yes ☐ No ☐................

Global impression of improvement

For Incontinence		For Prolapse	
	0 – Unanswered		0 - Unanswered
	1 - Very much worse		1 - Very much worse
	2 – Much worse		2- Much worse
	3 – A little worse		3 – A little worse
	4 – No change		4 – No change
	5 – A little better		5 – A little better
	6 – Much better		6 – Much better
	7 – Very much better		7 – Very much better

Residual symptoms POP Q

Post-operative examination

Anterior wall......................

Posterior wall.................................

Cervix.............................

Cuff.................................

Graft problems: ....

Tape related problems:..

Voiding difficulty:...

Name:...

Score:...

Plan:

Signature stamp....................................... Date of follow-up................................

CHAPTER 21

Body Dysmorphic Disorder and Its Implications in Cosmetic Gynecology

Manvi Verma

INTRODUCTION

Body dysmorphic disorder (BDD) is a psychiatric disorder characterized by preoccupation with an imagined defect in physical appearance or a distorted perception of one's body image **(Fig. 1)**.[1] Body image refers to the perceptions, thoughts, and feelings about the body. Four components of body image have been described, which are the factors influencing one's perception of appearance include the significance attributed to physical looks, the level of discontentment with one's appearance, the objective reality of one's physical features, and the subjective interpretation of one's appearance.[2] People experiencing BDD fixate on perceived flaws in their appearance, which may not be noticeable or only appear minor to others. Perception can be shaped by a multitude of factors, including expectations, motivations, knowledge, and memory. BDD is one such disorder in which perception becomes discordant with reality.

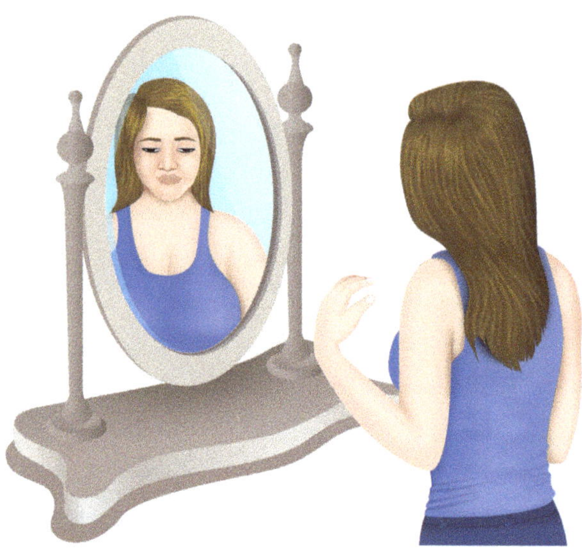

Fig. 1: Body dysmorphic disorder (BDD): Person is preoccupied with imagined defect in physical appearance with distorted perception of one's body image.

SYNONYMS

The syndrome is also known by the names dysmorphophobia,[3] "Dermatologic hypochondriasis", Schönheitshypochondrie ("beauty hypochondria"), Hässlichkeitskümmerer ("one who is worried about being ugly").[4,5]

EPIDEMIOLOGY

The prevalence of BDD has been found to vary according to the setting. In the general population, it varies from 0.7% to 5.8%. A higher prevalence is noted in dermatology and cosmetic surgery settings.[6] Among the different age groups, BDD is commonly seen among adolescents.[7] Generally, a higher prevalence in women is noted.[8]

DIAGNOSIS

Body dysmorphic disorder is diagnosed by the "The Diagnostic and Statistical Manual of Mental Disorders," 5th edition (DSM-V) criteria as described below **(Fig. 2)**.

- Individuals with BDD obsess over one or more imagined imperfections in their appearance, which typically remain unnoticed or seem trivial to others.
- The fixation on appearance prompts individuals to engage in repetitive behaviors such as checking, correcting, concealing, or seeking reassurance regarding perceived flaws.
- The appearance of preoccupations and resulting repetitive behaviors must cause clinically significant distress or impairment in social, occupational, or other important areas of functioning.

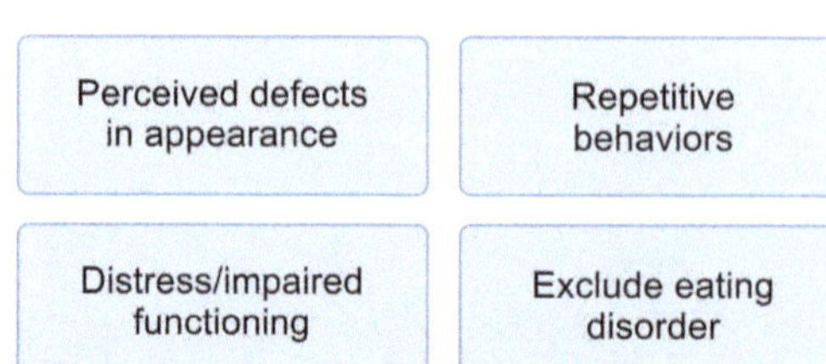

Fig. 2: Diagnostic criteria for body dysmorphic disorder (BDD).

- If appearance preoccupations center around perceived excessive body fat or weight and meet the criteria for an eating disorder diagnosis, they should be classified and diagnosed as an eating disorder rather than as BDD.[9]

SCREENING TOOLS FOR BODY DYSMORPHIC DISORDER

Various screening tools for BDD are available; the most common ones are listed in **Table 1**. The gold standard for diagnosing BDD involves conducting a structured clinical interview consisting of 24 questions designed to assess DSM-IV Axis I Disorders. However, it is time-consuming and not validated for cosmetic surgery settings.[10]

Apart from the above survey measures, the National Institute for Health and Clinical Excellence suggests five questions that could aid in diagnosing BDD:

1. Do you frequently fret about your appearance and wish you could dwell on it less?
2. What particular worries do you harbor regarding your appearance?
3. On an average day, how much time do you spend thinking about your appearance? (More than 1 hour/day is regarded as excessive.)
4. How does this preoccupation impact your daily life?
5. Does it interfere with your work or social interactions?[11]

ETIOLOGY

Unfavorable childhood experiences, increased exposure to social media, problems in the family environment, and social support are some of the risk factors associated with.[12,13]

TABLE 1: Screening tools for body dysmorphic disorder (BDD).

Survey	*Number of questions*	*Self-administered/ clinician*
Structured clinical interview for diagnosis for DSM-IV Axis I Disorders	24	Clinician
BDD questionnaire	4 sets	Self
Yale-Brown scale for BDD	12	Clinician
BDD symptoms scale	10	Self
Dysmorphic concern questionnaire	7	Self
Multidimensional body self-relations questionnaire	69 or 34	Self
Multidimensional body self-relations questionnaire-appearance scales	34	Self
Rosenberg self-esteem scale	10	Self

CLINICAL FEATURES

The characteristic behaviors of BDD comprise repetitive mirror checking, incessant comparison with others, excessive grooming, skin picking, concealing actions, frequent wardrobe changes, and believing that others are equally troubled by the perceived flaws (referred to as referential thinking). The symptoms of BDD have been graded into mild, moderate, and severe **(Table 2)**.[6]

EFFECT OF BODY DYSMORPHIC DISORDER ON PERCEPTION OF GENITALIA

The individual may think that her genitalia are too small, too large, or otherwise flawed. A distorted view of the size and shape of genitalia may exist. Patients may be overly concerned with the appearance of their pubic hair or labia.

TABLE 2: Grading of body dysmorphic disorder (BDD) by severity.

Mild/moderate	*Severe*	*Both*
No notable decline in overall functioning	Avoidant behavior	Checking mirror frequently
Localized appearance concerns	Impairment in global functioning	Comparing constantly with others
Realistic psychosocial concerns	Young	Need reassurance with the perceived flaws
	Significantly depressed	Unnecessary dermatological treatments or cosmetic procedures sought
	Significantly anxious	*Referential thinking:* Thinking that others are equally troubled by the perceived flaws
	Extreme preoccupation with defect	Camouflaging behavior
	Compulsive behaviors which are debilitating	Behavior that is unusual or requires extra attention towards the surgeon or staff
	Social isolation	
	Unemployment	
	Excessive or impractical anticipations concerning the cosmetic result	

They experience a notable hindrance in their job, social interactions, and intimate relationships, and may exhibit delusional beliefs regarding their appearance.

Body Dysmorphic Disorder and Cosmetic Gynecology Surgery

People with BDD often seek cosmetic surgery in an attempt to "fix" their perceived flaws, to improve self-esteem and body image, and to be able to engage in sexual activity or intimacy. However, it is important to note that cosmetic surgery is not usually an effective treatment for BDD. This is because people with BDD often have unrealistic expectations about what surgery can achieve and are frequently dissatisfied with the outcome.[14] Additionally, in the realm of body image distress, cosmetic procedures offer minimal enhancement.[15]

Surgery can sometimes make a person's BDD worse, as they may become more focused on their appearance and dissatisfied with their body. Postsurgery complications are likely to be more common in this subgroup of patients. This is because they are more likely to focus on their appearance and less likely to follow the surgeon's instructions.

If the patient is dissatisfied with the results of the surgery, they may sue the surgeon or even press charges against them. Also, in extreme cases, patients may develop suicidal tendencies. Furthermore, discontented patients might respond toward the surgeon through legal action, physical aggression, or even violence, leading to fatal consequences.[14] By screening for BDD, doctors can help to ensure that patients are making informed decisions about cosmetic surgery and that they are receiving the best possible care.

Setting realistic expectations and making the patient well informed about the risks of cosmetic gynecological surgery, psychiatric evaluation, and treatment in cases diagnosed with the disorder prior to surgery are of paramount importance.

Management of Body Dysmorphic Disorder in Cosmetic Gynecology Settings

- *Screening for BDD:* It is important to screen patients for BDD before considering cosmetic gynecological surgery.
- *Treatment of BDD:* If a patient is diagnosed with BDD, they should be treated for the underlying disorder. This can be done with psychotherapy, medication, or a combination of both.
- *Delaying surgery:* If a patient is considering cosmetic gynecological surgery, it is often recommended to delay surgery until the BDD has been treated. This will help to ensure that the patient is making a decision based on their true needs and desires and not on their distorted body image.
- *Multidisciplinary approach:* The management of BDD in cosmetic gynecology is often best approached from a multidisciplinary perspective. This means that a team of healthcare professionals, including a doctor, therapist, and surgeon, should work together to provide the best possible care for the patient.

It is important to note that there is no one-size-fits-all approach to the management of BDD in cosmetic gynecology. The best approach will vary depending on the individual patient.

Treatment Options in Body Dysmorphic Disorder

Serotonin reuptake inhibitors (SRIs) along with cognitive behavioral therapy (CBT) are considered the treatment of choice. The medications include selective serotonin reuptake inhibitors (SSRIs) such as fluoxetine, sertraline, paroxetine, citalopram, escitalopram, and fluvoxamine, and one tricyclic antidepressant (TCA) clomipramine.[16] CBT for BDD is aimed at helping patients build an alternative understanding of their difficulties, wherein patients are guided through graded exposure or behavioral experiments to test out their fears.[17]

Clinical Case

Mona, a 26-year-old unmarried woman residing with her parents and currently not employed, was accompanied by her parents for a gynecological consultation. Mona had let down 29 marriage proposals till date and was not in any committed heterosexual relationship. Her mother believed that she had some preconceived wrong notion about her genital area. Nevertheless, Mona doubted this assessment and was hesitant to attend the evaluation. She believed that she was truly ugly down there. Mona believed that her labia were too long and would interfere with sexual penetration. On examination, measurements were normal (Right: 1.8 cm) (Left: 1.65 cm). She held the belief that her vagina was malformed and undersized. Seeking relief, Mona consulted with 11 surgeons nationwide, seeking a labiaplasty to address her concerns. After numerous attempts, one surgeon agreed to perform the procedure, which Mona promptly scheduled. Convinced of her physical deformity, she fixated on these perceived flaws for 8–10 hours daily, spending an additional 6–8 hours scrutinizing her genital area in the mirror and comparing it with others, often celebrities online. Seeking validation, she frequently sought her elder sister's opinion on the appearance of her labia and extensively researched cosmetic surgery online. Mona's distress impeded her ability to work and deterred her from pursuing heterosexual relationships. She often expressed thoughts of passive suicidal ideation, citing her dissatisfaction with life due to her perceived genital appearance.

Case description and course:

- Mona was diagnosed with BDD due to the severity of her symptoms. Consequently, she underwent a comprehensive treatment plan comprising medication and specially tailored CBT for BDD, administered in an intensive outpatient setting.
- Although she was unwilling to cancel the scheduled labiaplasty, she consented to postpone it until after she underwent evidence-based treatments for BDD to ensure she received adequate care.
- Mona underwent treatment with fluoxetine, gradually increasing the dosage to 80 mg/day over 6 weeks. This dosage was well tolerated, and previous lower doses had not shown any improvement in symptoms.
- Following 12 weeks of fluoxetine treatment, the dosage was incrementally raised to 120 mg/day, which Mona tolerated well. Concurrently, Mona engaged in intensive CBT sessions for BDD 3 days/week. After 6 months of this combined treatment approach, her BDD symptoms were nearly in remission, her mood had significantly improved, suicidal ideation had ceased, she had begun actively seeking employment, and she had lost interest in pursuing cosmetic surgery.

CONCLUSION

Body dysmorphic disorder (BDD) is an important clinical entity that can significantly impact a person's self-esteem and quality of life. As highlighted, BDD is an important clinical entity that necessitates thorough evaluation before considering any cosmetic procedure. Proper diagnosis and treatment are imperative to prevent patient dissatisfaction, negative surgical outcomes, and potential legal complications. Clinicians, especially cosmetic gynecologists, should be aware of BDD and its presentations to ensure the best possible care for their patients. Early diagnosis and treatment with medications like SSRIs and cognitive behavioral therapy (CBT) can be very effective in managing BDD symptoms. By working together with a team of healthcare professionals, including therapists and psychiatrists, cosmetic surgeons can ensure that patients with BDD receive the best possible care and avoid the potential negative consequences of cosmetic surgery.

REFERENCES

1. Ribeiro RVE. Prevalence of body dysmorphic disorder in plastic surgery and dermatology patients: a systematic review with meta-analysis. Aesthetic Plast Surg. 2017;41: 964-70.
2. Sarcu D, Adamson P. Psychology of the facelift patient. Facial Plast Surg. 2017;33:252-9.
3. Phillips KA. Body dysmorphic disorder: Recognizing and treating imagined ugliness. World Psychiatry. 2004;3(1):12-7.
4. Janet P. Les obsessions et la psychasthenie. Paris: Felix Alcan; 1903.
5. Kraepelin E. Psychiatrie, 8th edition. Leipzig: Barth; 1909-1915.
6. Higgins S, Wysong A. Cosmetic surgery and body dysmorphic disorder—An update. Int J Womens Dermatol. 2018;4(1):43-8.
7. Anderson RC. Body dysmorphic disorder: Recognition and treatment. Plast Surg Nurs. 2003;23:125-8.
8. Danesh M, Beroukhim K, Nguyen C, Levin E, Koo J. Body dysmorphic disorder screening tools for the dermatologist: a systematic review. Pract Dermatol 2015;2:44-9.
9. American Psychiatric Association, DSM-5 Task Force. *Diagnostic and Statistical Manual of Mental Disorders: DSM-5™*, 5th edition. USA: American Psychiatric Publishing, Inc.; 2013.
10. Joseph AW, Ishii L, Joseph SS, Smith JI, Su P, Bater K, et al. Prevalence of body dysmorphic disorder and surgeon diagnostic accuracy in facial plastic and oculoplastic surgery clinics. JAMA Facial Plast Surg. 2016;19:269-74.
11. Veer V, Jackson L, Kara N, Hawthorne M. Pre-operative considerations in aesthetic facial surgery. J Laryngol Otol. 2014;128:22-8.
12. de Brito MJ, de Almeida Arruda Felix G, Nahas FX, et al. Body dysmorphic disorder should not be considered an exclusion criterion for cosmetic surgery. J Plast Reconstr Aesthet Surg. 2015;68:270-2.
13. Patchin JW. New national bullying and cyberbullying data. [online] Available from https://cyberbullying.org/new-national-bullying-cyberbullying-data [Last accessed June, 2024].
14. Sweis IE, Spitz J, Barry Jr DR, Cohen M. A review of body dysmorphic disorder in aesthetic surgery patients and the legal implications. Aesthetic Plast Surg. 2017;41:949-54.
15. Bouman TK, Mulkens S, van der Lei B. Cosmetic professionals' awareness of body dysmorphic disorder. Plast Reconstr Surg. 2017;139:336-42.
16. Singh AR, Veale D. Understanding and treating body dysmorphic disorder. Indian J Psychiatry. 2019;61 (Suppl 1):S131-135.
17. Veale D, Bewley A. Body dysmorphic disorder. BMJ. 2015;350:h2278.

CHAPTER 22

Platelet-rich Plasma for Ovarian Rejuvenation

Preeti Jindal, Sumitu Sahdev, Muskaan Mittal

BACKGROUND

In recent years, there has been a notable shift in societal patterns as an increasing number of women choose to postpone childbirth. Thus, they are more likely to face the problem of ovarian insufficiency by the time they are ready to conceive. Hence, the need of some therapy to restore ovarian function is crucially important, and this is where platelet-rich plasma (PRP) for ovarian rejuvenation comes into play **(Fig. 1)**.

INTRODUCTION

Women are born with a fixed reserve of eggs, which start getting depleted from the time they are born. At birth, a female has close to 1–2 million eggs, and by the time she achieves puberty, she is left with only 25–30% of her original reserve, which is around 300,000–400,000. This pool slowly gets depleted until the time she achieves

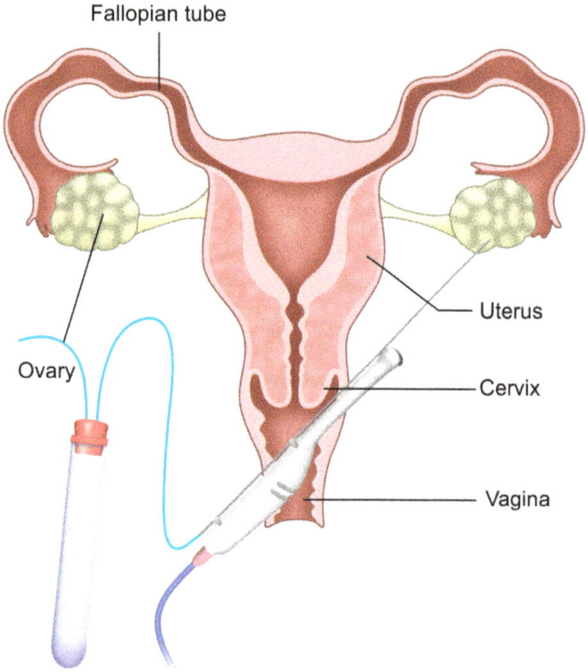

Fig. 1: Platelet-rich plasma for ovarian rejuvenation.

menopause by the age of 45–50 years. It is also important to appreciate that thousands of senescent eggs still persist even at the inception of perimenopause. These eggs may have a potential to be activated and hence may result in follicular growth, fertilization, pregnancy, and live birth.

Aging of the female reproductive system is directly associated with the disruption of ovarian function and jeopardizes fertility potential, ultimately leading to menopause—a stage identified hitherto as irreversible.[1-3] The ovary in a female's body has very important reproductive and endocrine roles.[4] In today's era, where the number of females planning a pregnancy in their 30s and 40s has increased exponentially, the problem of diminished ovarian reserve (DOR) is unmasking itself and bringing into light various strategies that can help these females produce their own genetic offspring.

There are currently few therapy options available to help women with their ovarian reserve and oocyte quality, like Coenzyme Q10, Dehydroepiandrosterone, vitamins, including vitamins C and D, or dietary or supplement isoflavones. No study has categorically validated the routine administration of these bioactive substances, despite the possibility that they have some therapeutic effects on DOR. Normally, most of the females with DOR resort to artificial reproductive techniques, such as intrauterine insemination (IUI), in vitro fertilization (IVF), oocyte donation programs, surrogacy, and also adoption in some cases. However, oocyte donation appears to be the last resort for these females. PRP appears to be one of the very few techniques that can help tide over this problem of DOR.

OVARIAN REJUVENATION WITH PLATELET RICH PLASMA

Ovarian PRP is a newly developing technique that uses PRP to stimulate the ovaries and improve female fertility. PRP is produced by centrifugation and separation of its various components from the patient's own blood, which contains plasma (55%), red blood cells (RBCs) (41%), platelets, and white blood cells (WBCs) (4%). RBCs are removed during the centrifugation and separation process, and plasma is created with a 5–10 times higher concentration of growth factors.[5,6] Alpha granules, which are found in platelets in PRP, produce a variety of substances that promote angiogenesis, cell proliferation, and growth.[7] Specific growth factors and cytokines, including transforming growth factor beta, fibroblast growth factor, insulin-like growth factors 1 and 2, vascular endothelial growth factor, and epidermal growth factor, are released **(Fig. 2)**.[8]

When injected into the ovaries, PRP releases these growth factors, which can stimulate cellular rejuvenation, improve ovarian blood flow, and promote the recruitment and maturation of healthy eggs, thereby naturally and effectively enhancing fertility.[9] Studies have shown PRP has a positive effect on the survival and growth of follicles.[10] A case series has also shown biochemical pregnancy following autologous PRP intraovarian infusion.[11] Also, there have been reports of live births in poor-responder patients following autologous PRP intraovarian infusion.[12] To ascertain whether autologous intraovarian PRP injection is advantageous in female reproduction, particularly for women with poor ovarian reserve (POR), primary ovarian insufficiency (POI), and early menopause, it needs to be researched on a larger scale in a clinical trial setting with standardized preparation, injection, and follow-up techniques.

Ovarian rejuvenation using PRP is not a cure for infertility, but it can be a helpful option for women who are struggling to conceive due to very low anti-Müllerian hormone (AMH) and POR. It is a safe and desirable option for many couples, as there is no need to go for donor eggs. The procedure is generally safe and well-tolerated, and it can be performed on an outpatient basis **(Fig. 3)**.

Indications for Ovarian Platelet-rich Plasma

The following are the indications for ovarian PRP:

- Menopausal or perimenopausal women <50 years
- Infertile women >35 years having low egg reserve and low AMH levels
- Women with premature ovarian failure
- Primary ovarian insufficiency (POI)
- Loss of ovarian function due to chemotherapy
- Ovarian dysfunction

Contraindications for Ovarian Platelet-rich Plasma

The following are the contraindications for ovarian PRP:

- Acute infectious or systemic diseases
- Viral hepatitis B and C
- Allergic reactions to anticoagulants
- Immunosuppressive conditions
- Blood-clotting disorders
- Pregnancy and lactation
- Mental disorders
- History of oncology
- Age under 18 years

Platelet-rich Plasma Preparation Procedure

Platelet-rich plasma is prepared by a differential centrifugation process. Around 10–15 mL of venous blood is obtained by venipuncture in Acid Citrate Dextrose

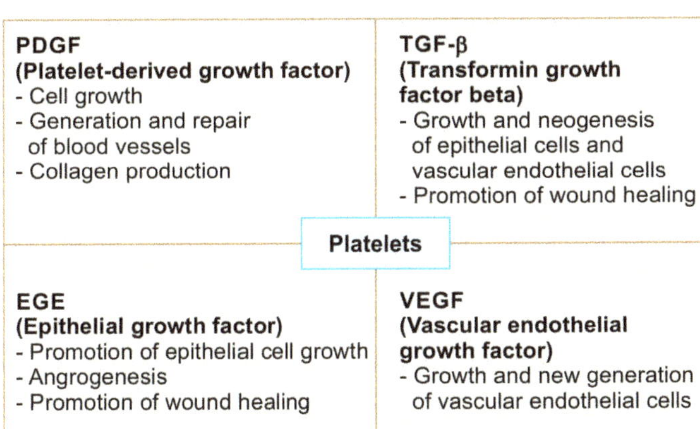

Fig. 2: Growth factors released by platelets.
Source: Annals of Burns and Fire disasters-vol. XXV-n. 4-December 2012.

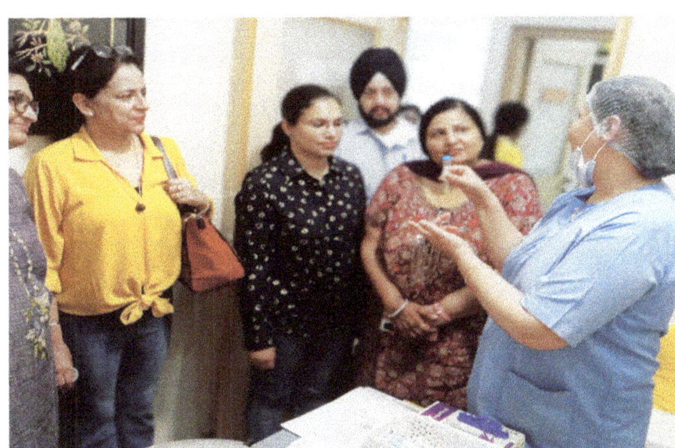

Fig. 3: Platelet-rich plasma (PRP) preparation procedure being demonstrated to the candidates for the cosmetic gynecology course organized at The Touch Clinic, Mohali.

Solution A (ACDA) prefilled syringe. The blood is not chilled at any time before or during platelet separation. The ideal temperature during centrifugation is 21–24°C. Centrifuge the blood using a "soft spin" at 1,200 rpm for 12 minutes. Three layers are formed because of its density. The bottom layer consists of RBCs, the middle layer has platelets and WBCs, and the top layer consist of platelet-poor plasma (PPP) layer. The top and middle layers are transferred to an empty sterile tube and centrifuged at a higher speed of 3,300 rpm for 7 minutes (a hard spin) to obtain platelet concentrate. The lower one third is PRP, and the upper two third is PPP. PPP is discarded, and PRP is now ready for injection **(Fig. 4)**.[11,12]

Platelet-rich Plasma Instillation Procedure

For ovarian rejuvenation, we require 4 mL (2–2 mL, each ovary), so dilution of the pellet is done accordingly. Patient is subjected to day-care total intravenous anesthesia. Once the PRP is prepared and activated, it is filled in the egg retrieval needle so as to remove any air which is present in the channel of the needle. A 17-gauge single lumen needle is usually employed, moving across from the peripheral to central part of the ovary and forth, carefully covering the distance from one side to the other. Activated PRP is then introduced via a syringe attached to the transvaginal probe transducer. Once the channel is filled with PRP and all the air is removed, a transvaginal ultrasonography (TVUS) probe is inserted in the vagina, the ovary is visualized, and the needle is inserted through the biopsy guide needle attached to the TVUS probe and then into the ovary under ultrasonography guidance. Extreme caution is exercised so as to avoid penetrating the outer wall of the ovary into the peritoneal cavity. Around 2 mL PRP is injected into each ovary at two or three sites. The duration of the intraovarian injection procedure is in the range of approximately 4–7 minutes.

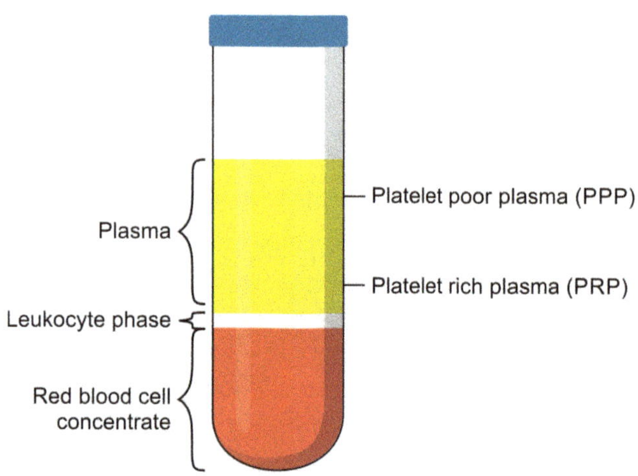

Fig. 4: Different fractions obtained after centrifugation of anticoagulated blood.

For patients whose ovaries are too small and felt inaccessible by the TVUS, a laparoscopic instillation of PRP is done into both the ovaries. For these patients, the blood is taken on admission to the hospital, after which they are prepared for and subjected to a therapeutic hysterolaparoscopy, wherein the visualization of the small ovaries becomes much easier, and the instillation of PRP is done by the egg retrieval needle inserted through the ancillary 5 mm trocar, where it can be injected at the hilum of the ovaries. The laparoscopic approach was chosen in order to get a better judgment about the instillation; it gives a precise location and the opportunity to check whether it is leaking. While performing sonography, the leakage cannot be checked, and there is difficulty in making out the hilum of the ovaries. Moreover, when done laparoscopically, identifying other factors like any deformity in the uterus or endometriosis can be checked easily **(Fig. 5)**.

Postprocedure Care

After the PRP injections, the patient is monitored for a short period to ensure that there are no immediate complications or adverse reactions.

Follow-up

Follow-up appointments help to monitor response to the treatment, assess changes in ovarian response, and evaluate the need for additional cycles of ovarian rejuvenation.

The number of sessions needed for ovarian rejuvenation therapy with PRP can vary from patient to patient. The major factors to be considered in deciding the number of sessions often depend on the patients' age, current ovarian reserve, and response to treatment. Since PRP therapy for ovarian rejuvenation is still an evolving technique, there is no standardized protocol regarding the number of sessions.

The time taken for ovarian rejuvenation therapy with PRP to start acting can vary from patient to patient, and the exact timeline is still being studied. In general, it may take several weeks for the effects of ovarian rejuvenation with PRP to become apparent. This is because the PRP is

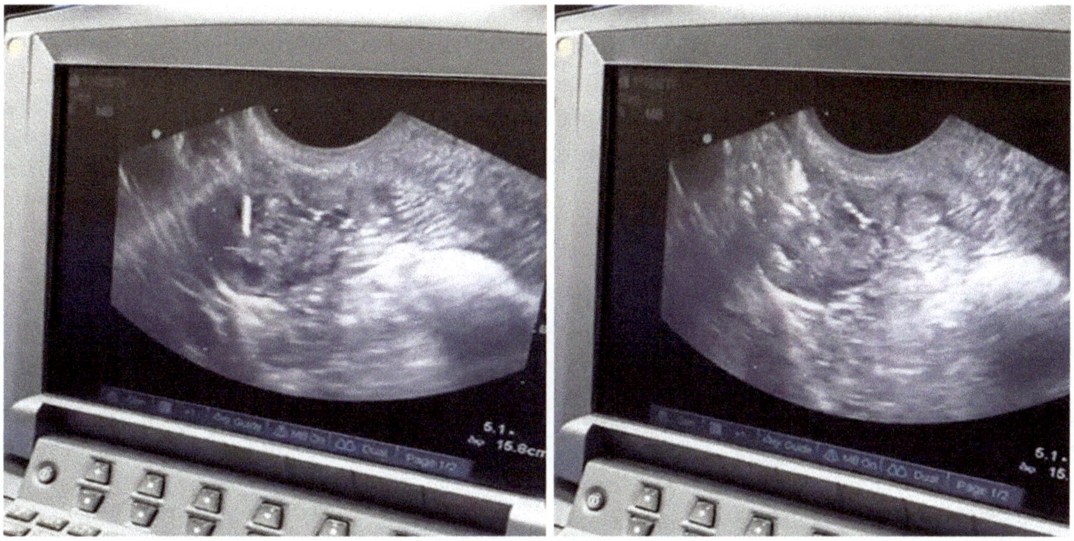

Fig. 5: Ovarian platelet-rich plasma (PRP) instillation procedure being performed at The Touch Clinic, Mohali.

intended to stimulate and regenerate ovarian tissue and ovarian germ cells, which may require time for cellular changes and tissue repair to occur.

The two tests done commonly to assess ovarian reserve are AMH and transvaginal sonography for antral follicle count. After 4–6 weeks, if ovarian rejuvenation has been effective, there will be an increase in AFC and AMH values, indicating an improvement in the ovarian reserve.

Risks and Side-effects

Ovarian PRP is a safe and minimally invasive procedure. The primary risks or side effects are minor discomfort, bruising, or spotting after the procedure. The complications, such as post-procedural pain, bleeding, and hematoma formation, are negligible. Allergies, hypersensitivity reactions, or anesthesia-related complications are rarely observed. It has been hypothesized that PRP promotes the development of isolated human primordial and primary follicles to the preantral stage.[13] Studies have revealed that autologous intraovarian infusion of PRP with a considerable amount of growth factors and cytokines has shown to enhance ovarian regeneration as well as reactivation of folliculogenesis[14] and has led to new horizons of hope in the field of reproductive gynecology.

Advantages of Platelet-rich Plasma Therapy for Ovarian Rejuvenation

- *Higher antral follicles*—chances of retrieving a larger number of mature oocytes after ovarian stimulation during an IVF cycle.
- *Higher AMH values*—chances of improving AMH values, indicative of improved ovarian reserve
- *Spontaneous resumption of menstrual cycles* in women with premature menopause.
- *Improvement in intracytoplasmic sperm injection (ICSI)/IVF cycle outcome*—in poor responders with increased number and quality of oocytes, leading to better embryos.
- *Higher number of retrieved oocytes in IVF cycle* resulting in higher and better quality of embryos in the IVF cycle.

Other Benefits of Platelet-rich Plasma

The benefits of PRP will continue to be seen as they are used in more areas of medicine for regenerative procedures.[15] PRP is a safe and effective alternative treatment modality for patients with stress urinary incontinence.[16]

Regarding the timing between ovarian rejuvenation and ovarian stimulation for IVF, there is no standard consensus or established guideline. However, at least a 6-week gap should be given between ovarian PRP injection and ovarian stimulation for IVF. Patients should take multivitamins and antioxidants during this period.

CONCLUSION

Ovarian rejuvenation by autologous intraovarian infusion of PRP can be conceived as one of the newer potential treatments or aids to partly restore the reproductive and endocrine functions of the ovary, which can help a female conceive and reproduce her own genetic offspring and avert the possibility of using a donor program for the same. Though this procedure has given us good results, multiple studies with different geographic populations and more robust data would be required to stamp an affirmative and build an overall positive consensus for this procedure.

REFERENCES

1. Leidal AM, Levine B, Debnath J. Autophagy and the cell biology of age-related disease. Nature Cell Biol. 2018;20:1338-48.
2. Hamet P, Tremblay J. Genes of aging. Metabolism. 2003;52:5-9.
3. Finch CE. The menopause and aging, a comparative perspective. J Steroid Biochem Mol Biol. 2014;142:132-41.
4. Faddy MJ. Follicle dynamics during ovarian ageing. Mol Cell Endocrinol. 2000;163:43-8.
5. Sills ES, Wood SH. Autologous activated platelet-rich plasma injection into adult human ovary tissue: molecular mechanism, analysis, and discussion of reproductive response. Biosci Rep. 2019;39(6):20190805.
6. Dhurat R, Sukesh MS. Principles and methods of preparation of platelet-rich plasma: a review and author's perspective. J Cutan Aesthet Surg. 2014;7:189-97.
7. Pavlovic V, Ciric M, Jovanovic V, Stojanovic P. Platelet rich plasma: a short overview of certain bioactive components. Open Med (Wars). 2016;11(1):242-47.
8. Marx RE. Platelet-rich plasma (PRP): What is PRP and what is not PRP? Implant Dent. 2001;10(4):225-8.
9. Seckin S, Ramadan H, Mouanness M, Kohansieh M, Merhi Z. Ovarian response to intraovarian platelet-rich plasma (PRP) administration: hypotheses and potential mechanisms of action. J Assist Reprod Genet. 2022;39(1):37-61.
10. Sills ES, Rickers NS, Li X, Palermo GD. First data on in vitro fertilization and blastocyst formation after intraovarian injection of calcium gluconate-activated autologous platelet rich plasma. Gynecol Endocrinol. 2018;34(9):756-60.
11. Everts PA, Mahoney CB, Hoffmann JJ, Schönberger JP, Box HA, Zundert A, et al. Platelet-rich plasma preparation using three devices: implications for platelet activation and platelet growth factor release. Growth Factors. 2006;24(3):165-71.
12. Sfakianoudis K, Simopoulou M, Nitsos N, Rapani A, Pantou A, Vaxevanoglou T, et al. A case series on platelet-rich plasma revolutionary management of poor responder patients. Gynecol Obstet Invest. 2019;84(1):99-106.
13. Hosseini L, Shirazi A, Naderi MM, Shams-Esfandabadi N, Boroujeni SB, Sarvari A, et al. Platelet-rich plasma promotes the development of isolated human primordial and primary follicles to the preantral stage. Reprod BioMed Online. 2017;35(4):343-50.
14. Anitua E, Andia I, Ardanza B, Nurden P, Nurden AT. Autologous platelets as a source of proteins for healing and tissue regeneration. Thromb Haemost. 2004;91(01):4-15.
15. Jindal P, Malhotra N, Joshi S (Eds). Aesthetic and Regenerative Gynaecology, 1st edition. USA: Springer; 2022.
16. Jindal P, Sahdev S, Gulati R, Kundal I. Non surgical management of stress urinary incontinence (SUI). Acta Sci Women's Health. 2020;2(11):51-4.

CHAPTER 23

Dermatological Changes in Pregnancy

Nutan Upadhaya

INTRODUCTION

The skin, hair, and nails may undergo many changes in a woman during the entire duration of pregnancy, some of which can persist postpartum. Pregnancy can also have profound effects on preexisting maternal and skin diseases. Hence, diagnosis counseling and management of dermatological changes in pregnancy are of utmost importance.

ENDOCRINE CHANGES IN PREGNANCY

With the establishment of pregnancy, corpus luteum is rescued by human chorionic gonadotropin (hCG) produced by the trophoblast of the developing gestation sac. By the seventh to eighth week of pregnancy, the placenta takes over (luteal to placental shift) and starts producing other hormones such as human placental lactogen (HPL) and relaxin. Other important endocrine alterations are increases in adrenocorticotropic hormone (ACTH) (which causes a rise in free serum cortisol's), prolactin, antidiuretic hormone (ADH), and thyroid hormones (in the first trimester).

IMMUNOLOGICAL CHANGES IN PREGNANCY

Maternal tolerance to the fetus is a result of various immunologic mechanisms, including the hormone-meditated suppression of immune response to the maternal-fetal barrier; the lack of expression of human leukocyte antigen (HLA) class II, and the expression of HLA-G by the trophoblast.

Another important immunologic change is the shift in Th1 to Th2 cytokine production that results from an interplay between hormones and the immune system; skin diseases that are Th2-mediated, such as autoimmune disorders and atopic dermatitis (AD), tend to exacerbate, whereas Th1-mediated processes, such as psoriasis and rheumatoid arthritis tend to improve during gestation.

VARIETY OF PHYSIOLOGICAL SKIN CHANGES SEEN IN PREGNANCY

Pigmentary Changes

Pigmentary changes can be seen in up to 90% of pregnant women:

- Hyperpigmentation and melasma are the most common pigmentary changes. Hyperpigmentation may manifest as an accentuation of naturally pigmented areas such as the nipples, areolae, genital skin, axillae, and inner thighs. There may be the pigmentation of nonpigmented skin such as Linea nigra, which results from the pigmentation of Linea alba. There may be generalized hypermelanosis or vulvar melanosis, the presence of pigmented macules on the vulvar mucosa.
  The physiology of hyperpigmentation may be related to elevated serum levels of melanocyte-stimulating hormone, estrogen, and possibly progesterone. Pigmentation typically normalizes in the postpartum period.
- Melasma-chloasma or mask of pregnancy is a hypermelanosis that presents with light to dark brown symmetric patches most commonly located on the face. It varies among different races and populations (75% in Caucasian, 31% in Asian population).[1] Melasma is classified by distribution—centrofacial, malar, mandibular, or by depth of pigment—predominantly epidermal versus predominantly dermal but a combination of types may occur.
- Pigmentation of scars and benign skin lesions
- Darkening of preexisting pigmentation
- Less common pigmentary changes such as pseudoacanthosis nigricans, dermal melanocytosis, pigmentary demarcation lines, idiopathic eruptive macular pigmentation, and nevoid hyperkeratosis of the nipple and/or areola.
- *Postinflammatory hyperpigmentation (PIH):* Inflammatory dermatoses occurring in pregnancy,

such as the polymorphic eruption of pregnancy, pemphigoid gestations, impetigo herpetiformis, AD, and others, may cause PIH. In some instances, hypopigmentation rather than hyperpigmentation follows the inflammatory process.

- *Jaundice:* Yellowish discoloration of the skin, conjunctiva, and mucous membranes due to hyperbilirubinemia may be seen in cholestasis of pregnancy, acute fatty liver of pregnancy, preeclampsia-associated hemolysis, elevated liver enzymes, low platelet count (HELLP) syndrome, hepatitis, and other liver diseases. Treatment of the underlying cause of jaundice resolves the yellow discoloration of the skin.

Treatment of Pigmentary Changes

Although the pigmentary changes cannot be totally prevented, good skin care can to some extent help in minimizing the pigmentary changes in pregnant women.

Melasma Management

- Protection from ultraviolet (UV) and visible light by application of a broad-spectrum sunscreen in pregnancy.
- Permanent treatment measures are delayed till postpartum preferably 6 months.
- Treatment depends on the depth of melanin pigment deposition.
- Topical applications work by inhibiting tyrosinase enzyme, leading to decreased production of melanin.
- Triple combination is preferred in topical medication for melasma. Hydroquinone is the current standard[2,3] in melasma treatment and is often combined with a topical retinoid and a mild topical steroid. But its used is deferred to postpartum period.
- Azelaic acid and kojic acid[4,5] are used in mild melasma and are safer in pregnant and nursing mothers.

Procedures for postpartum melasma treatment can be grouped into three categories:

1. *Chemical peels:* Glycolic acid, salicylic acid, trichloroacetic acid, and amino fruit acid promote exfoliation of stratum corneum and dispersion of melanin pigment. All common treatments of pigmentation usually work in one or more of the following ways:
   - The reduction of melanin synthesis (often through the inhibition of tyrosinase)
   - The increase of melanin transfer and shedding
   - Skin resurfacing and pigment-selective lasers

   The chemical peels carry the risk of PIH or hypopigmentation.
2. Types of lasers used for melasma treatment:
   - *Ablative:* Ablative skin resurfacing:
     - CO_2[6,7]
     - Erbium[8]
   - *Q-switched:* Disrupts pigment using short pulse, high power delivery:
     - Alexandrite[6,7]
     - Neodymium-doped:yttrium aluminum garnet (Nd:YAG)[9]
   - *Fractionated:*[10] Produces microscopic areas of thermal necrosis
3. Other devices, e.g., intense pulsed light,[11] which converts light energy to heat energy and destroys melanin.

Counseling in melasma treatment is very important as patients need to be aligned about the need for multiple sessions, the high rate of recurrence, and the importance of using sunscreen skin applications regularly. Triple combination skin application should be continued with laser and other device treatments.

VASCULAR CHANGES

Vascular changes have been reported as being more common in Caucasian (83%)[12] than in Indians (26%),[1] Pakistani (34%),[13] and African American pregnant women.[14] They occur secondarily to the production of placental hormones, such as hCG, ACTH-like substances, and thyrotropin-releasing hormone (TRH) as well as maternal hormones. Plasma volume increases to 149% of normal levels by the end of gestation and blood flow to the skin increases 4–16 times in the first 2 months of pregnancy and doubles again during the third month.[15]

Vascular changes occur as early as the fourth week of pregnancy with increased vascularity and softening of the vaginal portion of the cervical mucosa.

Patients often develop spider angiomas and other vascular proliferations, palmar erythema, edema of the extremities and face, venous abnormalities such as varicose veins and hemorrhoids, gingival edema/hyperemia, and occasionally pyogenic granulomas.[16]

Vasomotor instabilities present as purpura and petechiae over the lower extremities. Cutis marmorata is a transient bluish mottling of the skin on cold exposure.

Granuloma gravidarum is a pedunculated vascular growth that arises from the gingiva in approximately 2% of patients; it can ulcerate, cause pain, bleed profusely, and interfere with eating, thus necessitating removal.

Management

Most vascular changes fade or resolve spontaneously postpartum. Most of the vascular changes can be managed by a conservative approach and reassurance to the patient. Definitive treatment of vascular problems with pulsed dye laser,[4,17-19] intense pulsed light,[5] electrodessication,[20,21] cryosurgery,[22,] etc., is done 6 months postpartum.

CONNECTIVE TISSUE CHANGES

Nearly 65% of pregnant patients develop connective tissue changes such as striae gravidarum (SG), skin tags, keloids, and hypertrophic scars.

Striae Gravidarum

Striae gravidarum or linear gravidarum are atrophic scars of the dermis that appear during pregnancies in 50–90% of cases **(Fig. 1)**.[1,23,24] SG can appear in primigravidas; they may also develop for the first time in subsequent pregnancies. In 43% of women, SG may appear prior to 24 weeks of gestation.[1,23,25] SG occur mainly on the abdomen, especially the lower half (92.7% of cases) and breasts but may also occur on the upper arms, lower back, hips, buttocks, inguinal regions, and thighs.[1] Initially SG are flat pink and red striae rubra and later they fade to become striae alba (mature striae). SG may cause symptoms such as pruritus, burning, and discomfort. SG are influenced by maternal and family history, race, ethnicity, genetics, and lifestyle factors.[23-29]

Management of Striae Gravidarum

- Striae gravidarum can to some extent be prevented by using Trofolastin[20] cream and verum[20] ointment and massage during pregnancy.
- Postpartum management of SG includes:
  - Application of creams with tretinoin and glycolic acid peels
  - Microdermabrasion using radiofrequency and UV light
  - Ablative and nonablative lasers.

Skin Laxity

Excessive skin laxity in the abdominal and flank skin is common.

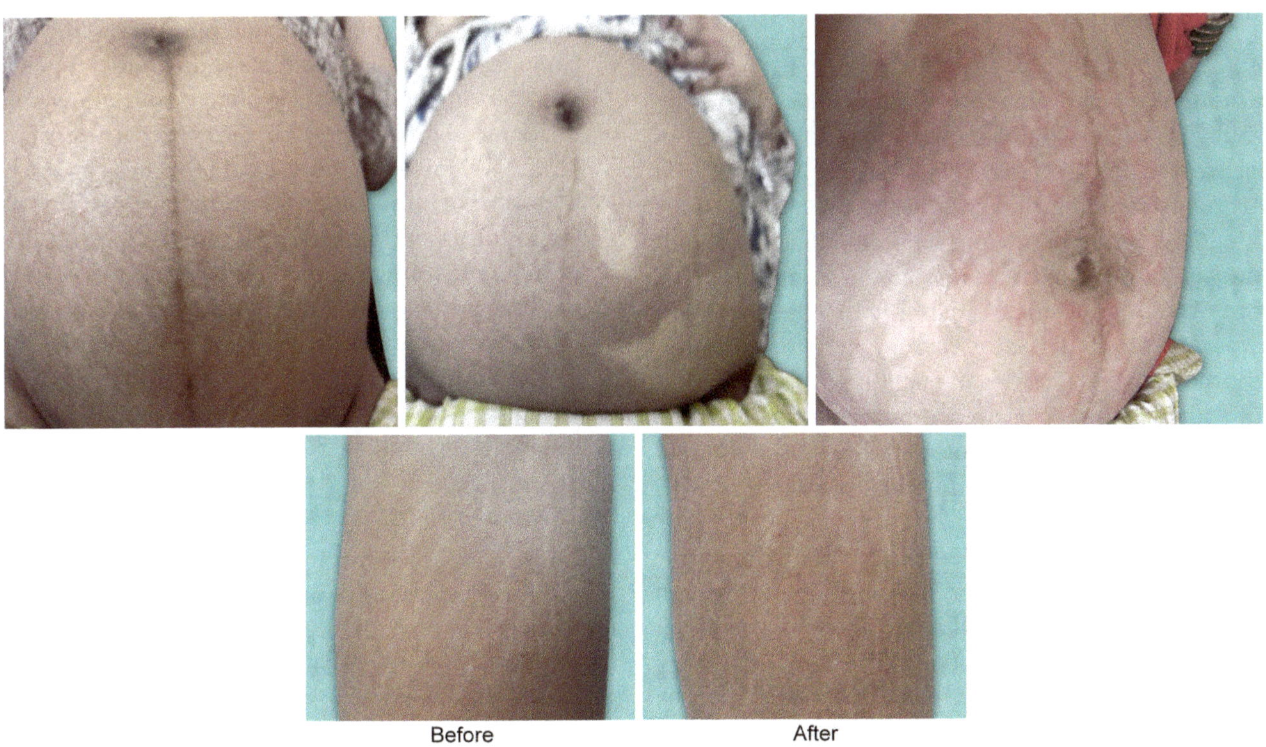

Fig. 1: Various presentations of striae gravidarum in pregnancy.

Skin laxity and localized fat deposition can be treated postpartum by noninvasive body contouring,[30] using monopolar/bipolar radiofrequency or combination treatment with infrared light, vacuum, and mechanical massage. Surgical options are liposuction, abdominoplasty, and brachioplasty.[31]

Mommy Makeover

Possible procedures in a mommy makeover include breast augmentation, breast lift, buttock augmentation, labiaplasty, liposuction, and tummy tuck.

- Molluscum gravidarum are the skin tags, which usually appear in the second or third trimesters. Treatment is scissor excision, electrodessication, radiofrequency, and cryosurgery.
- Pregnancy-associated hyperkeratosis of the nipple has been recently reported,[32] which is typically bilateral, can be symptomatic, and commonly persists postpartum, when it can be treated by using tretinoin cream application, emollients, or surgical curettage.
- Hypertrophic scars and keloids are more common in pregnancy. Wound healing is altered in pregnancy. There is a higher incidence of keloids in pregnancy as the hormonal changes and neoangiogenesis[33] may cause abnormal wound healing.

Prevention of Hypertrophic Scars and Keloids

- Although hypertrophic scars and keloids cannot be wholly prevented, there are ways to reduce the risk of occurrence. In pregnancy-related surgery, the surgical technique should be atraumatic and precise; incisions should follow skin lines and be perpendicular to joint surfaces in order to decrease wound tension.
- Hemostasis and closure using skin edge eversion are warranted. It has been reported that women who underwent a cesarean section with absorbable subcuticular stitch closure had better cosmetic results and less pain at 6 weeks compared to surgical staple closure, although the latter was associated with decreased operating times.
- Infections should be avoided at all costs, and proper wound care and debridement should be performed. After wound closure, avoiding tension and stretching of the areas should be practiced. The use of massage, greasy ointments, and occlusive materials such as bandages, compressive garments, silicone gel sheeting, and taping may be used.
- Obesity is a risk factor for complicated wound infections after a cesarean section. To minimize risk, there is some evidence to support the use of prophylactic antibiotics, the closure of any subcutaneous space over 2 cm, and the maintenance of procedural normothermia. Primary or secondary wound closure is encouraged over healing by a secondary intention.

Treatment of Keloids and Hypertrophic Scars

- Simple excision and primary closure of the scar
- Intralesional application of triamcinolone acetate may be done after surgical excision of keloids and hypertrophic scars. These may require repeated injections of triamcinolone acetate and the wound side.
- Daily topical silicone gel sheeting over the scar for 2 or more months
- Pressure therapy daily for 6 months
- Postexcisional radiation or laser therapy
- Use of pulsed dye, fractional or erbium:yttrium aluminum garnet (Er:YAG) laser over the scar.

HAIR AND NAIL CHANGES

- Hair cycle changes include an increase in anagen and thick hairs of the scalp, the former possibly related to the prolongation of the anagen phase.
- Changes in hair growth during pregnancy have been reported in 2.6–12.8% of patients, with many women noticing vigorous growth and thickening of scalp hair.[1,13,34] However, diffuse hair thinning and a male pattern-like hair loss (frontoparietal recession) in the later months of pregnancy have been reported.
- Mild hirsutism is observed in the majority of pregnant patients and is expected to improve or resolve within 6 months postpartum; if hirsutism is severe and/or in an abnormal distribution, polycystic ovary disease, androgen-secreting tumors of the ovary, luteomas, and lutein cysts should be ruled out.

Treatment of Hirsutism

- Counsel about the transient nature and postpartum improvement/resolution
- Search for other etiologies, such as polycystic ovary syndrome, androgen-secreting tumors, luteomas, and lutein cysts in cases of severe hirsutism
- Delay postpartum treatment for 6 months, because fine hair is expected to resolve spontaneously

- Consider hair removal postpartum for persistent terminal hairs by lasers or electrolysis
- Telogen effluvium occurs as a significant percentage of anagen hairs convert to telogen at or immediately after delivery and usually resolves spontaneously within 15 months postpartum; hair regrowth may not be complete, especially in cases with concomitant pattern hair loss.

Treatment of Telogen Effluvium (Telogen Gravidarum)

Patients should be counseled about the transient nature and postpartum improvement/resolution of the condition. We can consider postpartum treatment, such as topical minoxidil, in patients with concomitant male pattern hair loss. Mesotherapy using platelet-rich plasma (PRP) or various prepared solutions is also becoming popular in the postpartum period. If the above treatment options fail, the patient may need a hair transplant.

Nail changes are noticed in 0.66–2.1% of patients[1,13] and resolve postpartum; they include faster growth, softening, transverse grooving, brittleness, distal onycholysis, and subungual hyperkeratosis; longitudinal melanonychia with onset in gestation has been reported. Nail changes improve postpartum and no specific treatment is usually required. The use of solvent-based nail products should be reduced and nails should be kept short. The use of moisturizer on nails and cuticles may be helpful.

GLANDULAR CHANGES

During pregnancy, there are changes in the functions of eccrine, apocrine, and sebaceous glands. Glandular changes may occur in up to 36% of pregnant patients.[30,34]

Breast changes during pregnancy include enlargement, tenderness, nipple erection, secondary areolae, and hypertrophy of the areolar sebaceous glands. Eccrine sweating tends to increase, particularly in the last trimester of pregnancy, which can result in an increased incidence of hyperhidrosis and miliaria, both of which require wearing of light clothes and better personal hygiene.

Acne vulgaris runs a variable course in pregnancy. In one study, pregnancy affected acne in approximately 70% of women, with 41% reporting improvement and 29% reporting worsening in pregnancy.[31]

Treatment requires better skin care with liquid cleansers. In mild cases, topical applications using antibiotics such as erythromycin, clindamycin, and azelaic acid; dapsone and benzoyl peroxide (not recommended in pregnancy category C). Oral antibiotics may be needed for moderate to severe acne. Postdelivery α-hydroxy acid peels, microdermabrasion, narrowband UVB, laser, or intense pulsed light therapy may be used.[35]

Acne rosacea is a chronic inflammatory disease that primarily affects pilosebaceous units and blood vessels of the face. In management apart from the treatments used in acne vulgaris, corticosteroids may be required for severe flares.

Perioral dermatosis is a common dermatosis in which there are erythematous, variably scaly papulopustules around the mouth, chin, and upper lip. It may require treatment similar to acne vulgaris.

Hidradenitis suppurativa (HS) is a chronic, relapsing, inflammatory skin disease that affects intertriginous areas, especially the axillary and anogenital regions.[36] Management requires cessation of smoking and wearing loose clothes. Topical or oral antibiotics may be required. In severe cases, intralesional steroids[37] or surgical modalities[38] may be needed.

Inflammatory skin disease can worsen or, less often, improve during gestation.[39] Diseases that may develop and/or often worsen in gestation include AD, urticarias, and erythema annulare centrifugum (EAC).[39-41] Chronic plaque psoriasis may improve in pregnancy, whereas generalized pustular psoriasis (impetigo herpetiformis) can be triggered by pregnancy.

Dermatosis of Pregnancy

Most of the skin changes in pregnancy as mentioned above may be physiological. However, some dermatoses are specific to pregnancy, while others are altered by pregnancy. These changes occur as a result of an interaction of multiple factors in the body during pregnancy. The dermatoses which are specific to pregnancy include gestational pemphigoid (also known as pemphigoid gestationis), pruritic and urticarial papules and plaques of pregnancy (PUPPP, also known as pruritic eruption of pregnancy and toxemic rash of pregnancy), intrahepatic cholestasis of pregnancy, and impetigo herpetiformis. Atopic eruption of pregnancy encompasses atopic eczema in pregnancy, prurigo of pregnancy, as well as pruritic folliculitis of pregnancy as in earlier classifications.[42]

Skin Surgery in Pregnancy

- A biopsy of suspicious lesions should not be delayed because of pregnancy.

- Defer nonessential surgical procedures until at least the second trimester or postpartum.
- Minimize radiation exposure, especially in the first trimester.
- Use of pregnancy category B medications, such as lidocaine and penicillin family antibiotics, is recommended.
- Position the patient in left lateral decubitus position to prevent aortocaval compression syndrome.
- The removal of benign lesions, such as nevi, skin tags, and seborrheic keratoses, for cosmetic or medical reasons, using procedures such as shaving, electro-dessication, cryotherapy, and radiosurgery, is safe in pregnancy.
- Laser treatments for symptomatic lesions, such as granuloma gravidarum, and genital warts can be performed with standard safety precautions.
- Only procedures which are safe and necessary should be carried out in pregnant woman.
- Electrocautery, radiofrequency, cryotherapy, and laser for warts, particularly genital, surgical interventions for skin malignancies, and other small growths should be performed.
- Safe but cautions outlook is required for intralesional steroid injections, aesthetic procedures such as chemical peeling, botulinum toxin, microdermabrasion, and biopsies for questionable lesions.
- Absolutely contraindicated procedures include fillers, sclerotherapy, and liposuction.

CONCLUSION

The profound endocrine, immunologic, vascular and metabolic alterations occurring during pregnancy cause wide spectrum of physiological changes on the skin of the pregnant woman. Pigmentary changes are the commonest occurring in about 90% of pregnant women followed by connective tissue changes commoner in Indian women and vascular changes commoner in Caucasian women. Glandular, hair and nail changes are also seen in lesser proportion of pregnant women. A variety of treatment options are now available for addressing the persistent postpartum pigmentary, connective tissue, hair and other skin changes. The treating clinicians should be well aware of various available treatment options so that patient can be counselled and referred to the treating specialists accordingly.

REFERENCES

1. Rathore SP, Gupta S, Gupta V. Pattern and prevalence of physiological cutaneous changes in pregnancy: a study of 2000 ante-natal women. Indian J Dermatol Venereol Leprol. 2011;77(3):402.
2. Arefiev KLB, Hantash BM. Advances in the treatment of melasma: a review of the recent literature. Derm Surg. 2012;38:971-84.
3. Haddad AL, Matos LF, Brunstein F, Ferreira LM, Silva A, Costa Jr D. A clinical, prospective, randomized, double-blind trial comparing skin whitening complex with hydroquinone vs. placebo in the treatment of melasma. Int J Dermatol. 2003;42:153-6.
4. Scheepers J, Quaba A. Treatment of nevi aranei with the pulsed tunable dye laser at 585 nm. J Pediatr Surg. 1995;30:101-4.
5. Schroeter C, Neumann H. An intense light source. The photoderm VL-flashlamp as a new treatment possibility for vascular skin lesions. Dermatol Surg. 1998;24:743-8.
6. Goldman MP, Gold MH, Palm MD, Colón LE, Preston N, Johnson LA, et al. Sequential treatment with a triple combination cream and intense pulsed light is more efficacious than sequential treatment with an inactive (control) cream and intense pulsed light in patients with moderate to severe melasma. Dermatol Surg. 2011;37:224-33.
7. Kunachak S, Leelaudomlipi P, Wongwaisayawan S. Dermabrasion: a curative treatment for melasma. Aesthetic Plast Surg. 2001;25:114-7.
8. Kauvar AN. Successful treatment of melasma using a combination of microdermabrasion and Q-switched Nd:YAG lasers. Lasers Surg Med. 2012;44:117-24.
9. Snell RS, Bischitz PG. The effect of large doses of estrogen and estrogen and progesterone on melanin pigmentation. J Invest Dermatol. 1960;35:73-82.
10. Kroumpouzos G, Avgerinou G, Granter SR. Acanthosis nigricans without diabetes during pregnancy. Br J Dermatol. 2002;146:925-8.
11. Stone OJ. Acanthosis nigricans-decreased extracellular matrix viscosity: cancer, obesity, diabetes, corticosteroids, somatotrophin. Med Hypotheses. 1993;40:154-7.
12. Estève E, Saudeau L, Pierre F, Barruet K, Vaillant L, Lorette G. Physiological cutaneous signs in normal pregnancy: a study of 60 pregnant women. Ann Dermatol Venereol. 1994;121:227-31.
13. Muzaffar F, Hussain I, Haroon TS. Physiologic skin changes during pregnancy: a study of 140 cases. Int J Dermatol. 1998;37:429-31.
14. Bean W, Cogswell R, Dexter M. Vascular changes of the skin in pregnancy: vascular spiders and palmar erythema. Surg Gynecol Obstet. 1949;88:739-52.

15. Papoutsis J, Kroumpouzos G. Dermatologic disorders. In: Gabbe SG, Niebyl JR, Simpson JL (Eds). Obstetrics: Normal and Problem Pregnancies, 5th edition. Churchill Livingstone: Elsevier; 2007. pp. 1178-92.
16. Murad M, Coto-Yglesias F, Zumaeta-Garcia M. A systematic review and meta-analysis of the treatments of varicose veins. J Vasc Surg. 2011;53:49S-65S.
17. Polla L, Tan Q, Garden J. Tunable pulsed dye laser for the treatment of benign cutaneous vascular ectasia. Dermatologica. 1987;174:11-7.
18. Geronemus R. Treatment of spider telangiectasias in children using the flashlamp-pumped pulsed dye laser. Pediatr Dermatol. 1991;8:61-3.
19. Tan E, Vinciullo C. Pulsed dye laser treatment of spider treatment of spider telangiectasia. Austral J Dermatol. 1997;38:22-5.
20. Robinson J. Electrodessication of nevi aranei ("spiders") and senile angiomas. J Dermatol Surg Oncol. 1980;6: 794-5.
21. Henry F, Quatresooz P, Valverde-Lopez J. Blood vessel changes during pregnancy: a review. Am J Clin Dermatol. 2006;7:65-9.
22. Thai K, Sinclair R. Cryotherapy of benign skin lesions. Australian J Dermatol. 1999;40:175-84.
23. Ghasemi A, Gorouhi F, Rashighi-Firoozabadi M, Jafarian A, Firooz A. Striae gravidarum: associated factors. J Eur Acad Dermatol Venereol. 2007;21:743-6.
24. Murphy KW, Dunphy B, O'Herlihy C. Increased maternal age protects against striae gravidarum. J Obstet Gynecol. 1992;12:297-300.
25. Chang AL, Agredano YZ, Kimball AB. Risk factors associated with striae gravidarum. J Am Acad Dermatol. 2004;51:881-5.
26. Atwal GS, Manku LK, Griffiths CE, Polson DW. Striae gravidarum in primiparae. Br J Dematol. 2006;155: 965-9.
27. Kelekci KH, Kelekci S, Destegul E, Aksoy A, Sut N, Yilmaz B. Prematurity: is it a risk factor for striae distensae? Int J Dermatol. 2011;50:1240-5.
28. J-Orth R, Titapant V, Chuenwattana P, Tontisirin P. Prevalence and associate factors for striae gravidarum. J Med Assoc Thai. 2008;91:445-51.
29. Kluger N. Body art and pregnancy. Eur J Obstet Gynecol Reprod Biol. 2010;153:3-7.
30. Rathore SP, Gupta S, Gupta V. Pattern and prevalence of physiological cutaneous changes in pregnancy: a study of 2000 antenatal women. Indian J Dermatol Venereol Leprol. 2011;77:402.
31. Shaw JC, White LE. Persistent acne in adult women. Arch Dermatol. 2001;137:1252-3.
32. Higgins HW, Jenkins J, Horn TD, Kroumpouzos G. Pregnancy-associated hyperkeratosis of the nipple: a report of 25 cases. JAMA Dermatol. 2013;149:722-6.
33. Oluwasanmi JO. Keloids in the African. Clin Plast Surg. 1974;1:179-95.
34. Kumari R, Jaisankar TJ, Thappa DM. A clinical study of skin changes in pregnancy. Indian J Dermatol Venereol Leprol. 2007;73:141.
35. Zeichner JA. Narrowband UV-B phkototherapy for the treatment of acne vulgaris during pregnancy. Arch Dermatol. 2011;147:537-9.
36. Yu CC, Cook MG. Hindradenitis suppurativa: a disease of follicular epithelium, rather than apocrine glands. Br J Dermatol. 1990;122:763-9.
37. Alikhan A, Lynch PJ, Eisen DB. Hidradenitis suppurativa: a comprehensive review. J Am Acad Dermatol. 2009; 60:539-61.
38. Yazdanyar S, Jemec GBE. Hidradenitis suppurative: a review of cause and treatment. Curr Opin Infect Dis. 2011; 24(2):118-23.
39. Kroumpouzos G, Cohen LM. Dermatoses of pregnancy. J Am Acad Dermatol. 2001;45:1-19.
40. Koutroulis I, Papoutsis J, Kroumpouzos G. Atopic dermatitis in pregnancy: current status and challenges. Obstet Gynecol Surv. 2011;66:654-63.
41. Rosina P, D'Onghia FS, Barba A. Erythema annulare centrifugum and pregnancy. Int J Dermatol. 2002;41:516-7.
42. Kurien G, Badri T. Dermatoses of Pregnancy. Treasure Island: StatPearls Publishing; 2023.

CHAPTER 24

Sexual Pain in Women

Anita Shyam, AV Raveendran, Avinash Desousa

INTRODUCTION

Pain is defined as an "unpleasant sensory and emotional experience associated with, or resembling that associated with, actual or potential tissue damage."[1] Pain that persists or recurs for longer than 3 months is considered chronic pain.[2] Pain is influenced by varying degrees of biological, psychological, and social factors. Pain causes unpleasant consequences. Sex is an important component of any successful, happy, intimate relationship and it improves intimacy and has a positive effect on physical and psychological well-being. But when sex is painful, women will try to avoid sexual contact and it reduces sexual interest, arousal, and sexual pleasure and causes negative psychological impact. In this chapter, we briefly describe various conditions that can cause pain associated with sexual activity in women.

DEFINITIONS

The common condition described as sexual pain in women includes dyspareunia and vaginismus. Dyspareunia is defined as a recurrent and/or persistent genital pain (GP) associated with sexual intercourse causing marked distress or interpersonal difficulty.[3] Dyspareunia or painful intercourse is an underreported sexual problem among women. Pain can be localized to the vulva or vaginal entrance (i.e., superficial dyspareunia) or inside the vagina or lower pelvis (i.e., deep dyspareunia—usually associated with deep penetration). Dyspareunia is a provoked pain.

Vulvodynia is defined as persistent vulvar pain lasting longer than 3 months where there is no recognizable organic cause of the disease and with several potential associated factors.[4] In other words, vulvodynia is a chronic GP disorder localized to the vulva and vaginal introitus; which occurs with or without provocation. Diagnosis of vulvodynia is a diagnosis of exclusion. Vulvodynia can be generalized or localized, provoked or unprovoked, primary, or secondary. Depending upon the pain character it can be intermittent, persistent, or constant and depending upon the onset it can be immediate or delayed.[5] Rule out other infections, and inflammatory, neurologic, traumatic, or hormonal problems producing vulvar pain before making a diagnosis of vulvodynia.

Vaginismus is defined as "a recurrent or persistent involuntary spasm of the musculature of the outer third of the vagina, which interferes with coitus and causes distress and interpersonal difficulty."[6] The sexual pain disorders previously differentiated as dyspareunia and vaginismus are merged into a single entity as genito-pelvic pain/penetration disorder (GPPPD) in the latest DSM-5 classification.[7]

DSM-5 DIAGNOSTIC CRITERIA FOR GENITO-PELVIC PAIN/PENETRATION DISORDER[7]

"Genito-pelvic pain/penetration disorder is characterized by persistent or recurrent difficulties with one (or more) of the following:

A. *Persistent or recurrent difficulties with one (or more) of the following:*
   - *Vaginal penetration during intercourse.*
   - *Marked vulvovaginal or pelvic pain during vaginal intercourse or penetration attempts.*
   - *Marked fear or anxiety about vulvovaginal or pelvic pain in anticipation of, during, or because of vaginal penetration.*
   - *Marked tensing or tightening of the pelvic floor muscles during attempted vaginal penetration.*

B. *The symptoms in criterion A have persisted for a minimum duration of approximately 6 months.*

C. *The symptoms in criterion A cause clinically significant distress in the individual.*

D. *The sexual dysfunction is not better explained by a nonsexual mental disorder or because of severe relationship distress (e.g., partner violence) or other significant stressors and is not attributable to the effects of a substance/medication or another medical condition."*

Almost 50% of women with GPPPD have other pain disorders such as fibromyalgia, irritable bowel syndrome, or interstitial cystitis.[8]

PREVALENCE OF FEMALE SEXUAL PAIN

The occurrence of dyspareunia ranges widely, spanning from 1.2 to 56%, although most studies indicate a prevalence of 10–20%.[9] Vulvodynia is reported to have a prevalence between 3 and 7%. GPPPD affects approximately 14–34% of premenopausal women and 6.5–45% of postmenopausal women.[10]

CLASSIFICATIONS OF SEXUAL PAIN IN FEMALES

- Genito-pelvic pain/penetration disorder:
  - *Dyspareunia:* (a) Superficial dyspareunia and (b) Deep dyspareunia
  - *Vaginismus:* (a) Primary vaginismus and (b) Secondary vaginismus
- Nonsexual pain disorder

Introital Dyspareunia

Introital dyspareunia refers to discomfort experienced during vaginal penetration and intercourse, which can stem from factors such as insufficient arousal, mild vaginismus, conditions such as vulvar vestibulitis or vulvar dystrophy, discomfort resulting from certain vulvar treatments, perineal surgeries (such as episiotomy or colporrhaphy), pudendal nerve entrapment syndrome or pudendal neuralgia, as well as Sjögren's syndrome.[11]

Deep Vaginal Pain

The primary causes of deep vaginal pain often include endometriosis and pelvic inflammatory disease (PID), with less common culprits being pelvic radiotherapy or radical vaginal surgery. Additionally, varicocele, adhesions, abdominal muscle referred pain, and abdominal cutaneous nerve entrapment syndrome should also be taken into account during the diagnostic process.[12]

Midvaginal Pain

Midvaginal pain, as outlined by Binik et al. (1999),[13] presents with different characteristics:

Lateral pain: Typically attributed to levator ani myalgia, early identification of pelvic floor hyperactivity in adolescents might mitigate the risk of developing vulvodynia and dyspareunia later in life.

Anterior pain: This type of pain is linked to urological issues including bladder and urethral damage related to postcoital cystitis, recurring cystitis, symptoms of an irritable bladder such as frequency, urgency, and urge incontinence, and instances where pelvic floor contractions may be prompted to reinforce bladder control.

Posterior pain: This category of pain is associated with anorectal issues such as anismus, hemorrhoids, and constipation.

Classification of Vaginismus[14]

Lamont categorized vaginismus in 4° depending upon severity, the fifth degree was later added by Pacik.[15] They are as following:

- *First degree:* The contraction of the pelvic floor muscles, specifically the levator ani, relaxes upon reassurance from the physician, enabling them to carry out the examination fully.
- *Second degree:* Persistent and widespread pelvic floor muscle spasm persists despite reassurance, resulting in an inability to relax for the examination.
- *Third degree:* The patient experiences severe pelvic floor muscle spasms, leading her to involuntarily raise her buttocks in an attempt to evade the examination.
- *Fourth degree:* The most severe manifestation of vaginismus results in mild to moderate neurovegetative arousal, accompanied by spasms of the levator ani muscles, dorsal arching, adduction of the thighs, and defensive retraction to prevent examination.
- *Fifth degree (by Pacik):* Extreme defense and profound visceral reaction, along with severe neurovegetative arousal, patients may exhibit refusal of gynecological examination, characterized by increased heart rate, palpitations, hyperventilation, trembling, shaking, nausea or vomiting, uncontrollable crying, dizziness, fainting sensation, an urge to flee the examination table, escape the situation, or even display aggressive behavior toward the doctor.[15]

ETIOLOGY

Differentiating dyspareunia as superficial and deep dyspareunia helps to narrow down the etiological diagnosis. Common causes of dyspareunia are given in **Table 1**.

TABLE 1: Causes of dyspareunia.

Superficial dyspareunia	***Deep dyspareunia***
• Provoked vulvodynia • Genitourinary syndrome of menopause • Dermatologic disorders (e.g., lichen sclerosis, vulvar dystrophies) • Congenital malformations • Genital herpes simplex • Vaginitis • Bartholin gland abscess • Radiation fibrosis • Postsurgical introital narrowing • Recurrent tearing of the posterior fourchette • Large labia minora • Size of the penis • Hymenal remnants • Episiotomy/rupture/neuritis	• Pelvic floor muscle hypertonicity • Uterine or ovarian disorders • Fibroids • Chronic pelvic inflammatory disease • Endometriosis • Adnexal pathology • Urethral disorders • Retroverted uterus • *Postpartum:* Allen-Masters syndrome (broad ligament laceration) • Genital prolapse • Inflammatory bowel disease

Flowchart 1: Pathophysiological mechanisms of vulvar vestibulitis syndrome.

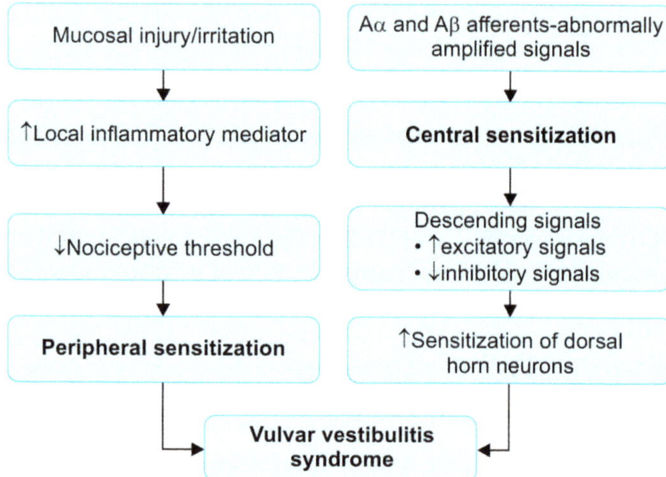

PATHOLOGY

Dividing the causes of sexual pain as superficial and deep dyspareunia helps to differentiate the etiology and pathophysiological mechanisms. Risk factors for the development of vulvodynia include nerve irritation, increased number, and sensitivity of nerve fibers, inflammation, pelvic floor muscle abnormalities, genetic susceptibility, and abnormal response to environmental stimuli.[16] In vulvar vestibulitis syndrome, peripheral and central sensitization leads to hyperalgesia and allodynia **(Flowchart 1)**.[17] The cause of initial sensitization is due to an inflammatory response believed to be due to infection by fungus or abnormal bacteria.[18] Various conditions producing deep dyspareunia usually produce pain during deep penetration.

Stress-induced central nervous system dysregulation increases pain perception.[19] The pelvic floor is considered an emotional organ because anxiety causes reflex contraction of pelvic floor muscles.[20] Negative cognition about pain also influences its intensity.[21] Sexual pain disorders are multifactorial, multisystemic, and complex.

Sexual pain of any type or etiology will result in a vicious cycle of pain, fear, anticipation, and avoidance. Women with dyspareunia reported decreased sexual frequency, relationship distress, decreased quality of life (QoL), social isolation, depression, and anxiety.[9] Female sexual pain is associated with other sexual dysfunctions, like female sexual interest/arousal disorder and low satisfaction with sexual activities.

CLINICAL ASSESSMENT OF SEXUAL PAIN

Women with GP usually get referred to gynecologists who look for organic causes which may not exist. Sexual functioning in GP is complex which needs proper investigation and evaluation. Besides investigating pain (quality and duration), the clinician should also inquire about QoL, psychological burden, and complexities in the relationship.[22] Focusing on the physical, psychological, sociocultural, and interpersonal factors, using the interaction model based on biopsychosocial approach is important to improve knowledge in the topic and provide better clinical care to the group of women with GP.[22]

The following steps are vital in the clinical assessment of the patient:

1. Validation of the patient's pain and establishing rapport and trust between the patient and provider foster openness, comfort, trust, and confidence with the patient through communication skill.[23]
2. A comprehensive history should encompass the following aspects: Pain characteristics including its location, duration, and factors that worsen it, any associated symptoms such as bowel, bladder, or musculoskeletal issues, sexual history and behavior, along with relationship and psychological history, existing medical conditions that may coexist, previous treatments attempted and any history of physical or sexual abuse.[9,23]

3. Medical and surgical history including pelvic floor assessment before progressing to gynecologic examination.

The overall goal of the medical interview should be to validate the patient's symptoms while gathering relevant information, excluding other diagnoses, and educating and reassuring the patient **(Box 1)**.

BOX 1: Useful questions to ask when obtaining a sexual pain history.[9,22,23]

Clinical evaluation of dyspareunia would involve a detailed clinical history and performing a physical examination:

Detailing the specifiers:

- Focusing on duration—lifelong versus acquired
- Focusing on context, physical or relational—generalized versus situational
- Focusing on etiology—organic, psychogenic, mixed, or unknown
- Focusing on intensity of distress—highly distressing, moderately distressing, or nondistressing, how intensely the woman experiences her coital pain.

Functional and anatomical details:

- Musculoskeletal history
- Any surgery, injury/accidents
- Any falls to the lumbo-pelvic-hip region and/or the tailbone and sacrum

Bowel and bladder function history:

- Urinary urgency, frequency, hesitancy, or incomplete emptying
- Chronic constipation or rectal fissures

Sexual history:

- Issues with sexual desire
- Issues with sexual arousal
- Issues with orgasm, frequency of and satisfaction with sex
- Sexual repertoire
- Sexual distress
- Decreased libido or decreased vaginal lubrication before the onset of dyspareunia

Relationship history:

- Quality of the relationship
- Sexual and nonsexual intimacy
- Romantic factors and emotions
- Couple interactions that accompany the pain in particular, avoidance, aversion, fear, adaptive, conflict, and negative conditioned response

Other important aspects in history:

- Comorbid medical or mental health conditions and treatments, for example anxiety and depression which can induce and exacerbate pain
- Past treatments that have been taken
- Expectations from the assessment and treatment
- History of neglect, physical, sexual, emotional abuse, and/or trauma, especially during childhood and any negative sexual experience
- Use of validated self-report questionnaires

Independent contributors for sexual distress:

- Negative self-image cognitions about vaginal penetration
- Negative body image
- Negative genital self-image

Other useful clinical pointers:

- Low back or hip pain
- Oral contraceptive pill use
- Ovarian suppression by medical agents
- Menopausal and perimenopausal symptoms such as hot flashes and night sweats
- Infection and inflammation—contact allergies or skin sensitive to chemicals recurrent (culture positive) yeast infections
- Persistent vaginal discharge

Contd...

Contd...

- Severe burning or an allergic reaction to a topical medication on the vulva or vagina
- Burning after intercourse
- Avoidance of intercourse
- Pain since first attempt at intercourse without any pain-free sex
- Pain with first tampon use
- Postcoital spotting or bleeding
- Vulvar itching
- Night-time scratching
- Diarrhea
- Midcycle spotting or pain
- Worsening pain in a sexual position with deep thrusting
- Vulvar ulcerations, tears, and fissures
- Painful periods
- Chronic pelvic pain
- Feeling an obstruction in the vagina
- Pain beginning after childbirth
- Dribbling after urination
- Changes in coloration or architecture of the labia or vulva
- Decreased clitoral sensation
- Frequent bicycle riding
- Aggressive abdominal muscle strengthening or pilates
- Pain mainly at the clitoris
- Since pain during intercourse began, has there been any pain-free intercourse
- Do you have oral lesions or bleeding gums
- Do you have a history of high-risk human papillomavirus or cervical dysplasia

PAIN AND PSYCHOSOCIAL ASSESSMENT GUIDE[9]

- Questions about the properties of the pain (e.g., onset, duration, location, quality, pattern, severity, and if pain is primary or secondary).
- Asking about pain mediators (i.e., whether any factors improve or exacerbate the pain; predisposing, precipitating, maintain factor, relieving factors).
- Activities have been affected by the pain and any comorbid issues (e.g., problems with sexual function, relationship distress, and psychological issues) allow for a comprehensive understanding of the problem.
- Questions related to previous treatments and their outcomes can be useful in further planning of treatment.

Pain Map

The location of pain during intercourse and how it manifests at the onset of an episode are highly indicative of whether it is organic or not. A thorough clinical examination can accurately replicate the site and nature of pain in about 90% of cases. Conversely, an insufficient examination may overlook biological factors contributing to coital pain, potentially leading to a misdiagnosis of a psychological issue, such as attributing the pain solely to the patient's mental state or labeling it as psychogenic.[24]

CLINICAL HISTORY[25]

Focusing on the presenting symptom of dyspareunia and keeping the sensitivity of the issue in mind, the key questions can be summarized as follows:

- *Timing and location of pain:* Pain may occur before, during, or after intercourse. It could indicate conditions, such as vaginismus, vulvar vestibulitis, or vulvodynia. Location and timing are crucial for diagnosis.
- *Duration of pain:* Understanding how long the pain has been present helps differentiate between lifelong and acquired conditions.
- *Severity of pain:* Keeping a pain diary can aid in understanding pain flares, their timing in relation to the menstrual cycle, and the impact of circadian rhythm. This information assists in tailoring treatment and evaluating its effectiveness.[26]
- *Provoked pain in sexual activities:* Provoked pain during vaginal penetration is common in women with provoked localized vulvodynia (PLVD). It is typically described as sharp or burning and localized to the vaginal entrance.[27]

- *Generalized unprovoked vulvodynia (GVD):* GVD pain is often described as burning, irritating, and sore. It affects the entire vulva and can worsen with contact to the affected area.[27]
- *Questionnaire:* The International Society for the Study of Vulvovaginal Disease offers a comprehensive questionnaire for patients to complete before their appointment, aiding in gathering relevant information for diagnosis and treatment planning.[28]

EVALUATION

Physical Examination

- *Examination of the external genitals:* Appearance, color, and condition, with attention to signs of inflammation or dystrophy.
- It is vital to plot the pain map as mentioned earlier.
- Assess the strength of the pelvic floor and its tone.
- Vaginal pH
- Neuromusculoskeletal referred pain
- Postoperative pelvic or perineal surgery (episiotomy) or radiotherapy

Gynecological Examination[29]

The goal of the physical examination is to gather data to help determine the etiology of vulvodynia and offer specific treatment for pain. Information gathered by a comprehensive, meticulous, methodical, and well-informed physical examination is invaluable.[29] Women with sexual pain have high levels of anxiety in response to any pelvic examination. A common strategy used to minimize anxiety, discomfort, and encourage cooperation is the educational examination process, which includes:

No rush strategies: Do not rush for gynecological examination right away, be slow and gentle while still being very detailed.

Inform and educate: Inform and educate the patient before, during, and after the assessment and examination; the use of internal and/or use of speculum or internal devices will not be necessary.

Teamwork: The patient and physician work together. Encourage and assure the patient that no examination will be pushed or forced. Describe each step and permit her to stop and interrupt the examination at her will doing. Encourage her to suggest and advise anything which can facilitate the examination and impart confidence and control.

Mirror test: The patient is given the choice to watch the process using a mirror to enable the patient to visualize her anatomy and the examination. An interactive process of explaining the genital anatomy, clarifying normal (or abnormal) structures, and constant reassurance is a must before and throughout the test. This can also alleviate misinformation and negative self-image and explain how sexual problems can be related to physical changes.[30]

Physical examination of patients with GP should include an external musculoskeletal evaluation, followed by external visual and sensory examination, as well as internal single digit palpation of the pelvic floor muscles.

If tolerated by the patient, proceed to a bimanual examination and a speculum examination can be performed to evaluate the uterus and adnexa. The purpose is to assess the uterus, cul-de-sac, and adnexa regions for any masses or tenderness. If the patient tolerates this portion of the examination, then the provider can proceed to an internal examination using a small-sized Graves or Pederson speculum.

It is essential to insert the speculum slowly to allow for the patient's comfort and to prevent any discomfort by avoiding contact with sensitive areas like the urethra or vulvar vestibule. During the speculum examination, the internal vaginal tissue, cervix, and vaginal secretions are assessed. This is also an opportune moment to gather cultures or biopsies to rule out infections, dermatoses, or abnormal cellular dysplasia, which could contribute to dyspareunia or vulvodynia.[29]

The superficial visual examination involves observing for signs of various conditions, such as inflammation, erythema, induration, excoriation, fissure, ulceration, lichenification, hypo-/hyperpigmentation, infection, scarring, atrophy, dermatitis, neoplasia, or architectural changes on the vulva. These findings may indicate dermatological diseases of the vulva, warranting further consultation with a dermatologist and possibly a pathological study through a punch biopsy. While erythema is a nonspecific finding, particularly intense redness at the ostia of the Bartholin and Skene glands suggests PLVD.[29]

Assessment of the Pelvic Floor Musculature[31]

- An assessment of the pelvic floor, trunk, and lower extremity musculature is very crucial in patients presenting with vulvar pain.

- Dysfunctional, dissymmetrical, or misaligned pelvis or restricted and overactive pelvic floor neuromuscular system can cause chronic vulvar pain.
- Women diagnosed with provoked vestibulodynia (PVD) typically exhibit heightened pelvic floor muscle tone, particularly at the superficial level. Additionally, they tend to demonstrate weaker pelvic floor muscle strength and control compared to individuals without this condition.
- Pelvic floor excursion testing should be performed along with biofeedback to objectively measure pelvic floor muscle coordination, strength, and tonicity. By using external perianal pads or internal sensors, the therapist can teach the patient to relax or activate the muscles.
- Positive findings will support the likelihood of bladder, bowel, and/or sexual dysfunction and abdominopelvic pain.
- The internal musculoskeletal and vaginal single-digit examination is the most reliable method for evaluating pelvic muscle tenderness.
- Using the index finger, the examiner can palpate the lateral, anterior, and posterior walls of the vagina, the urethra, and pelvic floor muscles (levator ani, coccygeus, piriformis, and obturator internus). The purpose is to access the specific areas for tone, tenderness, or involuntary spasms of the muscles of the introitus and pelvic floor.
- Tenderness during minimal or moderate palpation is considered abnormal; pelvic and vaginal structures can tolerate approximately 2 kg of pressure without pain.
- The patient is then asked to squeeze or contract around the single digit to assess their muscle strength. An effort should also be made to identify any scars from previous surgeries, episiotomy, or trauma.

Sensory Examination

Cotton swab test: A systematic sensory examination of the vulva involves using a moistened cotton swab to map the pain response. This process begins from nonpainful areas and gradually progresses to painful areas, allowing the patient to adapt gradually to the palpation method. Various areas of the anogenital region including the labia majora, clitoral prepuce, perineum, and intralabial sulci, as well as bilateral musculoskeletal structures such as the thighs, pelvis, and mons pubis, should be gently palpated. Pain experienced in these regions may indicate a condition affecting the entire anogenital region, such as vulvar dermatoses or vulvovaginal infections.

Special attention should be given to gently palpating the labia minora, especially medially, which lies lateral to the Hart line and lateral to the vestibule, at specific locations, including the ostia of the Skene glands (lateral to the urethra), the ostia of the Bartholin glands (at 4 and 8 o'clock positions at the vestibule), and at the fossa navicularis (at 6 o'clock position). Patients with provoked vestibulodynia (PVD) typically experience allodynia during cotton-swab palpation of the tissue of the vulvar vestibule, while perceiving normal sensation lateral to the Hart line.

In cases where pain is localized to the vestibule, it is important to determine whether the pain affects the entire vestibule or just the posterior portion. Pain throughout the entire vestibule may be associated with intrinsic pathology within the mucosa of the vestibular endoderm, whereas pain confined to the posterior vestibule suggests that the pain might be associated with extrinsic pathology, most commonly hypertonic pelvic floor muscle dysfunction.[32]

Capturing "Real-time" Pain

Vulvalgesiometer: The method described involves quantitative sensory testing using a seven-set vulvalgesiometer designed for women both with and without provoked vestibulodynia (PVD). This device allows for the standardization of pressure applied to the vestibule, enabling the quantification of sensitivity levels in the area.[33]

Tampon test: It is a real-life experience test with excellent construct validity. It is innovative, accurate, easy, and cost-effective with minimum participant burden but with strong methodologic properties.[15]

Speculum Examination

During speculum examination of the vagina, it is important to use a pediatric-sized Graves speculum and insert it through the hymeneal ring without touching the vulvar vestibule. While visualizing the vagina, key findings to note include atrophy (loss of rugae), erythema, erosions, ulcerations, abnormal discharge, or synechiae. Manual examination should be conducted with one finger, inserted through the hymen without touching the vestibule. The urethra and bladder trigone should be gently palpated, followed by examination of the levator ani muscles. The ischial spine should be located, and the pudendal nerve palpated as it enters the Alcock canal. Subsequently, a bimanual examination is performed to assess the uterus and adnexa (ovaries and fallopian tubes). Finally, a rectovaginal examination is conducted to assess the rectovaginal septum and posterior cul-de-sac.[34]

Wet Mount and Culture

A cotton swab should be used to collect abnormal vaginal discharge for pH testing, wet mount, and potassium hydroxide (KOH) preparation. In addition, a culture should be obtained and sent for speciation and sensitivity for candidiasis and immunochromatographic assay for trichomonas.[17]

Vulvoscopy/Colposcopic Examination

This is very useful in the evaluation of women with vulvodynia. A video colposcope or a handheld mirror can allow the patient to visualize all aspects of the examination, should she wish to be involved in this way.[35]

Histology

If specific findings suggestive of dermatoses, intraepithelial neoplasia, or neoplasia are observed during visual inspection or colposcopy examination of the vulva, it is recommended to obtain a biopsy sample from the vulva or vagina. This biopsy can provide further diagnostic clarity and guide appropriate management.[36]

Serum Testing

Serum hormone testing can be beneficial in evaluating women with vulvodynia, as hormonal abnormalities may play a role in this condition. It is recommended to obtain blood samples for serum levels of estradiol, total testosterone, free testosterone, albumin, sex hormone-binding globulin (SHBG), follicle-stimulating hormone (FSH), and prolactin. In women with provoked vestibulodynia (PVD), who are on hormonal contraceptives, elevated SHBG levels along with decreased free testosterone and estradiol levels are frequently observed.[37]

Additional testing/Investigations, such as radiography, ultrasonography, and detail pelvic floor musculature should depend upon the findings of history taking and physical examinations.

CASE VIGNETTE

A 24-year-old, Mary, came to the clinic with chief complaint of pain during sex saying "I have pain during penetrative sex. My boyfriend loves me a lot but does not understand my pain. Every time we have sex, my vagina is dry and tight. I hate to have sex and feel bad for him and it is affecting our relationship."

Clinical evaluation was done with the following in mind:

- *Predisposing factors:* Vaginismus and pain during penetration
- *Precipitating factors:* Attempt of penetration/intercourse
- *Maintaining factors:* Fear and anxiety about pain (systemic anxiety)

Clinical history revealed predisposing, precipitating, and maintaining factor. She reported the following: (1) She could not use tampons during menstruation due to pain; (2) She longs for intimacy but fears penetration; and (3) No history of abuse or trauma.

Observations suggested that she could have a hyperactive pelvic floor and acquired vaginismus causing dyspareunia.

Clinical examination and her body language indicated a systemic anxiety and fear of being examined. She was trembling in spite of her physician reassuring. Exquisite pain was elicited at entry of the vaginal opening in the lower right and left portions at the 4 o'clock and 8 o'clock positions of the vaginal introitus. Palpable Bartholin gland was felt; it is a mucus-secreting gland which plays a role in vaginal lubrication.

The diagnosis was acquired dyspareunia, comorbid with Bartholin gland abscess and a tightened, myalgic pelvic floor. Acquired vaginismus could be the predisposing factor. Acquired genital arousal disorder and acquired loss of sexual desire were the comorbid female sexual dysfunctions (FSDs).

A detailed and thorough clinical history is crucial to identify various factors and assess comorbidities. Comorbidities are common among FSDs including associations between lower urinary tract symptoms and dyspareunia, as well as between FSDs and other medical conditions. In one case, the natural progression of the complaint involved vaginismus as a likely predisposing factor, with intercourse serving as the precipitating factor. Biological factors, such as a Bartholin gland abscess, and psychosexual factors including systemic fear and anxiety about pain, contributed to the maintenance of symptoms.

Acquired desire and arousal disorders further increased vulnerability to mechanical trauma of the introital mucosa due to inadequate lubrication in response to sexual stimulation. Postcoital cystitis and subsequent abscess formation may have been precipitated by the mechanical trauma of intercourse with a dry (nonaroused) vagina and a tightened pelvic floor.[9]

MANAGEMENT OF FEMALE SEXUAL PAIN

Managing sexual pain in women involves a multidisciplinary approach that may include medical, psychological, and lifestyle interventions. It is important for women experiencing sexual pain to consult with healthcare professionals to determine the underlying cause and develop an appropriate treatment plan.[9] Here are some general strategies that may be considered:

Medical evaluation: Consult with a gynecologist or healthcare provider to identify any underlying medical conditions causing sexual pain. Rule out infections, hormonal imbalances, pelvic floor disorders, and other physical issues.

Pelvic floor physical therapy: Pelvic floor physical therapy can be helpful for women experiencing sexual pain. This therapy focuses on relaxing and strengthening the pelvic floor muscles.[38]

Lubricants and moisturizers: Using water-based or silicone-based lubricants can help reduce friction and improve comfort during sexual activity. Vaginal moisturizers may also be recommended to address dryness and discomfort.[39]

Hormone therapy: For women experiencing hormonal imbalances, hormone therapy may be recommended to address issues such as vaginal dryness.[37]

Psychological support: Consultation with a sex therapist or mental health professional can be beneficial for addressing any psychological factors contributing to sexual pain, such as anxiety or past trauma.[40]

Counseling and communication: Open communication with a partner is crucial. Couples counseling may be recommended to address relationship issues or improve communication regarding sexual intimacy.[40]

Education and relaxation techniques: Learning about sexual anatomy and function can help women understand their bodies better. Relaxation techniques, such as deep breathing and mindfulness, can also be beneficial.[41]

Medications: Depending on the underlying cause, your healthcare provider may prescribe medications such as pain relievers, muscle relaxants, or medications to address specific medical conditions.

Surgical intervention: In some cases, surgical interventions may be considered for conditions such as endometriosis or certain structural abnormalities contributing to sexual pain.

Alternative therapies: Acupuncture, biofeedback, and other alternative therapies may be considered, but their effectiveness varies, and it is important to discuss these options with a healthcare professional.[42]

It is crucial to note that the approach to managing sexual pain varies depending on the individual case, and treatment plans should be tailored to address the specific causes and contributing factors. Women experiencing sexual pain should seek guidance from healthcare professionals who can conduct a thorough evaluation and provide appropriate recommendations for their specific situation.

Medications Used in the Management of Female Sexual Pain

The medications used in the management of sexual pain in women can vary depending on the underlying cause of the pain. It is important to note that medication alone may not be sufficient, and a comprehensive approach involving medical, psychological, and lifestyle interventions is often necessary. Here are some medications that may be considered, depending on the specific situation:

Topical estrogens: For women experiencing vaginal dryness or atrophy due to hormonal changes (e.g., menopause), topical estrogen creams, rings, or tablets may be prescribed to restore moisture and elasticity to the vaginal tissues.[43]

Lidocaine cream or gel: Topical lidocaine can be used to numb the genital area temporarily, reducing pain and discomfort during sexual activity.[44]

Pain relievers (NSAIDs): Nonsteroidal anti-inflammatory drugs (NSAIDs), such as ibuprofen or naproxen, may be recommended to reduce inflammation and alleviate pain in cases where inflammation is a contributing factor.[45]

Muscle relaxants: In cases where pelvic floor muscle dysfunction or spasm contributes to sexual pain, muscle relaxants may be prescribed to help relax the muscles and reduce tension.[46]

Antidepressants: Certain classes of antidepressants, such as tricyclic antidepressants (TCAs) or selective serotonin reuptake inhibitors (SSRIs) may be prescribed for their pain-relieving properties. They can affect the perception of pain and may be used off-label in the management of chronic pain conditions.[47]

Gabapentin or pregabalin: These medications, originally developed for seizures and neuropathic pain, may be considered for their ability to modulate nerve signals and reduce pain sensations. They are sometimes used in cases where nerve-related issues contribute to sexual pain.[48]

Hormone therapy: In addition to topical estrogens, systemic hormone therapy may be considered for women experiencing hormonal imbalances affecting sexual function. This involves the use of estrogen or a combination of estrogen and progestin, but it is important to discuss the risks and benefits with a healthcare provider.[37]

Botulinum toxin injections: In some cases of pelvic floor dysfunction or spasm, botulinum toxin injections may be used to temporarily paralyze the muscles and alleviate pain.[38]

CONCLUSION

It is essential for women experiencing sexual pain to consult with a healthcare professional who can conduct a thorough evaluation, identify the underlying causes, and recommend appropriate medications or a combination of interventions. The choice of medication will depend on the specific diagnosis and individual factors, and the guidance of a healthcare provider is crucial to ensure safe and effective management. A team-based multidisciplinary approach with patient psychoeducation is the key to success in most cases.

REFERENCES

1. Raja SN, Carr DB, Cohen M, Finnerup NB, Flor H, Gibson S, et al. The revised International Association for the Study of Pain definition of pain: concepts, challenges, and compromises. Pain. 2020;161(9):1976-82.
2. World Health Organization. International Classification of Diseases, Eleventh Revision (ICD-11). Geneva: World Health Organization; 2021.
3. American Psychiatric Association. Diagnostic and Statistical Manual for the Classification of Psychiatric Disorders, 4th edition text revised (DSM-IV-TR). Washington, DC: American Psychiatric Association; 2000.
4. Bornstein J, Goldstein AT, Stockdale CK, Bergeron S, Pukall C, Zolnoun D, et al. 2015 ISSVD, ISSWSH, and IPPS Consensus Terminology and Classification of Persistent Vulvar Pain and Vulvodynia. J Sex Med. 2016;13(4):607-12.
5. Dias-Amaral A, Marques-Pinto A. Female Genito-Pelvic Pain/Penetration Disorder: Review of the Related Factors and Overall Approach. Rev Bras Ginecol Obstet. 2018;40(12):787-93.
6. American Psychiatric Association. Diagnostic and Statistical Manual for the Classification of Psychiatric Disorders, 4th edition (DSM-IV). Washington DC: American Psychiatric Association; 1994.
7. American Psychiatric Association. Diagnostic and Statistical Manual for the Classification of Psychiatric Disorders, 5th edition (DSM-5). Washington, DC: American Psychiatric Association; 2022.
8. Weijenborg PT, Ter Kuile MM, Stones W. A cognitive behavioural based assessment of women with chronic pelvic pain. J Psychosom Obstet Gynaecol. 2009;30(4):262-8.
9. Sorensen J, Bautista KE, Lamvu G, Feranec J. Evaluation and Treatment of Female Sexual Pain: A Clinical Review. Cureus. 2018;10(3):e2379.
10. Meana M, Fertel E, Maykut C. Treating genital pain associated with sexual intercourse. In: Peterson ZD. The Wiley Handbook of Sex Therapy. Malden, MA: John Wiley & Sons Ltd.; 2017. pp. 98-114.
11. Graziottin A. Dyspareunia and vaginismus: Review of the literature and treatment. Curr Sex Health Rep. 2008;5(1):43-50.
12. Flanagan E, Herron KA, O'Driscoll C, Williams AC. Psychological treatment for vaginal pain: does etiology matter? A systematic review and meta-analysis. J Sex Med. 2015;12(1):3-16.
13. Binik YM, Meana M, Berkley K, Khalifé S. The sexual pain disorders: is the pain sexual or is the sex painful? Annu Rev Sex Res. 1999;10:210-35. Erratum in: Annu Rev Sex Res. 2000;11:286.
14. Lahaie MA, Boyer SC, Amsel R, Khalifé S, Binik YM. Vaginismus: a review of the literature on the classification/diagnosis, etiology and treatment. Womens Health (Lond). 2010;6(5):705-19.
15. Pacik PT, Babb CR, Polio A, Nelson CE, Goekeler CE, Holmes LN. Case Series: Redefining Severe Grade 5 Vaginismus. Sex Med. 2019;7(4):489-97.
16. Vieira-Baptista P, Lima-Silva J, Pérez-López FR, Preti M, Bornstein J. Vulvodynia: A disease commonly hidden in plain sight. Case Rep Womens Health. 2018;20:e00079.
17. Weijmar Schultz W, Basson R, Binik Y, Eschenbach D, Wesselmann U, Van Lankveld J. Women's sexual pain and its management. J Sex Med. 2005;2(3):301-16.
18. Nyirjesy P. Vulvar vestibulitis syndrome: a post-infectious entity? Curr Infect Dis Rep. 2000;2:531-5.

19. Basson R. The recurrent pain and sexual sequelae of provoked vestibulodynia: a perpetuating cycle. J Sex Med. 2012;9(8):2077-92.
20. Both S, van Lunsen R, Weijenborg P, Laan E. A new device for simultaneous measurement of pelvic floor muscle activity and vaginal blood flow: a test in a nonclinical sample. J Sex Med. 2012;9(11):2888-902.
21. Nobre PJ, Pinto-Gouveia J. Cognitions, emotions, and sexual response: Analysis of the relationship among automatic thoughts, emotional responses, and sexual arousal. Arch Sex Behav. 2008;37:652-61.
22. Nimbi FM, Rossi V, Tripodi F, Luria M, Flinchum M, Tambelli R, et al. Genital Pain and Sexual Functioning: Effects on Sexual Experience, Psychological Health, and Quality of Life. J Sex Med. 2020;17(4):771-83.
23. Goldstein AT, Pukall CF, Brown C, Bergeron S, Stein A, Kellogg-Spadt S. Vulvodynia: Assessment and Treatment. J Sex Med. 2016;13(4):572-90.
24. Rosen NO, Bergeron S, Pukall CF. Recommendations for the Study of Vulvar Pain in Women, Part 1: Review of Assessment Tools. J Sex Med. 2020;17(2):180-94.
25. Althof SE, Rosen RC, Perelman MA, Rubio-Aurioles E. Standard operating procedures for taking a sexual history. J Sex Med. 2013;10(1):26-35.
26. Kingsberg SA. Taking a sexual history. Obstet Gynecol Clin North Am. 2006;33(4):535-47.
27. Arnold LD, Bachmann GA, Rosen R, Kelly S, Rhoads GG. Vulvodynia: characteristics and associations with comorbidities and quality of life. Obstet Gynecol. 2006;107(3):617-24.
28. Erekson EA, Yip SO, Wedderburn TS, Martin DK, Li FY, Choi JN, et al. The Vulvovaginal Symptoms Questionnaire: a questionnaire for measuring vulvovaginal symptoms in postmenopausal women. Menopause. 2013;20(9):973-9.
29. Rossi MA, Vermeir E, Brooks M, Pierce M, Pukall CF, Rosen NO. Comparing Self-Reported Pain During Intercourse and Pain During a Standardized Gynecological Exam at 12- and 24-Month Postpartum. J Sex Med. 2022;19(1):116-31.
30. Hill DA, Taylor CA. Dyspareunia in Women. Am Fam Physician. 2021;103(10):597-604.
31. Shafik A, El-Sibai O. Study of the pelvic floor muscles in vaginismus: a concept of pathogenesis. Eur J Obstet Gynecol Reprod Biol. 2002;105(1):67-70.
32. Dargie EE, Chamberlain SM, Pukall CF. Provoked Vestibulodynia: Diagnosis, Self-Reported Pain, and Presentation During Gynaecological Examinations. J Obstet Gynaecol Can. 2017;39(3):145-51.
33. Cardaillac C, Levesque A, Riant T, Mortier A, Neunlist M, Perrouin-Verbe MA, et al. Evaluation of a scoring system for the detection of central sensitization among women with chronic pelvic pain. Am J Obstet Gynecol. 2023;229(5):530.e1-530.e17.
34. Bates CK, Carroll N, Potter J. The challenging pelvic examination. J Gen Intern Med. 2011;26(6):651-7.
35. Gagné HM. Colposcopy of the vagina and vulva. Obstet Gynecol Clin North Am. 2008;35(4):659-69; x.
36. Jannini EA, d'Amati G, Lenzi A. Histology and immunohistochemical studies of female genital tissue. In: Goldstein I, Meston CM, Davis S, Traish A (Eds). Women's Sexual Function and Dysfunction: study, diagnosis and treatment. London: Taylor and Francis. 2006; pp. 125-33.
37. Smith NK, Jozkowski KN, Sanders SA. Hormonal contraception and female pain, orgasm and sexual pleasure. J Sex Med. 2014;11(2):462-70.
38. Rosenbaum TY. Pelvic floor involvement in male and female sexual dysfunction and the role of pelvic floor rehabilitation in treatment: a literature review. J Sex Med. 2007;4(1):4-13.
39. Potter N, Panay N. Vaginal lubricants and moisturizers: a review into use, efficacy, and safety. Climacteric. 2021;24(1):19-24.
40. O'Donohue W, Dopke CA, Swingen DN. Psychotherapy for female sexual dysfunction: A review. Clin Psychol Rev. 1997;17(5):537-66.
41. Brotto LA, Basson R, Luria M. A mindfulness-based group psychoeducational intervention targeting sexual arousal disorder in women. J Sex Med. 2008;5(7):1646-59.
42. Spadt SK, Fariello JY. Complementary and Alternative Treatments for Female Sexual Pain. In: Bartlik B, Espinosa G, Mindes J (Eds). Integrative Sexual Health. Oxford, England: Oxford University Press; 2018;395-407.
43. Santoro N, Worsley R, Miller KK, Parish SJ, Davis SR. Role of Estrogens and Estrogen-Like Compounds in Female Sexual Function and Dysfunction. J Sex Med. 2016;13(3):305-16.
44. Morin M, Dumoulin C, Bergeron S, Mayrand MH, Khalifé S, Waddell G, et al. Multimodal physical therapy versus topical lidocaine for provoked vestibulodynia: a multicenter, randomized trial. Am J Obstet Gynecol. 2021;224(2):189.e1-189.e12.
45. Zahradnik HP, Hanjalic-Beck A, Groth K. Nonsteroidal anti-inflammatory drugs and hormonal contraceptives for pain relief from dysmenorrhea: a review. Contraception. 2010;81(3):185-96.
46. Victoria K, Jha S. Female sexual dysfunction. Obstet Gynaecol. 2022;24(1):12-23.
47. Leo RJ, Dewani S. A systematic review of the utility of antidepressant pharmacotherapy in the treatment of vulvodynia pain. J Sex Med. 2013;10(10):2497-505.
48. Philippsohn S, Kruger TH. Persistent genital arousal disorder: successful treatment with duloxetine and pregabalin in two cases. J Sex Med. 2012;9(1):213-7.

CHAPTER 25

Understanding Varicose Veins: Causes, Management, and Complications

Ravul Jindal, Piyush Chaudhary, Muneer Ahmad Para, Taranvir Kaur, Shabjot Dhillon

INTRODUCTION

Varicose veins refer to enlarged, twisted veins, usually found in the legs; however, they can also occur in other parts of the body. They occur when the valves within the veins weaken or fail to function properly, causing blood to pool, thus leading to varicose veins leg swelling and discomfort. These veins often appear blue or dark purple and may be accompanied by symptoms such as heaviness, aching, or itching.

CAUSES OF VARICOSE VEINS

Varicose veins can be caused by various factors such as *genetic predisposition*, *lifestyle factors*, and *physiological changes*. While the exact cause may vary among individuals, several key factors contribute to their development.

Understanding these underlying causes is essential for effective management and prevention strategies. This section sheds light on genetic influences, occupational hazards, lifestyle choices, and physiological changes that lead to this vascular disorder.

Varicose veins can develop due to various factors:

Genetic Predisposition

Genetic predisposition refers to the likelihood of inheriting varicose veins from family members due to shared genetic traits. Family history is a significant determinant, indicating an increased risk for individuals with relatives affected by the condition.

Understanding these hereditary factors is crucial for assessing an individual's susceptibility to varicose veins and implementing preventive measures.

Prolonged Standing or Sitting

Occupations or lifestyles that involve prolonged periods of standing or sitting can increase pressure on the veins, which can lead to varicose veins. When someone spends a long time standing or sitting, especially without moving much, it puts extra pressure on the veins. This increased pressure can make it harder for blood to flow properly through the veins in the legs, leading to the development of varicose veins over time.

Obesity

Excess weight puts additional pressure on the veins, particularly in the lower extremities, which increases the risk of varicose vein formation. When someone carries extra weight, it adds more pressure on their veins, especially in their legs and feet. This added pressure makes it harder for the veins to work properly, leading to a higher chance of developing varicose veins.

Hormonal Changes

Hormonal fluctuations, such as those occurring during puberty, menopause, or hormone therapy, can affect vein elasticity and contribute to varicose veins. When the veins lose elasticity, they can become weak and varicose veins might develop. These hormonal shifts play a role in making the veins more prone to developing this condition.

Pregnancy

Hormonal changes and increased blood volume during pregnancy can weaken vein walls and valves, leading to the development of varicose veins. These changes can weaken the walls and valves of her veins, especially in her legs. As a result, varicose veins may develop during pregnancy due to the added strain on the circulatory system.

Aging

With age, vein walls may lose elasticity and valves may weaken, leading to varicose veins. This makes it more likely for varicose veins to form because the veins cannot work as well as they used to in keeping the blood flowing properly back to the heart.

Thus, people with a family history of varicose veins, those in jobs requiring lots of standing or sitting, overweight individuals, older adults, and women going through hormonal changes are at the most risk for developing varicose veins.

CEAP CLASSIFICATION OF VARICOSE VEINS

The clinical, etiological, anatomical, and pathophysiological (CEAP) classification system is a method used to categorize varicose veins according to their clinical severity, providing healthcare professionals with a structured approach to assess and manage this vascular condition **(Table 1)**.

C0: No Visible or Palpable Signs of Venous Disease

This category includes individuals who do not exhibit any outward signs or symptoms of varicose veins upon examination. Despite the absence of visible indicators, underlying venous abnormalities may still be present.

C1: Telangiectasias or Reticular Veins

Varicose veins in this category are characterized by the presence of *telangiectasias*, commonly known as *spider veins* or *reticular veins*. In this case, small and dilated blood vessels are visible beneath the skin's surface, often appearing as red or blue lines.

C2: Varicose Veins

Individuals in this category display visible varicose veins, which are enlarged, twisted veins typically found on the legs or feet. These veins may be lumpy, bulging, or twisted in appearance, causing discomfort or cosmetic concerns.

C3: Edema

Edema refers to swelling caused by the accumulation of fluid in the tissues, commonly observed in the lower extremities. In the context of varicose veins, edema may result from impaired venous circulation and increased pressure within the veins.

TABLE 1: CEAP classification of varicose veins.

CEAP class	*Description*
C0	No visible symptoms
C1	Telangiectasias or reticular veins
C2	Varicose veins
C3	Edema
C4	Skin changes (pigmentation, eczema)
C5	Healed venous ulcer
C6	Active venous ulcer

(CEAP: clinical, etiological, anatomical, and pathophysiological)

C4: Skin Changes, Such as Pigmentation or Eczema

Skin changes associated with varicose veins include pigmentation alterations, such as darkening or discoloration of the skin, and *eczema*, a chronic inflammatory skin condition. These changes often occur due to chronic venous insufficiency (CVI) and inadequate tissue perfusion.

C5: Healed Venous Ulcer

Venous ulcers are open wounds or sores that develop on the skin, usually around the ankles, as a result of CVI and poor wound healing.

Individuals with a history of venous ulcers that have healed fall into this category.

C6: Active Venous Ulcer

This category includes individuals with active venous ulcers, indicating ongoing tissue damage and impaired wound healing due to severe venous insufficiency. Active venous ulcers require prompt medical attention and comprehensive wound care to facilitate healing and prevent complications.

Understanding the CEAP classification system enables healthcare providers to accurately assess the severity of varicose veins, tailor treatment strategies to individual patient needs and monitor disease progression effectively.[1]

COMPLICATIONS OF UNTREATED VARICOSE VEINS

When varicose veins are left untreated, they can give rise to several complications, posing risks to an individual's health and well-being. Following are some of the complications of untreated varicose veins:

Chronic Venous Insufficiency

Venous hypertension, i.e., persistent pressure elevation within the veins, can lead to *CVI*. This condition is characterized by symptoms, such as leg pain, swelling, and skin changes, such as discoloration or thickening. CVI results from impaired venous circulation and can significantly impact a person's quality of life.[2]

Venous Ulcers

Chronic venous hypertension and associated skin changes can lead to the development of venous ulcers, particularly in the lower leg area. Venous ulcers are open wounds or sores that occur when the skin fails to heal properly due to poor circulation and tissue damage. These ulcers can be painful, prone to infection, and challenging to treat, requiring comprehensive wound care.

Thrombophlebitis

Thrombophlebitis is a condition that occurs due to inflammation of the veins, often accompanied by the formation of blood clots. This condition leads to redness, warmth, swelling, and tenderness along the affected vein.

Superficial Thrombosis

Superficial thrombosis typically presents as a tender, firm lump beneath the skin, accompanied by redness and swelling in the affected area. While usually not life-threatening, superficial thrombosis can lead to complications if the blood clot migrates to deeper veins. Blood clots formed within superficial veins can also cause inflammation and pain.

Deep Vein Thrombosis

In rare cases, untreated varicose veins may lead to deep vein thrombosis (DVT), a serious condition characterized by the formation of blood clots in deep veins, typically in the legs. DVT poses a significant risk of complications including *pulmonary embolism (PE)* or *post-thrombotic syndrome*, if not promptly diagnosed and treated.

Pulmonary Embolism

If a blood clot dislodges from a deep vein and travels to the lungs, it can cause a *PE*, a potentially life-threatening condition. PE can obstruct blood flow to the lungs, leading to chest pain, difficulty breathing, rapid heart rate, and in severe cases, cardiac arrest or death.

Prompt recognition and management of varicose veins are essential to prevent these complications and minimize their impact on an individual's health and quality of life.

MANAGEMENT OF VARICOSE VEINS

Varicose veins can be effectively managed by focusing on alleviating symptoms, preventing complications, and enhancing the overall quality of life.

Various treatment options are available, catering to individual needs and preferences. Some of the methods of management of varicose veins are as follows:

Conservative Methods

- *Lifestyle modifications:* Implementing lifestyle changes such as regular exercise, elevating the legs when resting, maintaining a healthy weight, and avoiding prolonged periods of standing or sitting can play a pivotal role in managing varicose veins. These measures help reduce symptoms and prevent the progression of the condition by improving blood circulation and relieving pressure on the veins.
- *Compression therapy:* Wearing *compression stockings, wraps,* or *bandages* is a cornerstone of conservative management for varicose veins. Compression stockings exert graduated pressure on the legs, which helps in reducing swelling. This noninvasive approach helps alleviate discomfort and prevents complications associated with venous insufficiency.

Surgical and Minimally Invasive Interventions

- *Sclerotherapy: Sclerotherapy* involves the injection of a sclerosing agent directly into the affected vein, causing it to collapse and eventually fade away. This minimally invasive procedure is commonly used to treat smaller varicose veins and spider veins, yielding satisfactory cosmetic outcomes with minimal downtime.
- *Endovenous ablation techniques: Endovenous ablation techniques*, such as *endovenous laser treatment (EVLT), radiofrequency ablation (RFA)*, and *microwave* utilize thermal energy to seal off the diseased vein, redirecting blood flow to healthier vessels. These outpatient procedures offer effective, minimally invasive alternatives to traditional vein stripping surgery, with shorter recovery times and excellent clinical outcomes.
- *Surgical ligation and stripping:* In severe cases of varicose veins, *surgical ligation* and *stripping* may be needed to remove the diseased vein entirely. During this procedure, the affected vein is ligated (tied off) and then surgically removed through small incisions. Although more invasive than minimally invasive interventions, surgical ligation and stripping remain a viable option for patients with extensive varicose vein involvement or recurrent disease.
- *Phlebectomy: Phlebectomy* is a surgical procedure which is performed under local anesthesia to remove varicose veins in outpatient settings. It involves making

small incisions near the affected veins and extracting them using specialized instruments. This procedure is minimally invasive, leaving minimal scarring and allowing for quick recovery. It is effective for larger varicose veins that cannot be treated with other minimally invasive techniques.

By tailoring treatment strategies to individual patient needs and preferences, healthcare providers can effectively manage varicose veins, improving symptoms, and enhancing overall vascular health.

THERMAL AND NONTHERMAL TREATMENT METHODS

Within the spectrum of treatment modalities, thermal and nonthermal interventions emerge as prominent approaches, each offering distinct advantages and considerations. This section explores these methods in detail, providing insights into their mechanisms, benefits, and potential drawbacks.

Thermal Treatments

- *Endovenous laser treatment:* Endovenous laser treatment stands as a cornerstone in the management of varicose veins. This minimally invasive procedure involves the targeted application of laser energy to seal off diseased veins, thereby redirecting blood flow to healthier vessels. However, there is a risk of nerve injury and heat-related complications associated with this approach, if not done properly.[3]
- *Radiofrequency ablation:* Radiofrequency ablation represents another thermal-based intervention utilized in varicose vein management. By delivering radiofrequency energy to the affected vein, RFA achieves closure and subsequent redirection of blood flow. Similar to EVLT, RFA offers a minimally invasive alternative to surgical options, with favorable outcomes.
- *Microwave: Microwave ablation* is an emerging thermal treatment modality for varicose veins. During the procedure, microwave energy is delivered through a specialized catheter to heat and close off the diseased vein. This leads to the redirection of blood flow to healthier veins. Microwave ablation offers several advantages including shorter procedure times and potentially lower rates of nerve injury compared to other thermal techniques. It is performed as an outpatient procedure under local anesthesia, allowing for quicker recovery and minimal discomfort.

Nonthermal Treatments

- *Sclerotherapy:* Sclerotherapy emerges as a versatile option in the techniques available for varicose veins treatment. This technique involves the injection of a sclerosing agent into affected veins, inducing their collapse and subsequent absorption by surrounding tissues. Sclerotherapy is lauded for its efficacy in treating smaller varicose veins and spider veins, coupled with minimal downtime and satisfactory cosmetic results. However, there is a potential necessity for multiple sessions to achieve optimal outcomes.[4]
- *Mechanochemical ablation (MOCA):* Mechanochemical ablation represents an innovative approach that combines mechanical disruption of the vein wall with the infusion of a sclerosing agent. This synergistic mechanism effectively closes off diseased veins, offering patients a minimally invasive treatment option with low complication rates. MOCA is feasible under local anesthesia in an outpatient setting; however, its availability is limited compared to other interventions.
- *Glue ablation:* Glue ablation, also known as *cyanoacrylate adhesive closure,* is a novel nonthermal treatment method for varicose veins. In this procedure, a medical-grade adhesive is injected into the diseased vein, causing it to close off and redirect blood flow to healthier veins. The adhesive rapidly polymerizes upon contact with blood, forming a permanent seal within the vein. Glue ablation offers several advantages including rapid closure of the treated vein, minimal discomfort during the procedure, and quick recovery times. Additionally, it can be performed as an outpatient procedure under local anesthesia, making it a convenient option for patients.

In summary, thermal and nonthermal treatment methods present patients with a diverse array of options for managing varicose veins. By defining the mechanisms, benefits, and considerations associated with each approach, healthcare providers can engage in informed discussions with patients, facilitating the development of tailored treatment plans aligned with individual needs and preferences **(Table 2)**.

POSTOPERATIVE MEASURES

After undergoing surgical or minimally invasive interventions for varicose veins, it is important to take comprehensive postoperative care measures to optimize healing and minimize the risk of complications.

TABLE 2: Comparison of thermal and nonthermal treatment methods.

Treatment method	Procedure	Advantages	Disadvantages
Thermal	EVLT	Less invasive than surgery	Risk of nerve injury
	RFA	High success rate	Potential heat-related complications
	Microwave	Effective closure of veins and minimal discomfort	Limited availability compared to others
Nonthermal	Sclerotherapy	Suitable for smaller veins	Multiple sessions may be required
	MOCA	Minimally invasive	Limited availability compared to others
	Glue ablation	Fast closure of veins and little discomfort	Long-term effectiveness needs more research

(EVLT: endovenous laser treatment; MOCA: mechanochemical ablation; RFA: radiofrequency ablation)

Some of the key postoperative measures are as follows:

Compression Therapy

Patients are often advised to wear compression stockings or wraps following varicose vein treatment. These specialized stockings exert graduated pressure on the legs, promoting venous return and reducing swelling. Compression therapy helps maintain the integrity of the treated veins, prevents blood from pooling, and facilitates the healing process.[5]

Activity Restrictions

In the immediate postoperative period, individuals are advised to limit strenuous activities and avoid heavy lifting. Engaging in excessive physical exertion can exert undue stress on the treated veins, potentially compromising their integrity and delaying healing. Patients should prioritize gradual resumption of normal activities as guided by their healthcare provider post getting operated for varicose veins.

Follow-up Care

Regular follow-up appointments are essential components of postoperative management for varicose veins. These appointments allow healthcare providers to monitor the patient's recovery progress, assess treatment outcomes, and address any concerns or complications that may arise. Close communication between the patient and healthcare team facilitates timely intervention and ensures optimal long-term results.

Elevation of Legs

Encouraging patients to elevate their legs above heart level intermittently can aid in reducing swelling and promoting venous return. Elevating the legs helps counteract the effects of gravity, facilitating the drainage of excess fluid from the treated area and enhancing overall comfort.

Pain Management

Providing appropriate pain management measures, such as over-the-counter or prescribed painkillers, can help alleviate discomfort during the postoperative period. Patients should be educated on the safe and effective use of pain medications and encouraged to report any persistent or severe pain to their healthcare provider.

Wound Care

Proper wound care is essential for individuals who have undergone surgical interventions to prevent infection and promote healing. Patients should receive instructions on how to clean and dress any incisions or wounds as directed by their healthcare provider. Monitoring for signs of infection, such as increased redness, swelling, or discharge, is crucial for early detection and intervention.

By adhering to these postoperative measures, patients can facilitate a smooth recovery process, minimize discomfort, and achieve favorable outcomes following varicose vein treatment.

MANAGING RECURRENCE AFTER TREATMENT

Even after undergoing treatment for varicose veins, recurrence can occur over time. To minimize the risk of recurrence and maintain vein health, the following strategies are recommended:

Lifestyle Modifications

Encouraging patients to adopt healthy lifestyle habits plays a crucial role in preventing varicose vein recurrence.

Maintaining a healthy weight through balanced nutrition and regular exercise helps alleviate pressure on the veins and promotes overall vascular health. Additionally, practicing good vein health habits, such as avoiding prolonged periods of standing or sitting and elevating legs when possible, can further reduce the likelihood of recurrence.

Long-term Compression Therapy

For individuals at higher risk of varicose vein recurrence, long-term compression therapy may be beneficial. Compression stockings exert continuous pressure on the legs, supporting venous circulation, and reducing the risk of venous insufficiency.

Healthcare providers may recommend wearing compression stockings regularly, especially during periods of prolonged standing or sitting, to provide ongoing support to the veins.

Regular Follow-up

Scheduled follow-up appointments with healthcare providers are essential for monitoring post-treatment progress and detecting any signs of recurrence early on. During these evaluations, healthcare providers can assess the patient's vein health, review lifestyle habits, and intervene promptly if recurrence is suspected. By maintaining regular communication and adherence to follow-up appointments, patients can receive timely intervention and minimize the impact of recurrent varicose veins.

By incorporating these measures into post-treatment care plans, healthcare providers can empower patients to take proactive steps toward preventing varicose vein recurrence and maintaining optimal vascular health.

CONCLUSION

Varicose veins are a prevalent vascular issue with various causes and risk factors. This chapter has outlined the definition, causes, classification, complications, and management options for varicose veins. Understanding these aspects is crucial for effective treatment and prevention strategies.

REFERENCES

1. De Maeseneer MG, Kakkos SK, Aherne T, Baekgaard N, Black S, Blomgren L, et al.; ESVS Guidelines Committee. Editor's Choice-European Society for Vascular Surgery (ESVS) 2022 Clinical Practice Guidelines on the Management of Chronic Venous Disease of the Lower Limbs. Eur J Vasc Endovasc Surg. 2022;63(2):184-267.
2. Gloviczki P, Lawrence PF, Wasan SM, Meissner MH, Almeida J, Brown KR, et al. The 2023 Society for Vascular Surgery, American Venous Forum, and American Vein and Lymphatic Society clinical practice guidelines for the management of varicose veins of the lower extremities. Part II: Endorsed by the Society of Interventional Radiology and the Society for Vascular Medicine. J Vasc Surg Venous Lymphat Disord. 2024;12(1):101670.
3. Whiteley MS. Current best practice in the management of varicose veins. Clin Cosmet Investig Dermatol. 2022; 567-83.
4. Sassaki VS, Fukaya E. Varicose veins: Approach, assessment, and management to the patient with chronic venous disease. Med Clin North Am. 2023;107(5):895-909.
5. Gibson K, Nicolini P. Up to date guidance for the clinical management of chronic venous disease. Eur J Vasc Endovasc Surg. 2022;63(2):179-80.

APPENDIX

- *CEAP classification:* A system used to categorize varicose veins based on clinical severity including criteria, such as telangiectasias, varicose veins, edema, skin changes, and ulcer status.
- *Chronic venous insufficiency (CVI):* A condition characterized by persistent venous hypertension, leading to symptoms, such as leg pain, swelling, and skin changes.
- *Endovenous laser treatment (EVLT):* A minimally invasive procedure that uses laser energy to seal off varicose veins, redirecting blood flow to healthier vessels.
- *Radiofrequency ablation (RFA):* A thermal ablation technique that uses radiofrequency energy to close off varicose veins.
- *Sclerotherapy:* A procedure involving the injection of a sclerosing agent into varicose veins to collapse them and fade them away.
- *Compression therapy:* The use of compression stockings, wraps, or bandages to improve venous circulation and reduce swelling in varicose veins.
- *Deep vein thrombosis (DVT):* The formation of blood clots in deep veins, typically in the legs, which can lead to serious complications if not treated promptly.
- *Pulmonary embolism (PE):* A potentially life-threatening condition caused by a blood clot that travels to the lungs, obstructing blood flow.

CHAPTER 26

The Anatomy of a Smile: An Introduction to the Art and Science of Teeth Brightening

Shivani Jain, Gauri Sachdeva

INTRODUCTION

A great majority of the population is becoming increasingly aware and interested in dental aesthetics today. This is due to cosmetic reasons because many people prefer white teeth and a bright smile as it may also affect their quality of life.[1,2] Lifestyle habits like smoking or consumption of red wine or black tea can lead to darker teeth.[3] Tooth whitening procedures provide a conservative means to improve dental aesthetics. All types of tooth whitening procedures can be useful on their own or as an adjunct to other restorative procedures. Tooth whitening is a blanket term for a process resulting in a material becoming similar in color to a preferred or standard white regardless of the means used. Tooth bleaching has been defined as the lightening of the color of a tooth through the application of a chemical agent to oxidize the organic pigmentation in the tooth.[4] As the general population becomes more aware of dental aesthetics, this may be accompanied by an increase in the demand for aesthetic procedures as well as increased expectations for treatment outcomes. It is therefore pertinent for the dentist to understand different teeth whitening procedures, over-the-counter (OTC) products, their specific indications, and the potential risks of whitening treatment.

HISTORICAL OVERVIEW OF DENTAL BLEACHING

Dental bleaching is a cosmetic dental procedure aimed at lightening the shade of teeth. Its history traces back centuries, reflecting humanity's enduring quest for dental aesthetics and oral hygiene. This historical overview of dental bleaching spans millennia, showcasing the evolution of techniques and materials used to achieve brighter smiles. Ancient civilizations were among the first to explore teeth whitening methods. Egyptians, for instance, used a mixture of ground pumice stone and wine vinegar to scrub teeth, while Romans employed urine (which contains ammonia) for its bleaching properties. These early attempts, though crude by modern standards, laid the foundation for future developments in dental bleaching. In the 18th century, Europeans experimented with various abrasive substances such as alum, salt, and even sulfuric acid to whiten teeth. However, these abrasive methods often damaged tooth enamel and caused more harm than good.

In 1848, a breakthrough in dental bleaching came with the discovery of hydrogen peroxide by French chemist Louis Jacques Thénard. Its properties were soon recognized, and dentists began using it to whiten teeth. However, its corrosive nature led to tissue irritation and enamel damage when used in high concentrations. Throughout the 20th century, dental bleaching methods continued to evolve. In the 1960s, the "walking bleach" technique was introduced, involving the application of a paste containing hydrogen peroxide and sodium perborate inside the tooth, which was left for several days to achieve whitening. This method was primarily used to treat discolored nonvital teeth (teeth with damaged pulp).[5,6]

In the late 1980s and early 1990s, the introduction of carbamide peroxide as a bleaching agent revolutionized dental bleaching. Carbamide peroxide breaks down into hydrogen peroxide and urea, providing a controlled release of hydrogen peroxide, thus minimizing tissue irritation. This led to the development of at-home bleaching kits containing carbamide peroxide gel in custom-fitted trays, offering patients a convenient and effective whitening option. The turn of the 21st century witnessed the rise of in-office bleaching procedures using high-concentration hydrogen peroxide gels activated by light or laser. These procedures, often referred to as power bleaching or laser bleaching, promised quicker results compared to traditional at-home methods. However, concerns arose regarding the potential damage to tooth enamel and increased sensitivity associated with these high-intensity treatments.

In recent years, advancements in dental bleaching technology have focused on improving efficacy while minimizing adverse effects. Light emitting diode (LED) bleaching systems have gained popularity for their gentler approach, utilizing blue light to activate bleaching agents and accelerate the whitening process without causing significant damage to tooth structure.[7]

CLASSIFICATION OF DENTAL STAINING

Dental discoloration is generally classified as extrinsic or intrinsic staining. Extrinsic staining is of external origin and is often superficial in nature **(Table 1)**. Intrinsic discoloration can occur due to dental treatment such as pulp extirpation which induces hemorrhage into dentin, remaining pulpal tissue during root canal procedures, root canal irritants, or root canal restorative materials. Combining irritants containing sodium hypochlorite and chlorhexidine may lead to a reddish-brown precipitate. Some endodontic materials that contain tetracycline for example Ledermix, Endofill, zinc oxide eugenol, Tubliseal, gutta-percha, and gray mineral trioxide aggregate can lead to intrinsic discoloration.[4,8-17]

DEGREE OF TEETH WHITENESS

To assess the performance of a whitening agent, in vitro and in vivo methods have been developed to quantify the degree of whiteness and of staining (e.g., the pellicle cleaning ratio or PCR is a very prominent in vitro approach).[18] Staining solutions to determine the PCR in vitro often contain coffee or tea to imitate a natural staining process in the oral cavity.[19] Several methods can be used to evaluate the tooth color, e.g., a visual assessment using shade guides, spectrophotometry, colorimetry, or computer analysis of digital images.[20]

The Lobene stain index is commonly used and is based on a visual inspection of the tooth color.[21] It can only be used to assess extrinsic stains. Staining is classified regarding its intensity (no stain, light stain, moderate stain, and heavy stain) and area (no stain detected, stain covering up to one-third of the region, stain covering >1/3 to 2/3 of the region, and stain covering >2/3 of the region).[22] Tooth stain can be semiquantitatively assessed by color shade guides.[21] A more quantitative assessment of tooth color and brightness requires the measurement of optical reflection spectra as a function of the light wavelength and their interpretation with respect to different colors and their intensity. Quantitative methods are available, based on the CIEL* a *b* color tables, based on lightness (L*), red/green (a*), and blue/yellow (b*). The numbers can be combined in the CIEL *a *b* equation to give a relative change in tooth color ΔE.[18,23,24]

TABLE 1: Summary of common extrinsic and intrinsic causes of dental staining.

Extrinsic causes	***Intrinsic causes***
• Consumption of certain foods, beverages such as coffee and red wine, or tobacco products • Inadequate oral hygiene can also result in extrinsic staining	• Hemorrhage of the pulp which leads to blood entering the dentinal tubules. The blood then decomposes leading to deposition of chromogenic blood degradation products such as hemosiderin and hemin • Necrosis of the pulp • Calcification of the pulp through obliteration of dentinal tubules and buildup of tertiary dentin. Triggers for calcification are abrasion, erosion, or iatrogenic irritations • Systemic use of tetracycline antibiotics

MECHANISMS OF DENTAL BLEACHING

The process involves the use of bleaching agents to lighten the color of the teeth, resulting in a brighter and more attractive smile. Understanding the mechanisms behind dental bleaching is crucial for dental professionals to effectively carry out the procedure and for patients to achieve desired outcomes safely.

- *Oxidation:* One of the primary mechanisms behind dental bleaching is oxidation. Bleaching agents such as hydrogen peroxide or carbamide peroxide penetrate the enamel and dentin of the teeth, where they break down into oxygen radicals. These radicals then react with the pigmented molecules that cause discoloration, breaking them down into smaller, less pigmented molecules. As a result, the overall color of the teeth is lightened, and the appearance of stains is reduced.
- *Chemical degradation:* In addition to oxidation, dental bleaching also involves chemical degradation of pigmented molecules. Bleaching agents disrupt the chemical bonds within the chromophores responsible

for tooth discoloration. This process effectively breaks down the molecular structure of the pigments, leading to a reduction in their concentration and ultimately resulting in whiter teeth.

- *Diffusion:* Another mechanism involved in dental bleaching is diffusion. Bleaching agents diffuse into the tooth structure, reaching the discolored molecules within the enamel and dentin. This allows the bleaching agents to interact directly with the pigments, facilitating their breakdown and removal. Diffusion plays a crucial role in ensuring uniform whitening of the entire tooth surface.
- *Activation:* The effectiveness of dental bleaching is often enhanced using activation techniques. Activation methods, such as heat, light, or laser energy can accelerate the breakdown of bleaching agents, leading to faster and more efficient results. These activation techniques help to speed up the oxidation and chemical degradation processes, thereby improving the overall efficacy of the bleaching treatment.
- *Remineralization:* While dental bleaching primarily focuses on whitening the teeth, it can also lead to temporary demineralization of the enamel. However, remineralization mechanisms come into play following the bleaching treatment. Remineralization involves the deposition of minerals such as calcium and phosphate back into the enamel, restoring its strength and integrity. This helps to counteract any potential weakening of the enamel that may occur during the bleaching process.
- *pH balance:* Maintaining the proper pH balance is essential for the success of dental bleaching. Bleaching agents often have acidic properties, which can temporarily lower the pH of the oral environment. However, maintaining an optimal pH balance is crucial to minimize the risk of adverse effects such as tooth sensitivity and tissue irritation. Dental professionals may use pH-neutralizing agents or recommend post-treatment oral care products to help restore the natural pH of the oral cavity.[25,26]

TOOTH WHITENING PROCEDURES

There are various techniques of dental bleaching, each with its own advantages, disadvantages, and considerations.

Dental Prophylaxis

Professional hygiene procedures and polishing are performed to eliminate extrinsic staining by use of an abrasive paste and a rubber cup on a slow speed rotary instrument. Extrinsic stains can influence tooth color assessment and it has been shown that performing dental prophylaxis has a positive effect on patient's perception of the whiteness of their teeth.[27]

In-office Bleaching

It is a technique that involves the application of a high-concentration bleaching gel directly to the teeth by a dental professional. The gel usually contains hydrogen peroxide or carbamide peroxide as the active bleaching agent. A protective barrier is placed over the gums and soft tissues to prevent irritation. The bleaching gel is then activated using a special light or laser, which helps to accelerate the whitening process. In-office bleaching typically yields immediate results and can lighten teeth by several shades in a single session.[28-36] However, it may cause temporary tooth sensitivity or gum irritation in some patients.

At-home Bleaching

It involves the use of custom-made bleaching trays filled with a lower concentration bleaching gel. These trays are provided by a dentist and are designed to fit snugly over the teeth. Patients are instructed to wear the trays for a specified amount of time each day, usually for several hours or overnight, depending on the concentration of the bleaching gel. At-home bleaching may take longer time to achieve desired results compared to in-office bleaching, but it offers the convenience of being able to whiten teeth in the comfort of one's own home.[37-42] It is important for patients to follow their dentist's instructions carefully to avoid overuse of the bleaching gel, which can lead to tooth sensitivity or gum irritation.

Over-the-counter Products

Nowadays, there are also numerous OTC bleaching products available, such as whitening toothpaste, strips, and gels, which can be purchased without a prescription. These products typically contain lower concentrations of bleaching agents compared to professional-grade products and may take longer to produce noticeable results. Some dental professionals may recommend a combination of in-office and at-home bleaching for optimal results. This approach involves an initial in-office bleaching session followed by at-home maintenance using custom-made bleaching trays.[43-46] This combination technique allows for both immediate results and long-term maintenance, providing patients with a whiter, brighter smile that lasts.

Microabrasion

It is a minimally invasive technique used to remove surface stains and discoloration from teeth.[47] It involves the use of a mild abrasive compound, usually containing hydrochloric acid and pumice, which is applied to the surface of the teeth using a rotating rubber cup or brush. It was first introduced by Croll et al. in 1986.[47,48] He recommended the use of 18% hydrochloric acid with abrasives in a water-soluble mixture on a low rotational handpiece.[49] Microabrasion can be performed alone or in combination with other bleaching techniques to enhance the overall results.

POTENTIAL ADVERSE EFFECTS

The severity of the adverse effects of tooth whitening is dependent on the whitening technique followed, the concentration of whitening agent used, and the duration of the treatment. The most noticed adverse effects are:

- Tooth sensitivity is a common adverse effect. It is often transient lasting 2–3 days and moderate to mild in severity. It is believed to be a result of byproducts of bleaching agents diffusing through the dentinal tubules and inducing a transient pulpal reaction. Desensitizing agents such as potassium nitrate have been incorporated into bleaching agents to combat bleaching-induced tooth sensitivity. Application of a calcium phosphate-based desensitizer prior to in-office bleaching shown reduction in tooth sensitivity.[50-54]
- Gingival irritation is another potential adverse effect of bleaching. The incidence of gingival irritation during at-home bleaching ranged from 5 to 50%. The most common risk factor when using tray bleach is the use of an ill-fitting tray. When performing in-office bleaching, failed gingival barrier protection is the leading cause of gingival irritation. Gingival irritation can also occur when patients use excessive amounts of bleaching material that over-flow out of the tray.[55] When it occurs, the irritation is often tolerable, self-limiting, and is not a barrier to completing treatment.
- Bleaching has also been shown to alter the mineral content in enamel with laser-activated tooth bleaching being particularly damaging.[56,57] These alterations can be reversed by the application of remineralizing toothpastes that contain calcium phosphate.
- External cervical resorption (ECR) is a potential adverse effect of nonvital bleaching. 10% of teeth have natural anatomic defects in the cementum at the cementoenamel junction (CEJ) (Rotstein) which could allow hydrogen peroxide to reach the external tooth surface via dentinal tubules during intracoronal bleaching. Once the hydrogen peroxide encounters the periodontal tissues, dentin is denatured, and the host immune response is initiated. Younger patients may be more susceptible due to larger tubules. The number of reported cases has decreased over the years due to use of lower concentrations of bleaching agent and proper cervical seals.[58-64]

SAFETY IMPLICATIONS

While the desire for whiter teeth is understandable, it is crucial to consider the safety implications, particularly concerning women's oral health and overall well-being. Women may have specific safety concerns regarding dental bleaching due to hormonal fluctuations, pregnancy, breastfeeding, and oral health conditions. Hormonal changes, particularly during pregnancy, can affect gum sensitivity and increase the risk of oral health issues such as gingivitis and periodontal disease.

Additionally, the safety of bleaching agents during pregnancy and breastfeeding is still debated among dental professionals, emphasizing the need for caution. Before undergoing any dental bleaching procedure, women should consult with a qualified dental professional. Women who are pregnant or breastfeeding should exercise caution when considering dental bleaching. While there is limited research on the safety of bleaching agents during these periods, it is generally recommended to avoid elective procedures and opt for nonbleaching alternatives until after pregnancy.[65]

After dental bleaching, women should follow the recommended postcare instructions provided by their dentist. This may include avoiding certain foods and beverages that can stain teeth, using desensitizing agents to alleviate any sensitivity, and attending follow-up appointments for evaluation. Women who are concerned about the safety of dental bleaching may consider alternative whitening methods such as enamel microabrasion, which involves removing surface stains using a mild abrasive solution without the use of bleaching agents.[66]

FACTORS DETERMINING THE EFFECTIVENESS OF BLEACHING

While it is sought after by both men and women, various factors influence its effectiveness, particularly in women. Understanding these factors is crucial for dental professionals to tailor treatments effectively and achieve optimal results. Women undergo hormonal fluctuations throughout their lives, such as during puberty, menstruation, pregnancy, and menopause. These hormonal changes can affect the composition of dental tissues and impact the effectiveness of dental bleaching. For instance, increased estrogen levels during pregnancy may lead to greater susceptibility to tooth discoloration, requiring adjustments in bleaching protocols.[67]

The oral health status of women, including factors like dental caries, gum disease, and enamel defects, can influence the effectiveness of dental bleaching. Patients with underlying oral health issues may experience uneven whitening results or increased sensitivity during bleaching treatments. Therefore, addressing any oral health concerns before initiating bleaching procedures is essential for optimizing outcomes. Women's lifestyle choices, such as smoking, dietary habits, and oral hygiene practices, play a significant role in dental bleaching effectiveness. Smoking, for example, can contribute to tooth discoloration and hinder the bleaching process.[3,68] Additionally, consumption of highly pigmented foods and beverages like coffee, tea, and red wine can compromise the longevity of bleaching results if not managed appropriately.

Variations in tooth structure and composition among women can impact the penetration of bleaching agents and the overall effectiveness of treatment. Factors such as enamel thickness, dentin density, and presence of intrinsic stains influence the ability of bleaching agents to reach and whiten the underlying tooth structure. Dental professionals must assess these individual factors to determine the most suitable bleaching approach for each patient. Adherence to bleaching treatment protocols significantly influences its effectiveness. Women may face challenges in maintaining consistent treatment schedules due to various commitments, including work, family responsibilities, and social engagements. Lack of compliance with treatment instructions, such as wearing whitening trays for the prescribed duration or attending follow-up appointments, can compromise the desired bleaching outcomes.

Psychological factors, including patient expectations, satisfaction with dental appearance, and self-esteem, influence the perceived effectiveness of dental bleaching in women.[68] Unrealistic expectations or dissatisfaction with the results may lead to diminished treatment outcomes, despite achieving clinically acceptable whitening effects. Therefore, open communication between patients and dental professionals is crucial for managing expectations and ensuring patient satisfaction.

POST-BLEACHING MAINTENANCE

Whether done professionally in a dental office or through at-home kits, dental bleaching can effectively lighten the color of teeth. However, achieving a dazzling smile is just the beginning; maintaining the results of dental bleaching requires proper post-treatment care and maintenance. One common side effect of dental bleaching is tooth sensitivity. This sensitivity usually subsides within a few days to a week after the bleaching treatment. However, during this period, it is essential to avoid foods and drinks that may exacerbate sensitivity, such as ice-cold beverages or extremely hot foods.

Maintaining good oral hygiene is crucial for preserving the results of dental bleaching. Brushing at least twice a day with a fluoride toothpaste and flossing daily helps remove surface stains and prevent the buildup of plaque and tartar, which can dull the appearance of teeth. Additionally, using a whitening toothpaste or mouthwash formulated for maintaining bleached teeth can help prolong the whitening effects. One should minimize consumption of staining agents, such as coffee, tea, red wine, and dark-colored fruits and sauces.[3] If consuming these beverages or foods, using a straw can help minimize contact with the teeth, reducing the risk of staining. Routine dental check-ups are essential for monitoring oral health and ensuring the longevity of dental bleaching results. Additionally, professional dental cleanings help remove surface stains and plaque buildup, keeping the teeth looking bright and healthy.[69] Touch-up treatments may be necessary to restore the desired level of whiteness that can be performed either at home using OTC whitening products or in a dental office under professional supervision.

PATIENT SATISFACTION AND PSYCHOLOGICAL IMPACT OF DENTAL BLEACHING

While the primary goal of dental bleaching is to enhance aesthetic appeal, its impact on patient satisfaction and psychological well-being is a topic of growing interest and research within the dental community. Patient satisfaction is a crucial aspect of any medical or dental procedure, as it reflects the effectiveness of the treatment and its ability to meet the patient's expectations. In case of dental bleaching, patient satisfaction is often closely linked to the perceived improvement in the appearance of their teeth. Studies have shown that the majority of patients experience a significant improvement in the whiteness of their teeth, leading to increased confidence and self-esteem.[70,71]

The psychological impact of dental bleaching extends beyond mere satisfaction with the physical results. A bright, white smile is often associated with attractiveness, youthfulness, and overall well-being in many cultures. As a result, the psychological benefits of dental bleaching can be profound, with patients reporting increased self-confidence, improved social interactions, and even a more positive outlook on life. For individuals who may have felt self-conscious about the appearance of their teeth, dental bleaching can be a transformative experience, boosting their self-esteem, and quality of life. However, it is essential to recognize that the psychological impact of dental bleaching may vary from patient to patient. While many individuals experience a significant improvement in their psychological well-being following the procedure, others may have unrealistic expectations or underlying psychological issues that cannot be fully addressed through cosmetic dental treatments alone. In some cases, patients may experience temporary sensitivity or discomfort during or after the bleaching process, which can affect their overall satisfaction and psychological well-being.

Moreover, the long-term effects of dental bleaching on patient satisfaction and psychological well-being are still not fully understood. While the immediate results of the procedure are often positive, studies on the longevity of the whitening effects and their impact on patient satisfaction over time are limited.[71] Additionally, the potential for relapse, whereby the teeth gradually return to their original shade over time, can affect patient satisfaction and psychological well-being in the long term. It is also essential to consider the ethical implications of dental bleaching, particularly concerning patient autonomy and informed consent. Dentists have a responsibility to ensure that patients fully understand the potential risks and benefits of the procedure, as well as any alternative treatment options available. Additionally, dentists must consider the psychological impact of dental bleaching on vulnerable populations, such as individuals with body dysmorphic disorder or other mental health conditions, and exercise caution when recommending cosmetic dental procedures.[72]

DEVELOPMENTS IN WHITENING AGENTS

With more technology and advancements, a lot of brands like Perfora and Protouch have come up with many kinds of innovative and safe-to-use tooth whitening solutions. Some of them are tooth whitening pen, tooth whitening powder, tooth whitening serum, and tooth whitening strips.[41-44] Newer developments in tooth whitening include incorporation of sweet potato enzymes into hydrogen peroxide as they contain several antioxidant molecules which theoretically are free radical scavengers that target chromogens. In vitro studies on these enzymes are promising.[73] Other advancements involve the incorporation of chemical, bioactive and natural organic additives into hydrogen peroxide with the aim of elevating the pH and therefore delaying the decomposition of hydrogen peroxide. In vitro studies of these agents are also promising and open the field to more extensive clinical trials.[74-78]

CONCLUSION

Dental bleaching has emerged as a significant aspect of cosmetic dentistry, offering patients the opportunity to achieve brighter and whiter smiles. Throughout this chapter, we have explored various aspects of dental bleaching, including its history, mechanisms of action, different bleaching techniques, safety considerations, and future directions. The future of dental bleaching holds promising advancements in technology and techniques. Innovations such as light-activated bleaching systems, nanotechnology-based whitening agents, and personalized treatment regimens are likely to enhance the efficiency and outcomes of bleaching procedures. Furthermore, ongoing research into novel bleaching agents and delivery methods may lead to safer and more sustainable approaches to achieving whiter smiles. As we continue to advance our knowledge and technology in the field of dental bleaching, it is essential to prioritize patient safety and satisfaction. Through ongoing research, education, and collaboration among dental professionals, we can further improve the effectiveness, safety, and accessibility of dental bleaching treatments, ultimately empowering individuals to smile with confidence.

REFERENCES

1. Meireles SS, Goettems ML, Dantas RV, Bona ÁD, Santos IS, Demarco FF. Changes in oral health related quality of

life after dental bleaching in a double-blind randomized clinical trial. J Dent. 2014;42(2):114-21.

2. Pavicic DK, Kolceg M, Lajnert V, Pavlic A, Brumini M, Spalj S. Changes in Quality of Life Induced by Tooth Whitening are Moderated by Perfectionism: A Randomized, Double-Blind, Placebo-Controlled Trial. Int J Prosthodont. 2018;31(4):394-6.
3. Silva EMD, Maia JNDSMD, Mitraud CG, Russo JDES, Poskus LT, Guimarães JGA. Can whitening toothpastes maintain the optical stability of enamel over time? J Appl Oral Sci. 2018;26:e20160460.
4. Vernon-Sparks L. (2010). A history of tooth-whitening. [online]. Available from https://www.seattletimes.com/seattle-news/health/a-history-of-tooth-whitening/ [Last accessed June, 2024].
5. Kezian SA. The history of the dental profession—from ancient origins to modern day. Pacific J Health. 2020;3(1):1-31.
6. Walker L. (2022). Teeth whitening: Antiquated to present-day. [online] Available from https://dentalacademyofce.com/wp-content/uploads/2022/03/2202CEDwal.pdf [Last accessed June, 2024].
7. Arens D. The role of bleaching in esthetics. Dent Clin North Am. 1989;33(2):319-36.
8. Marin PD, Bartold PM, Heithersay GS. Tooth discolouration by blood: an in vitro histochemical study. Dent Traumatol. 1997;13(3):132-8.
9. Brown G. Factors influencing successful bleaching of the discoloured root-filled tooth. Oral Surg Oral Med Oral Pathol. 1965;20(2):238-44.
10. Faunce F. Management of discoloured teeth. Dent Clin North Am. 1983;27(4):657-70.
11. Basrani BR, Manek S, Sodhi RN, Fillery E, Manzur A. Interaction between sodium hypochlorite and chlorhexidine gluconate. J Endod. 2007;33(8):966-9.
12. Tay FR, Mazzoni A, Pashley DH, Day TE, Ngoh EC, Breschi L. Potential iatrogenic tetracycline staining of endodontically treated teeth via NaOCl/MTAD irrigation: a preliminary report. J Endod. 2006;32(4):354-8.
13. Van der Burgt TP, Mullaney TP, Plasschaert AJ. Tooth discolouration induced by endodontic sealers. Oral Surg Oral Med Oral Pathol. 1986;61(1):84-9.
14. Kim ST, Abbott PV, McGinley P. The effects of Ledermix paste on discolouration of mature teeth. Int Endod J. 2000;33(3):227-32.
15. Jacobovitz M, De Lima RK. Treatment of inflammatory internal root resorption with mineral trioxide aggregate: a case report. Int Endod J. 2008;41(10):905-12.
16. Bortoluzzi EA, Araújo GS, Tanomaru JM, Tanomaru-Filho M. Marginal gingiva discolouration by gray MTA: a case report. J Endod. 2007;33(3):325-7.
17. Joiner A, Luo W. Tooth colour and whiteness: A review. J Dent. 2017;67:S3-S10.
18. Stookey GK, Burkhard TA, Schemehorn BR. In vitro removal of stain with dentifrices. J Dent Res. 1982;61(11):1236-9.
19. Joiner A. Tooth colour: a review of the literature. J Dent. 2004;32:3-12.
20. Joiner A. Whitening toothpastes: a review of the literature. J Dent. 2010;38(Suppl 2):e17-e24.
21. Terezhalmy GT, Walters PA, Bartizek RD, Grender JM, Biesbrock AR. A clinical evaluation of extrinsic stain removal: a rotation-oscillation power toothbrush versus a dental prophylaxis. J Contemp Dent Pract. 2008;9:1-8.
22. Viscio D, Gaffar A, Fakhry-Smith S, Xu T. Present and future technologies of tooth whitening. Compend Contin Educ Dent Suppl. 2000;(28):S36-43; quiz S49.
23. Joiner A, Hopkinson I, Deng Y, Westland S. A review of tooth colour and whiteness. J Dent. 2008;36 Suppl 1:S2-7.
24. Price RB, Sedarous M, Hiltz GS. The pH of tooth-whitening products. J Can Dent Assoc. 2000;66(8):421-6.
25. Xu B, Li Q, Wang Y. Effects of pH values of hydrogen peroxide bleaching agents on enamel surface properties. Oper Dent. 2011;36(5):554-62.
26. Pereira R, Corado D, Silveira J, Alves R, Mata A, Marques D. Dental prophylaxis influence in tooth color assessment—Clinical study. J Esthet Restor Dent. 2020;32(6):586-92.
27. Bernardon JK, Sartori N, Ballarin A, Perdigão J, Lopes G, Baratieri LN. Clinical performance of vital bleaching techniques. Oper Dent. 2010;35(1):3-10.
28. da Costa JB, McPharlin R, Paravina RD, Ferracane JL. Comparison of at-home and in-office tooth whitening using a novel shade guide. Oper Dent. 2010;35(4):381-8.
29. Rezende M, Loguercio AD, Reis A, Kossatz S. Clinical effects of exposure to coffee during at-home vital bleaching. Oper Dent. 2013;38(6):E229-36.
30. Zekonis R, Matis BA, Cochran MA, Shetri SA, Eckert GJ, Carlson TJ. Clinical evaluation of in-office and at-home bleaching treatments. Oper Dent. 2003;28(2):114-21.
31. Acosta Gómez AP, Henao Giraldo GM, Henao Arango LG. Peróxido de hidrógeno al 35 por ciento y peróxido de carbamida al 10 por ciento para el blanqueamiento dental. Univ Odontol. 1999;14-20.
32. Kossatz S, Dalanhol AP, Cunha T, Loguercio A, Reis A. Effect of light activation on tooth sensitivity after in-office bleaching. Oper Dent. 2011;36(3):251-7.
33. Reis A, Tay LY, Herrera DR, Kossatz S, Loguercio AD. Clinical effects of prolonged application time of an in-office bleaching gel. Oper Dent. 2011;36(6):590-6.
34. De Geus JL, Wambier LM, Kossatz S, Loguercio AD, Reis A. At-home vs in-office bleaching: a systematic review and meta-analysis. Oper Dent. 2016;41(4):341-56.
35. Maran BM, Burey A, de Paris Matos T, Loguercio AD, Reis A. In-office dental bleaching with light vs. without light: a systematic review and meta-analysis. J Dent. 2018;70:1-3.
36. Sulieman M. An overview of bleaching techniques: 2. Night Guard Vital Bleaching and non-vital bleaching. Dent Update. 2005;32(1):39-46.

37. Nathoo SA, Richter R, Smith S, Zhang YP. Kinetics of carbamide peroxide degradation in bleaching trays. J Dent Res. 1996;75:286.
38. Matis BA, Gaiao U, Blackman D, Schultz FA, Eckert GJ. In vivo degradation of bleaching gel used in whitening teeth. J Am Dent Assoc. 1999;130(2):227-35.
39. Leonard RH Jr, Haywood VB, Caplan DJ, Tart ND. Nightguard vital bleaching of tetracycline-stained teeth: 90 months post treatment. J Esthet Restor Dent. 2003;15(3):142-53.
40. Martini EC, Favoreto MW, Coppla FM, Loguercio AD, Reis A. Evaluation of reservoirs in bleaching trays for at-home bleaching: a split-mouth single-blind randomized controlled equivalence trial. J Appl Oral Sci. 2020;28:e20200332.
41. Levrini L, Paracchini L, Bakaj R, Diaconu A, Cortese S. Dental bleaching during orthodontic treatment with aligners. Int J Esthetic Dent. 2020;15(1):44-54.
42. Soares CN, Amaral FL, Mesquita MF, Franca FM, Basting RT, Turssi CP. Toothpastes containing abrasive and chemical whitening agents: efficacy in reducing extrinsic dental staining. Gen Dent. 2015;63(6):e24-8.
43. Casado BG, Moraes SL, Souza GF, Guerra CM, Souto-Maior JR, Lemos CA, et al. Efficacy of dental bleaching with whitening dentifrices: a systematic review. Int J Dentist. 2018;2018:7868531.
44. Carey CM. Tooth whitening: what we now know. J Evid Base Dent Pract. 2014;14:70-6.
45. Jiang N, Zhang C, Agingu C, Attin T, Cheng H, Yu H. Comparison of whitening dentifrices on the effectiveness of in-office tooth bleaching: a double-blind randomized controlled clinical trial. Oper Dent. 2019;44(2):138-45.
46. Sundfeld RH, Franco LM, Gonçalves RS, de Alexandre RS, Machado LS, Neto DS. Accomplishing esthetics using enamel microabrasion and bleaching—a case report. Oper Dent. 2014;39(3):223-7.
47. Croll TP, Cavanaugh RR. Enamel color modification by controlled hydrochloric acid-pumice abrasion. II. Further examples. Quintessence Int. 1986;17(3):157-64.
48. Croll TP. Enamel microabrasion: the technique. Quintessence Int. 1989;20(6):395-400.
49. Eva K, Marijan M, Mira R, Ivan S, Katica P, Zrinka T. Surface changes of enamel and dentin after two different bleaching procedures. Acta Clinica Croatica. 2013;52(4):413-28.
50. West NX, Lussi A, Seong J, Hellwig E. Dentin hypersensitivity: pain mechanisms and aetiology of exposed cervical dentin. Clin Oral Investig. 2013;17(1):9-19.
51. Chemin K, Rezende M, Loguercio AD, Reis A, Kossatz S. Effectiveness of and dental sensitivity to at-home bleaching with 4% and 10% hydrogen peroxide: a randomized, triple-blind clinical trial. Oper Dent. 2018;43(3):232-40.
52. Maran BM, Vochikovski L, de Andrade Hortkoff DR, Stanislawczuk R, Loguercio AD, Reis A. Tooth sensitivity with a desensitizing-containing at-home bleaching gel—a randomized triple-blind clinical trial. J Dent. 2018;72:64-70.
53. Mehta D, Jyothi S, Moogi P, Finger WJ, Sasaki K. Novel treatment of in-office tooth bleaching sensitivity: a randomized, placebo-controlled clinical study. J Esthet Restor Dent. 2018;30(3):254-8.
54. Li Y, Greenwall L. Safety issues of tooth whitening using peroxide-based materials. Br Dent J. 2013;215(1):29-34.
55. Farawati FA, Hsu SM, O'Neill E, Neal D, Clark A, Esquivel-Upshaw J. Effect of carbamide peroxide bleaching on enamel characteristics and susceptibility to further discolouration. J Prosthet Dent. 2019;121(2):340-6.
56. Coceska E, Gjorgievska E, Coleman NJ, Gabric D, Slipper IJ, Stevanovic M, et al. Enamel alteration following tooth bleaching and remineralization. J Microsc. 2016; 262(3):232-44.
57. Rotstein I, Torek Y, Misgav R. Effect of cementum defects on radicular penetration of 30% H_2O_2 during intracoronal bleaching. J Endod. 1991;17(5):230-3.
58. Cate T, Nanci A. Oral Histology: development, structure, and function. St Louis, Missouri: Mosby; 1985.
59. Camps J, de Franceschi H, Idir F, Roland C, About I. Time-course diffusion of hydrogen peroxide through human dentin: clinical significance for young tooth internal bleaching. J Endod. 2007;33(4):455-9.
60. Pashley DH, Thompson SM, Stewart FP. Dentin permeability: effects of temperature on hydraulic conductance. J Dent Res. 1983;62(9):956-9.
61. MacIsaac AM, Hoen CM. Intracoronal bleaching: concerns and considerations. J Can Dent Assoc. 1994;60(1):57-64.
62. Rotstein I, Zyskind D, Lewinstein I, Bamberger N. Effect of different protective base materials on hydrogen peroxide leakage during intracoronal bleaching in vitro. J Endod. 1992;18(3):114-17.
63. Newton R, Hayes J. The association of external cervical resorption with modern internal bleaching protocols: what is the current evidence? Br Dent J. 2020;228(5):333-7.
64. Wrzosek T, Einarson A. Dental care during pregnancy. Can Fam Physician. 2009;55(6):598-9.
65. Favero V, Bacci C, Volpato A, Bandiera M, Favero L, Zanette G. Pregnancy and Dentistry: A Literature Review on Risk Management during Dental Surgical Procedures. Dent J (Basel). 2021;9(4):46.
66. Hassan GS, Helal MB, Ibrahim HF. Immunohistochemical expression of estrogen receptor alpha in the maxillary sinus, pulp, and periodontal ligament of adjacent teeth in late pregnancy in rats. Odontology. 2023;111(3):608-17.
67. Vt H, T M, T S, Nisha V A, A A. Dental considerations in pregnancy-a critical review on the oral care. J Clin Diagn Res. 2013;7(5):948-53.
68. Demarco FF, Meireles SS, Masotti AS. Over-the-counter whitening agents: a concise review. Braz Oral Res. 2009;23 Suppl 1:64-70.
69. Moldovan AM, Popescu V, Lonescu CV, Mesaros AS, Cuc S, Craciun A, et al. Various aspects involved in the study of

tooth bleaching procedures: a questionnaire-based study. Int J Environ Res Public Health. 2022;19(7):3977.
70. Goettems ML, Fernandez MDS, Donassollo TA, Henn Donassollo S, Demarco FF. Impact of tooth bleaching on oral health-related quality of life in adults: a triple-blind randomised clinical trial. J Dent. 2021;105:103564.
71. Bonafé E, Rezende M, Machado MM, Lima SNL, Fernandez E, Baldani MMP, et al. Personality traits, psychosocial effects and quality of life of patients submitted to dental bleaching. BMC Oral Health. 2021;21(1):7.
72. Gopinath S, James V, Vidhya S, Karthikeyan K, Kavitha S, Mahalaxmi S. Effect of bleaching with two different concentrations of hydrogen peroxide containing sweet potato extract as an additive on human enamel: an in vitro spectrophotometric and scanning electron microscopy analysis. J Conserv Dent. 2013;16(1):45-9.
73. Al Batayneh O. The clinical applications of Tooth Mousse TM and CPP-ACP products in caries prevention: evidence-based recommendations. Smile Dent J. 2009;8-12.
74. Somasundaram P, Vimala N, Mandke LG. Protective potential of casein phosphopeptide amorphous calcium phosphate containing paste on enamel surfaces. J Conserv Dent. 2013;16(2):152-6.
75. Farooq I, Moheet IA, Imran Z, Farooq U. A review of novel dental caries preventive material: Casein phosphopeptide-amorphous calcium phosphate (CPP-ACP) complex. King Saud Univ J Dent Sci. 2013;4(2):47-51.
76. Baldea I, Olteanu DE, Filip AG, Cenariu M, Dudea D, Tofan A, et al. Toxicity and efficiency study of plant extracts-based bleaching agents. Clin Oral Investig. 2017;21(4):1315-26.
77. Hyland BW, McDonald A, Lewis N, Tredwin C, Petrie A, Hall S, et al. A new three component formulation for the efficient whitening of teeth (Carbamide Plus). Clin Oral Investig. 2015;19(6):1395-404.
78. Kalyana P, Shashidhar A, Meghashyam B, Sreevidya KR, Sweta S. Stain removal efficacy of a novel dentifrice containing papain and bromelain extracts—an in vitro study. Int J Dent Hyg. 2011;9(3):229-33.

CHAPTER 27

Designer Smiles

Renu Datta, Tarika Datta

INTRODUCTION

A smile is an important social gesture and conveys a lot about the individual instantly. There is no definition of an "ideal" smile, but an attractive smile includes a sense of proportion and symmetry with the face and personality of the individual. It has also been shown that a balanced face and smile improve a person's self-esteem and self-worth as well.

THE IMPORTANCE OF FACIAL BEAUTY AND THE BEAUTIFUL SMILE

The smile conveys an individual's confidence and makes them attractive and pleasing to look at. One cannot deny that sometimes natural causes (such as irregular dental crowding or spacing, i.e., malocclusion) or neglect and decay of teeth can lead to an unattractive appearance and smile.[1]

Technological advances and the evolution of biomaterials in oral and dental science have combined to allow modification of an existing smile to create one that is more pleasing, aesthetic, and confident.[2]

An aesthetic analysis is an essential aspect of all dental treatment planning and is done to understand and define the outcome of any dental treatment or intervention, i.e., its influence on the patient's smile.[3]

Defining Beauty and Norms: Dental and Facial

Recognition of facial beauty is both inborn and learned through social discourse and exposure.[4]

A balanced face and smile are a beautiful and powerful tool. It is a scientifically proven fact that having a beautiful smile improves your self-esteem and self-worth.

Golden ratio of beauty is also known as Phi or Fibonacci, a mathematical algorithm that underlies our perception of attractiveness. Scientists made mathematical formulas to make their artwork scientifically perfect. The face serves as both the self's mirror and mask. This bodily part is significantly very powerful and influential, and we are the faces we wear. A key skill in conversational and communication skills is face reading. The facial expression is just as significant as the words themselves, as it has the power to contradict their meaning.

The attractiveness of a face is influenced by symmetry, averageness, and distinguishing features such as dental aesthetics or gender-specific characteristics. There is a shared concept of what constitutes an "ideal" face. Anthropometric methods are preferable to cephalometric methods in determining the "ideal" face's dimensions since anthropometric methods are valid, three-dimensional, noninvasive, suitable for a great variety of purposes, and easy to implement. Symmetry and averageness play important roles in determining the attractiveness of a face, although distinguishing features make it extraordinarily beautiful. Finally, allowance has to be made for the fact that the ideal of beauty is subject to certain fluctuations in fashion.

The literature mentions a few constellations that directly influence attractiveness: Crowding or gaps in the frontal area had a negative influence on facial aesthetics, while well-shaped, correctly inclined, or slightly protruding anterior teeth had a positive influence.

Dental Treatment and the Smile

An aesthetic analysis is an essential aspect of all dental treatment planning and is done to understand and define the outcome of any dental treatment or intervention, i.e., its influence on the patient's smile.

The goal of cosmetic dentistry is to replicate the natural world as much as possible. The foundation for this is knowledge of the natural tooth's organization, locations, dimensions, forms, hues, and morphology.

It was not until the latter half of the 20th century that aesthetic smiles were finally evaluated scientifically.

- *The relationship between the midline of the face and teeth:* The quantity of dental structure is visible when someone smiles. The average grin displays between 70% and 100% of the maxillary anterior teeth, the premolars, and the tips of the interproximal papillae. A smile that shows more gingiva is referred to as "high," while one that shows less tooth display is referred to as "low."

- *Harmony between the incisal line, or anterior teeth, and the curve of smile:*
  - Harmony between the lower lip's curvature and the anterior teeth, also known as the incisal line; these should be parallel.
  - Rectangular, triangular, and ovoid are the three basic forms of teeth.
- The application of strict norms and scientific procedures is complicated; there is no common concept of ideal aesthetics.
- Orthodontics was the first dental specialty to emphasize both function and aesthetics.
- Multidisciplinary planning and execution of sophisticated procedures in dentistry have been made easier by digital technology.

Diagnosis: Making a Problem List

- One aspect of the patient's overall condition vs. other significant problems. For example, diastema or spacing between teeth is part of the consideration for making a diagnosis.
- Priorities and patient concerns need to be part of the treatment plan for successful treatment.
- A comprehensive treatment plan requires a broad overview of the patient's problem list, considering both objective and subjective findings.
- In this method, diagnosis is carried out in logical steps to gather an adequate database.

BASIC COMPONENTS OF SMILE DESIGN

The basic components include:

- *Facial analysis:*
  - Frontal
  - Profile
  - Symmetry and asymmetry
  - Jaw proportions
- *Smile analysis:*
  - Lip shape and outline during smiling
  - Incisal edge relationship to lips
  - Midline symmetry
  - Gingival exposure and contour
- *Dental or tooth-level analysis:*
  - Tooth size
  - Tooth shape
  - Tooth proportions (height and width)
  - *Dental proportions:* Size and shape of adjacent teeth in relation to each other
  - Inclination or angulation from the midline
  - Color and texture of the teeth, including staining
- *Dentition analysis:*
  - Malocclusion (spacing and crowding)
  - Canting of the dentition
  - Asymmetry

Facial Analysis

This is done using photographs of the patient facing front and in profile.

A complete set of extraoral and intraoral photographs is taken to evaluate different aspects of the face, including the smile, jawline, vertical height of the face, and alignment of the teeth. The following facial photographs are recommended as part of the expected routine for each patient:

- *Frontal:*
  - Frontal at rest
  - Frontal view with the teeth in maximal intercuspation, with the lips closed, even if this strains the patient
  - Frontal dynamic (smile)
  - A close-up image of a posed smile

  Two profile images are used:

  1. *Profile at rest:* The lips should be relaxed.
  2. *Profile smile:* The profile smile image allows one to see the angulation of the maxillary incisors—an important aesthetic factor.
- Facial photographs offer a lot of information on soft tissue morphology and facial expression.
- Extra- and intraoral photographs are useful diagnostic aids.
- For extraoral photographs, the *Frankfort horizontal* (FH) plane should be parallel to the floor.

Uses:

- Useful in the assessment of facial symmetry, facial type, and profile.
- Serves as a diagnostic record.
- Helps in assessing the progress of the treatment.

There are a number of systems of facial analysis which help in the identification of the ratio and proportion of various parts of the face.

Horizontal Facial Proportions

- The width of the face should be the width of five "eyes."
- The distance between the eyebrow and chin should be equal to the width of the face.

Vertical Facial Proportions

The facial height is divided into three equal parts: From the forehead to the eyebrow line, from the eyebrow line to the base of the nose, and from the base of the nose to the base of the chin.

The lower part of the face, from the base of the nose to the chin, is divided into two parts: the upper lip forms one third of it, and the lower lip and the chin form two-thirds of it.

The basic shape of the face when viewed from the frontal aspect can be one of the following:

- Square
- Tapering
- Square tapering
- Ovoid

The lateral profile can be:

- Straight
- Convex
- Concave

Models

These are plasters or virtual replica of the patient's teeth for examination and calculation of the tooth width and arch perimeter analysis.

Radiographs

All comprehensive cases need intraoral periapical (IOPA) X-rays and orthopantomagram (OPG), whereas special X-rays such as cone-beam computed tomography (CBCT) and *posteroanterior* (PA) cephalograms are advised as per the patient's conditions. These radiographs are used to view the teeth and soft tissues around the teeth.

Profile Analysis

Goals

- Establishing whether the jaws are proportionately positioned in the AP plane of space.
- Evaluation of lip posture and incisor prominence.
- Re-evaluation of vertical facial proportions and evaluation of mandibular plane angle.

Establishing whether the jaws are proportionately positioned in the AP plane of space: Position the patient in natural head position (NHP), i.e., patient either sitting upright or standing but not reclining in a dental chair and looking at the horizon or a distant object.

Note the relationship between the maxilla and mandible with the help of two lines: The bridge of the nose to the base of the upper lip and the second line extending from that point to the chin.

Evaluation of lip posture and incisor prominence: Teeth protrude excessively if two conditions are met:

1. The lips are prominent and everted.
2. The lips are separated at rest by more than 3 or 4 mm.

Lip prominence is evaluated by observing the distance that each lip projects forward from a true vertical line through the depth of the concavity at its base. Lip prominence of 2–3 mm in the presence of lip incompetence indicates dentoalveolar protrusion.

Re-evaluation of vertical facial proportions and evaluation of mandibular plane angle: The mandibular plane is readily visualized by placing a finger or mirror handle along the lower border. A steep mandibular plane angle usually accompanies long anterior facial vertical dimensions and a skeletal open bite tendency **(Fig. 1)**.

Shape of the head:
Index = Maximum skull width/maximum skull length

Types and index values:

- *Mesocephalic:* Average: 76–80.9
- *Brachycephalic:* Short, broad skull 81–85.4
- *Dolichocephalic:* Long, narrow skull 75.9 and below

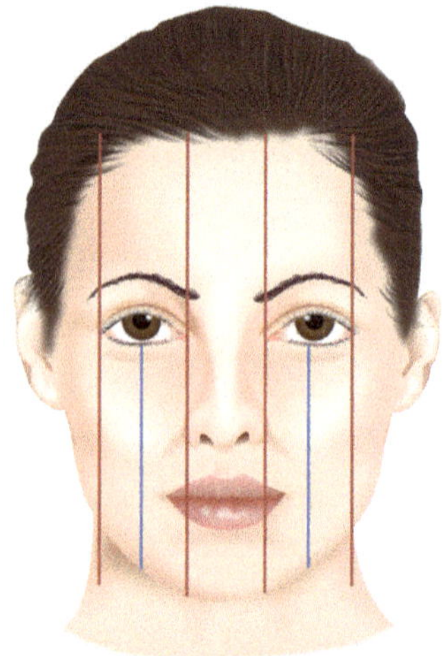

Fig. 1: Re-evaluation of vertical facial proportions and evaluation of mandibular plane angle.

Shape of the face:

I = Facial height/Bizygomatic width

- *Euryprosopic:* Broad and square arches, 79–83
- *Mesoprosopic:* Average 84–87.9
- *Leptoprosopic:* Narrow arches 88–92.9

Smile Analysis

This includes an evaluation of the lips in resting and smiling positions and their relationship to the facial symmetry and proportions externally and to the teeth internally **(Fig. 2)**.

Correct incisal edge position is crucial, because it is related to the pitch of the anterior teeth, labial contours, lip support, anterior guidance, lingual contours, and tooth display. The pitch of each anterior tooth is determined by the combination of correct lip support and the lingual labial position of the incisal edge. This location influences anterior guidance and the labial and lingual contours. In short, all these factors play a dominant role in both aesthetics and function.

Gingival Exposure and Contour

Figure 3 shows gingival exposure and contour.

Dental or Tooth-level Analysis

Figure 4 depicts dental or tooth-level analysis.

Tooth Dimensions

An aesthetically pleasing smile is largely dependent on having the right dental proportions, which are related to facial morphology. According to the principle of central dominance, the central teeth in a smile must be the dominant teeth and have aesthetically pleasing proportions. The secret to the smile lies in them. Both mathematically and aesthetically, the centrals' proportions must be correct. The centrals' width-to-length ratio should be roughly 4:5 (0.8–1.0); a range of 75–80% of their length is the most reasonable for their width. The appearance and placement of the laterals and canines are determined or influenced by the shape and location of the central.

Various guidelines for establishing correct proportions in an aesthetically pleasing smile are:

- Golden proportion (Lombardi)
- Recurring esthetic dental (RED) proportions (Ward)
- M proportions (Methot)
- Chu's aesthetic gauges

The important point to be noted here is that it is not the actual size, but instead the perceived size, that these proportions are based on when viewed from the facial aspect (in short, it is the distance between proximal line angles of the teeth).

- *Golden proportion (Lombardi):* When viewed from the facial, the width of each anterior tooth is 60% of the width of the adjacent tooth (mathematical ratio being 1.6:1:0.6). It is difficult to apply as patients have different arch forms, lip anatomy, and facial proportions. Strict adherence to golden proportion calculations limits creativity, and this may lead to cosmetic failure.
- *RED proportion:* The successive width proportion when viewed from the facial aspect should remain constant as we move posteriorly from the midline. This offers great flexibility to match tooth properties with facial proportions.
- *M proportions (Methot):* This method compares the tooth width with the facial width using software. The whole analysis is done on the computer and hence involves more mathematics rather than artistic analysis.

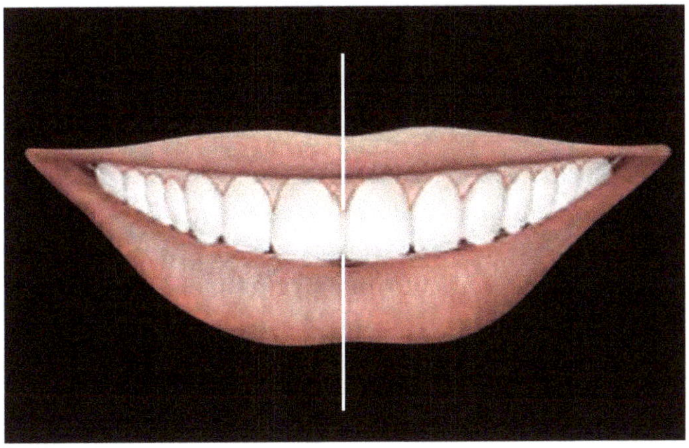

Fig. 2: Smile analysis.

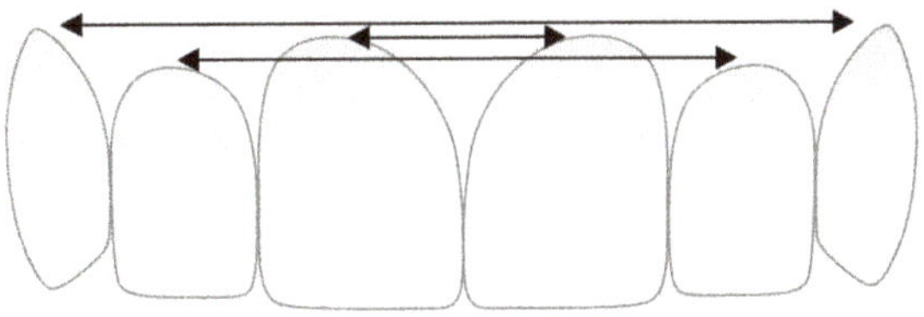

Fig. 3: Gingival exposure and contour.

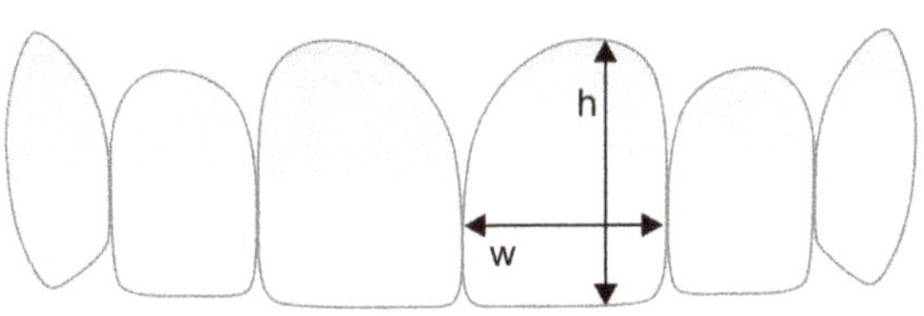

Fig. 4: Dental or tooth-level analysis.

- *Chu's aesthetic gauges:* Dr Chu's research supports Levin's RED concept and refutes the golden proportion. A series of gauges are available to make intraoral analysis easier. The gauges allow for fast, simple analysis and diagnosis of tooth width problems, tooth length problems, and gingival length discrepancies; color coding predefines desired tooth proportions, quicker and easier to read than any other instrument; they are used as a reference guide between clinician and laboratory technician, hence reduces the incidence of miscommunication errors.

These principles are used as a guide rather than a rigid mathematical formula.

The Proportional Size of the Anterior Teeth

Figure 5 shows the proportional size of the anterior teeth.

The factors guiding individual tooth dimensions are as follows:

Maxillary central incisor: The centrals are the focal point of an aesthetic smile and create the central dominance as described earlier. The approximate length of the central should be 10–11 mm, and the width is calculated accordingly so that the ratio falls between 75% and 80%.

Maxillary lateral incisor: These are the playful parts of the smile. They provide individuality, are never symmetrical, and influence gender characterization.

Maxillary canine: They play a critical role in creating a pleasing smile as they are the junction between the anterior and posterior dental segments; hence, only the mesial half of the canine is visible from the frontal view when the patient smiles; support the frontal muscles—the size and characteristics of the buccal corridor are determined by the size, shape, and position of the canine. The canine depicts the personality characterization (masculine: vigorous and aggressive; feminine: delicate and soft).

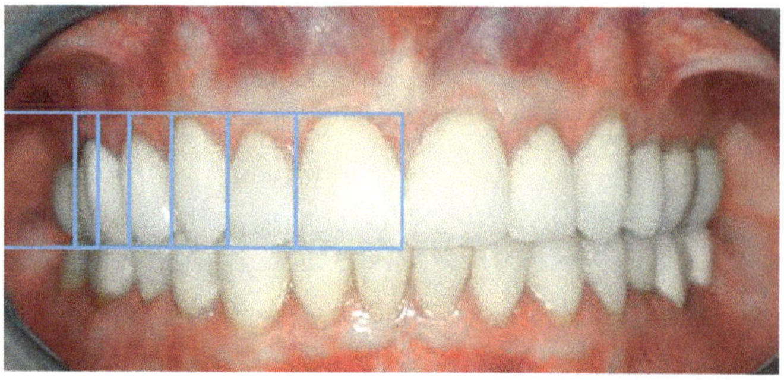

Fig. 5: The proportional size of the anterior teeth.

Buccal corridor refers to the dark space (negative space) visible during smile formation between the corners of the mouth and the buccal surfaces of the maxillary teeth. Its appearance is influenced by the following:

- The width of the smile and the maxillary arch
- The tone of the facial muscles
- The positioning of the labial surface of the upper premolars
- The prominence of the canines, particularly at the distal facial line angle
- Any discrepancy between the value of the premolars and the six anterior teeth

Tooth–lip relationship:

- Dental midline to skeletal midline
- Vertical relationship of teeth to the lips at rest and on the smile:
  - Incisor display
  - Recording lip height at the philtrum and the commissure, e.g., short upper lip or long face
- Transverse roll of the aesthetic line of the dentition/transverse cant of the occlusal plane:
  - Amount of incisor and gingival display
  - *Adolescent:* Ideal elevation of the lip on the smile—slightly below the gingival margin, so that most of the upper incisors can be seen.
  - A 4 mm of display of gingiva in addition to the crown of the tooth, or up to 4 mm of lip coverage of the incisor crown, is acceptable.
  - As age increases, the amount of incisor exposure decreases.
  - Transverse dimensions of the smile relative to the upper arch
- Buccal corridors/negative space
- The distance between the maxillary posterior teeth (especially premolars) and the inside of the cheek
- The relationship of the cheeks to the posterior teeth on smile is just another way of evaluating the width of the dental arches:
  - Percentage of black space of intercommissure width is 13–17%.
  - *The smile arc:* The smile arc is defined as the contour of the incisal edges of the maxillary anterior teeth relative to the curvature of the lower lip during a social smile.
  - The contour of these teeth should match that of the lower lip.

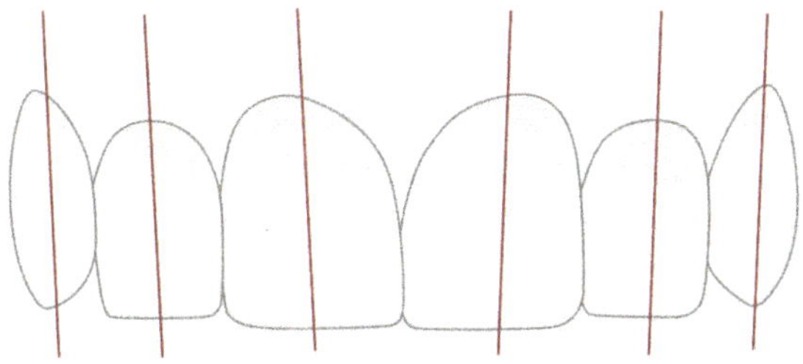

Fig. 6: Angulation.

- A flattened smile arc makes the patient less attractive and also makes the patient look older.
- If lip and dental contours match, they are said to be consonant.

Tooth Inclinations

To evaluate the axial inclination, a photograph of the front teeth in a frontal view can be used. A line is drawn on each tooth, starting from the middle of the incisal edge and extending through the midline of the tooth at its gum line. Additionally, axial inclination can also refer to the degree of tipping in any given reference plane **(Fig. 6)**.

The guide for labiolingual inclination is as follows:

- Maxillary central incisor—positioned vertically or slightly labial.
- Maxillary lateral incisor—cervical is tucked in, and the incisal edge is inclined slightly labially.
- Maxillary canine—cervical area positioned labially, cusp tip lingually angulated.

Gingival health plays a crucial role in the overall aesthetic outcome of dental treatments, as it serves as the framework for the teeth. Therefore, it is imperative that the gingival tissues are in a state of complete health before any treatment is initiated.

Healthy Gingiva

Healthy gingiva typically exhibits the following characteristics: It is pale pink in color, has a stippled appearance, is firm to the touch, and has a matte surface. In terms of location, the facial aspect of the gingiva should be positioned approximately 3 mm above the alveolar crestal bone, while the interdental aspect should be positioned approximately 5 mm above the intercrestal bone. Additionally, the papilla between the teeth should be pointed and fill the gingival embrasure up to the contact area.

Achieving the correct gingival levels for each individual tooth is essential for creating a harmonious smile. The cervical gingival height of the central incisors should be symmetrical, and it can also match that of the canines. While it is acceptable for the laterals to have the same gingival level, a more aesthetically pleasing result can be achieved by having a slight variation in the soft tissue contour. This can be achieved by positioning the gingival contour over the laterals slightly toward the incisal edge compared to the tissue level of the centrals and canines. Gingival health plays a crucial role in the overall aesthetic outcome of dental treatments, as it serves as the framework for the teeth. Therefore, it is imperative that the gingival tissues are in a state of complete health before any treatment is initiated.

The gingiva acts as the frame for the teeth; thus, the final aesthetic success of the case is greatly affected by the gingival health. It is of paramount importance that the gingival tissues are in a complete state of health prior to the initiation of any treatment.

Healthy gingiva is usually:

- Pale pink in color, stippled, firm, and it should exhibit a matte surface.
- Located facially—3 mm above the alveolar crestal bone
- Located interdentally—5 mm above the intercrestal bone papilla should be pointed and should fill the gingival embrasure right up to the contact area.

Gingival Level and Harmony

Establishing the correct gingival levels for each individual tooth is the key to the creation of a harmonious smile. The cervical gingival height (position or level) of the centrals should be symmetrical. It can also match that of the canines. It is acceptable for the laterals to display the same gingival level. However, the resultant smile may be too uniform, and it is preferable to exhibit a rise and fall in the soft tissue by having the gingival contour over the laterals located toward the incisal compared to the tissue level of the centrals and canines.

The gingival margin of the lateral incisor is 0.5–2.0 mm below that of the central incisors. The least desirable gingival placement over the laterals is for it to be apical to that of the centrals and/or the canines.

The gingival shape on the mandibular incisors and the maxillary laterals should exhibit a symmetrical half-oval or half-circular shape. The maxillary centrals and canines should exhibit a gingival shape that is more elliptical. Thus, as mentioned earlier, the gingival zenith is located distal to the long axis of the maxillary centrals and canines and coincides with the long axis of the maxillary lateral incisors.

Tooth Color

One of the greatest challenges in aesthetic dentistry is the analysis, selection, communication, and application of proper color when restoring or replacing teeth with dental materials.

The color of teeth is determined by intrinsic and extrinsic coloration.

There is a significant tendency of natural teeth to become darker and more yellow with an increase in age.[7]

The color is determined by the hue, chroma, and value of the tooth. Secondary optical properties such as translucency, opacity, iridescence, surface gloss, and luminescence determine the appearance of the tooth.

Instruments, including digital devices and light sources, have become useful in providing information regarding the appropriate color of tooth replacement materials when compared to natural teeth.[5]

Treatment Aspects

Tooth Whitening

Vital bleaching of teeth by the application of an oxidizing agent for the purpose of removing color-producing stains or chromogens from the tooth is the most cost-effective and least invasive procedure.

Office bleaching using hydrogen peroxide was predominant in the last century.

The nightguard vital bleach method was introduced by Haywood in 1989.

Trayless over-the-counter strip systems are now available and have been shown to be both safe and effective.

Bleaching procedures utilize hydrogen peroxide, sodium perborate, and carbamide peroxide, which are considered safe when used as instructed. Side effects include tooth sensitivity and gingival irritation.

Teeth can be lightened by one to two shades, and the effects can last for about 1 year.

Adhesive restorations: Adhesively bonded restorations can provide aesthetic and pleasing smiles with minimal invasiveness and a limited sacrifice of natural tooth structure.[4]

Acid etching was discovered by Michael Buonocore in 1955 and was used for pit and fissure sealants (1970).

This led to the evolution of enamel-resin adhesion and the onset of restorations using the "acid-etch" technique.

This was enabled by the development of tooth-colored restoratives by Ray Bowen (1963), who formulated the BIS-GMA (bisphenol A glycidyl methacrylate) resin, which could polymerize rapidly under oral conditions and could be filled with a variety of ceramic fillers. This led to the evolution of composite resin materials.

Composite resins and adhesive technologies have led to bonded ceramic restorations (such as onlays and inlays and laminate veneers) and resin-bonded fixed dental prostheses.

Prosthodontics

Observation and geometric assessments of facial features led to the definition of aesthetic guidelines for complete denture treatment, and these were also applied in fixed prosthodontics.

- Laminates and veneers
- Crown and bridge
- Dentures

Orthodontic Treatment

Orthodontics is the branch of dentistry concerned with skeletal and dental growth, the development of dentition, and occlusion, together with the prevention and correction of occlusal anomalies. Orthodontic treatment helps move teeth into the corrected position using fixed orthodontic appliances or removable appliances. The main aim of orthodontics is correction of functional, aesthetic, or structural imbalances. Malaligned teeth are aligned after creating space for them. Space can be created in a variety of ways, including extraction of appropriate teeth, arch expansion, interproximal enamel reduction, distalization, or a combination of these methods.

If the patient has a skeletal discrepancy, there are three main approaches to orthodontic treatment:

1. Growth Modification

This treatment approach is possible for growing patients. Skeletal discrepancies can be corrected to a large extent with the help of myofunctional and orthopedic appliances. Treatment is best done in the early and late mixed dentition stages **(Fig. 7)**.

2. Camouflage Treatment

Mild-to-moderate skeletal discrepancy after growing age can be disguised by moving teeth along with extraction or by using any other way for gaining space to improve the malocclusion.

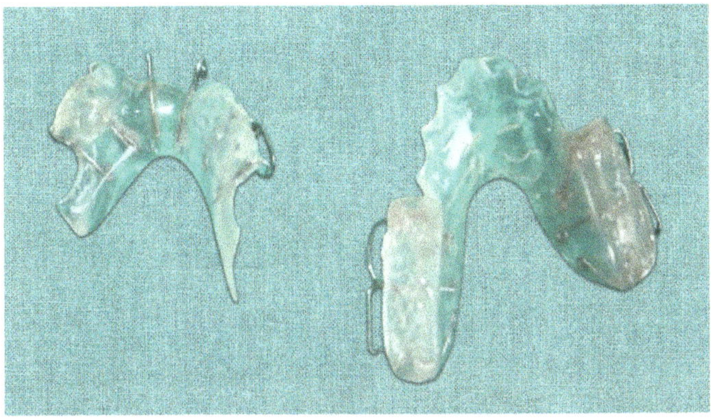

Fig. 7: Growth modification.

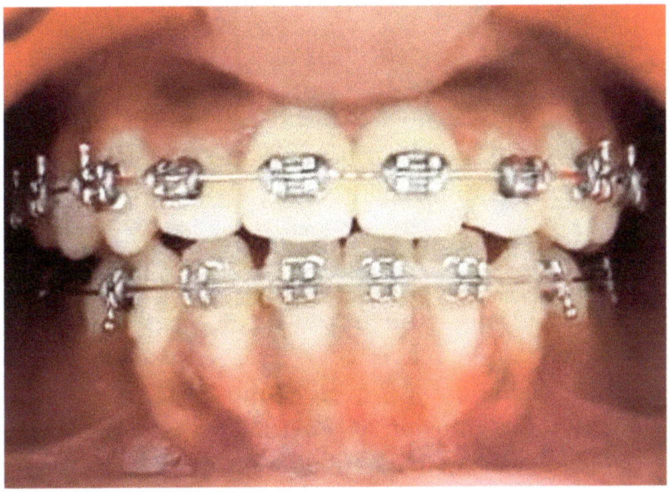

Fig. 8: A combination of orthodontic treatment and orthognathic surgery.

3. A Combination of Orthodontic Treatment and Orthognathic Surgery

In cases of severe skeletal discrepancy, a combination of jaw surgery and fixed orthodontic appliance therapy is useful to correct the patient's skeletal problem, which ultimately leads to a beautiful and confident smile **(Fig. 8)**.

Fixed orthodontic appliances can move the teeth in all three directions. These appliances are fixed to the teeth, and wires and other auxiliaries such as elastics and springs help apply force to align teeth. Brackets or fixed appliances can be made up of stainless steel or ceramic and can be placed on the buccal or lingual surfaces of teeth as per patient preference **(Fig. 9)**.[6]

Aligners: These are customized removable trays that can be used to correct the malocclusion. A digital scan is used, and customized trays are printed using specialized software.

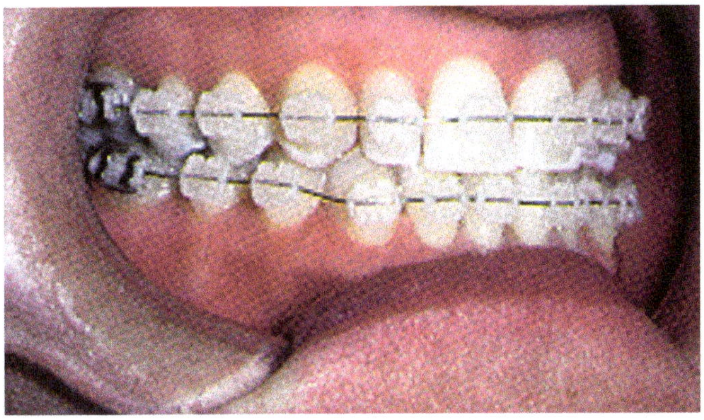

Fig. 9: Brackets or fixed appliances can be made of stainless steel.

CONCLUSION

Dentistry plays a significant role in improving one's smile. It is an art and science which needs creativity to design a natural looking and aesthetically pleasing smile. Most important step in selecting treatment is diagnosis and planning. It includes understanding of patient's needs, etiology of the problem and comprehensive knowledge of various treatment options. After understanding the cost benefit ratio, the treatment is meticulously selected which can include straightening of the teeth, professional teeth whitening, fillings, crowns, veneers and/or replacing missing teeth to give the patient a designer smile.

REFERENCES

1. Philips C, Bennett ME, Broder HL. Dentofacial disharmony: Psychological status of patients seeking treatment consultation. Angle Orthod.1998;68(6):547-56.
2. Proffit WR, Fields HW, Sarver DM. Etiology of orthodontic problems. Contemporary Orthodontics, 5th edition. India: Elsevier; 2012. pp. 114-46.
3. Van der Geld P, Oosterveld P, Van Heck G, Kuijpers-Jagtman AM. Smile attractiveness: self-perception and influence on personality. Angle Orthod. 2007;77(5):759-65.
4. Parrini S, Rossini G, Castroflorio T, Fortini A, Deregibus A, Debernardi C. Laypeople's perceptions of frontal smile esthetics: a systematic review. Am J Orthod Dentofacial Orthop. 2016;150(5):740-50.
5. Sands NB, Adamson PA. Global facial beauty: approaching a unified aesthetic ideal. Facial Plast Surg. 2014;30(2):93-100.
6. Bhuvaneswaran M. Principles of smile design. J Conserv Dent. 2010;13(4):225-32.
7. Joiner A. Tooth color: a review of the literature. J Dent. 2004:32(Suppl 1):3-12.

CHAPTER 28

Anesthesia for Cosmetic Gynecological Procedures

Jasmeet Kaur, Akashdeep Singh

INTRODUCTION

With the development of safe and modern anesthesia drugs and equipment, many procedures/surgeries (minor or major) have been made possible without undue risk. It is especially important for cosmetic procedures/surgeries to have no or minimal anesthesia-related risks, as these are mainly done to improve aesthetics or the quality of life.

Anesthesia for cosmetic procedures is tailored according to the requirements of the procedure and the medical needs of the patients. So, a thorough preoperative evaluation of the patients is necessary in terms of their medical and surgical history, physical examination, and relevant laboratory investigations.

ANESTHESIA FOR MINOR PROCEDURES

Hymenoplasty, labiaplasty, cliteroplasty, vaginoplasty, vaginal rejuvenation, etc., are some of the commonly performed minor cosmetic gynecological procedures. Some of the minimally invasive/noninvasive methods of treatment include laser therapy, radio frequency (RF), high-intensity focused ultrasound (HIFU), electromagnetic field therapy, chemical treatments, platelet-rich plasma (PRP) therapy, Labial fillers (hyaluronic acid and fat grafting), etc.

Local Anesthesia

These procedures are usually carried out in an outpatient clinic setting under local anesthesia. Local infiltration with an injection of 2% lignocaine or topical application of 2% lignocaine jelly to the genital mucosa is commonly used before the procedure. Also, EMLA cream can be used, which is the eutectic mixture of local anesthetics (prilocaine 2.5% and lignocaine 2.5%). It should be applied to the skin of the genital area around 45 minutes before the procedure. These give a good numbing effect for the procedure to be pain free.

Monitored Anesthesia Care

Supervision and watchful monitoring of the patient may be required by an experienced anesthesiologist if the patient falls under high-risk category [American Society of Anesthesiologists (ASA) grade III or IV patients].

Conscious Sedation

Some patients need sedation either because of preprocedural anxiety or because they just need to be more relaxed during the procedure.

Commonly used drugs for sedation are as follows:

- *Dexmedetomidine:* It is an alpha-2 agonist. It provides good sedation and analgesia. It does not cause respiratory depression. It is used as an intravenous bolus (0.5–1 µg/kg) over 10 minutes, followed by continuous infusion at 0.2–1 µg/kg/h. It may cause bradycardia and needs monitoring for that.
- *Benzodiazepines:* Midazolam is the most preferred agent. It is used as an intravenous bolus of 0.05–0.1 mg/kg as and when required. It provides good anxiolysis and sedation.
- *Opioids:* Short-acting opioids, such as fentanyl, can be used for sedation and analgesia. These may cause respiratory depression, especially when combined with benzodiazepines.
- *Ketamine:* It provides good sedation and analgesia, but it is not an agent of choice for day care procedures as it may cause emergence delirium, which may be undesirable in a clinic setting for day care procedures.

Laboratory investigations include basic workup: Complete blood count, coagulation profile, blood sugar, and renal function tests. Cardiac evaluation [echocardiography (ECG)], chest X-ray, liver function tests, thyroid profile, etc., need to be done, if seem relevant according to the patients' medical history.

Preprocedure Instructions

Patients are usually advised to take light meals around 3–4 hours before the procedure to be done under local anesthesia. If sedation is desired, patients are instructed to fast for 6 hours for solids and 2 hours for clear liquids before the procedure. They are instructed to take their regular medications for blood pressure, diabetes mellitus, cardiac disease, etc., if any, as per schedule.

Monitoring and Resuscitation

Basic monitoring of vitals [noninvasive blood pressure (NIBP) measurement] and heart rate should be checked in all patients undergoing any procedure. Additionally, continuous ECG, oxygen saturation, and respiration should be monitored in patients under sedation.

Regardless of whether sedation is used or not, resuscitative drugs and equipment should always be available at the place of procedure, which may be required in case of untoward events such as vasovagal syncope and anaphylactic reaction.

ANESTHESIA FOR MAJOR PROCEDURES

Some of the major cosmetic surgeries include:

- Perineoplasty and vaginoplasty
- Gender reassignment surgery (GRS)
- Mammoplasty, abdominoplasty, and liposuction

These procedures are done in the operation theater setting, where all the facilities such as an anesthesia workstation, multichannel monitor (NIBP, ECG, SpO_2, $EtCO_2$, and temperature), and resuscitation equipment are available. Patients need thorough preanesthesia check-up with their medical and surgical history, physical examination, and routine investigations, which include complete blood count, coagulation studies, renal/liver function tests, blood glucose, ECG, chest X-ray, thyroid function tests, and echocardiography, if required.

Preoperative optimization of comorbid medical illnesses and risk stratification are done. Accordingly, informed consent is taken, keeping in view the anticipated risks associated with the medical condition.

Preoperative Instructions

- Patients are kept fasting for 6 hours for solids and 2 hours for clear liquids before surgery.
- They are instructed to continue their routine medications according to the individual drug protocol.
- Antiplatelets and anticoagulant medications are routinely stopped for a few days before the surgery, according to the recommendation for the particular drug.

Choice of Anesthesia

Regional Anesthesia

Lower abdominal and perineal surgeries can be performed under neuraxial block, spinal anesthesia (subarachnoid block), epidural block, or combined spinal epidural anesthesia (CSEA). CSEA with an epidural catheter has the advantage of providing good postoperative analgesia.

Before performing a neuraxial block, one has to look for any contraindications, such as:

- *Absolute contraindications:*
  - Patient refusal
  - Deranged coagulation
  - Skin infection at the injection site
- *Relative contraindications*
  - Previous spine surgery
  - Neurological deficit
  - Patient on anticoagulant or antiplatelet treatment
  - Certain cardiac conditions, such as stenotic valvular heart disease and hypertrophic obstructive cardiomyopathy (HOCM)

Advantages of regional anesthesia include an awake patient, no airway instrumentation, avoiding sympathetic stimulation associated with intubation and extubation, and better postoperative analgesia.

One of the concerns with neuraxial block is postdural puncture headache (PDPH). However, with the use of small-gauge spinal needles (26G or 27G) and pencil-point spinal needles (Whitacre or Sprotte), the incidence of PDPH has significantly decreased.

Earlier neuraxial blocks were avoided in day care surgeries, but the latest guidelines suggest that patient can safely go home after the surgery under a neuraxial block once the discharge criteria are met, and sensory and motor blocks in the lower limbs are fully recovered.

General Anesthesia

Major surgeries like GRS, abdominoplasty, mammoplasty, and liposuction are usually done under general anesthesia.

Balanced anesthesia is usually practiced, which includes intravenous anesthetic agents such as propofol and etomidate; inhalational anesthetic agents such as desflurane, sevoflurane, and isoflurane; analgesics such as opioids (morphine and fentanyl) and nonopioids [nonsteroidal anti-inflammatory drugs (NSAIDs) and paracetamol]; and muscle relaxants such as atracurium, cis-atracurium, rocuronium, and vecuronium. The use of newer short-acting anesthetic agents is usually desirable so as to achieve rapid and clear-headed recovery from anesthesia, which is especially important in day care surgeries.

For postoperative analgesia, a multimodal approach is preferred, which includes:

- Intravenous analgesics (opioids, NSAIDs, and paracetamol)
- Patient-controlled analgesia (PCA)
- Epidural analgesia
- Regional blocks (nerve blocks and plexus blocks)

The use of ultrasound and nerve stimulator has increased the efficiency of regional blocks to a great extent.

Anesthetic Considerations in Specific Surgeries

Liposuction

A high volume of intravenous fluids with a dilute local anesthetic is infiltrated in the area desired for liposuction.

Problems anticipated are as follows:

- Fluid overload, which may cause cardiac complications in patients with borderline cardiac status
- Electrolyte imbalance
- Hypothermia because of large volume fluid infiltration and large surface area exposed

Close monitoring of vitals and the total fluid intake (intravenous and infiltration) and output (fat and saline aspirated, blood loss, and urine output) is important. Patients may require close observation in the intensive care unit (ICU) postoperatively.

Mammoplasty

It is usually done under general anesthesia. Nerve blocks, such as pectoral nerve 1 (PEC 1) and PEC 2 blocks, and paravertebral blocks can be combined with general anesthesia to achieve better analgesia and decrease the requirement for systemic medications.

Gender Reassignment Surgery

The transgender community has specific health risks and has special requirements during the perioperative period. GRS is a major surgery that involves multidisciplinary teamwork, involving a surgeon, endocrinologist, anesthesiologist, psychiatrist, and psychological counselor.

Preoperative assessment: Healthcare workers need to be sensitized regarding addressing the gender of the patient. Patient should be given the option to decline to answer questions related to gender.

Preoperative evaluation of the hormonal status and psychological counseling of the patient are very important. Patients are usually on hormone replacement therapy (HRT) for feminizing or masculinizing effects. Patients on feminizing HRT need to be screened for thromboembolism and dyslipidemias. Prophylaxis for such patients in the form of anticoagulants and compression stockings needs to be considered. Patients on masculinizing HRT need to be screened for liver disease and endometrial cancers. Withdrawal of HRT may lead to mood swings and hot flushes, which need to be monitored.

Intraoperative concerns:

- We must minimize the traffic and rotation of staff in the operating room, especially if the surgical procedure involves the exposure of the genitalia and chest area.
- Routine procedure for urinary catheterization can be challenging due to previous GRSs.
- Airway management may be complicated by previous vocal cord surgeries or laryngeal surgeries.
- Chest binders or chest wraps for transgender men need to be removed to avoid respiratory compromise.

Postoperative concerns: Although it is an elective surgery done after extensive psychiatric counseling, anxiety, fear, depression, and regret are common problems in the postoperative period. It may be worsened by awkward or negative interactions with healthcare workers. All sensitive information with respect to gender identity, preferred noun or pronoun has to be included in the staff handover. There is a compelling need for good community and social network support.

CONCLUSION

With the increasing awareness of availability of cosmetic procedures/surgeries in the present time, a greater number of people are opting for them. As we say that every procedure has some risk involved, however minor it may be, it is absolutely essential for the healthcare workers to ensure the safety of the patient. Thorough preoperative assessment and preparation, followed by adequate planning and communication among the treating physicians and the patient, is of utmost importance. Every step should be taken to prevent complications and improve patient outcomes and patient satisfaction.

CHAPTER 29

Extraperitoneal Laser Applications

Preeti Jindal, Cherry Malhi

INTRODUCTION

Laser can be used for various nonaesthetic treatments. A few are listed below:

- Vaginal atrophy, dryness, and rejuvenation
- Stress urinary incontinence
- Vaginal relaxation or hyperlaxity
- Vulvar lichen sclerosus
- Elimination of genital warts
- Vaporization of cervicitis, ectopia, and cervical dysplasia
- Genital prolapse
- Genital whitening
- Treatment of recurrent vaginal infections
- Intimate female surgery

VAGINAL ATROPHY, DRYNESS, AND REJUVENATION

The vaginal mucosa is very sensitive to changes in estrogen levels and pH. Various stages of life have different problems, like young women are more prone to vaginal infections due to sexual habits, pregnancy, and childbirth. Menopausal women are affected due to hypoestrogenism. These problems lead to vaginal mucosal damage, thinning, and atrophy. The vaginal laser and other energy-based devices are currently the most effective treatments for vaginal atrophy and dryness. The vaginal laser treatment is aimed at improving sensitivity, hydration, and elasticity in the vulvar, introital, and vaginal tissues.[1] The thermomodulation at 42–45°C, which is achieved by energy-based devices, helps in breaking microscopic fibrosis at the lamina propria level and leads to neocollagenogenesis, neoelastogenesis, and rejuvenation of the vagina. Increased vascularity shown in **Figure 1** (capillaries penetrating newly formed papillae underneath the epithelium) in connective tissue supports the renewed activity of fibroblasts and provides the metabolic support for epithelial cell proliferation and differentiation.[2,3]

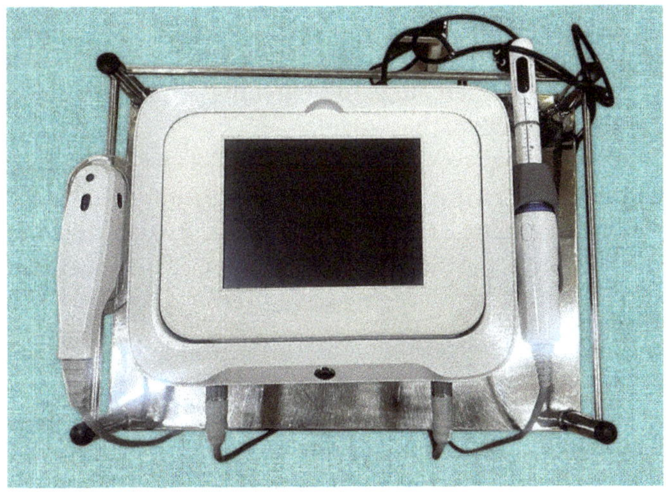

Fig. 1: *High-intensity focused ultrasound* (HIFU) for vaginal atrophy.

Vaginal atrophy and dryness are usually caused by a deficiency of estrogen hormone during perimenopause and menopause period, recurrent vaginal infections and post-pregnancy. It is accompanied by a number of important symptoms such as:

- Burning sensation
- Itching
- Pain during sexual intercourse
- Increased susceptibility to both urinary and vulvo-vaginal infections
- Uterovaginal prolapses
- Urinary incontinence

Three sittings of a vaginal laser, 1 month apart, provide relief in the majority of women. The long-term efficacy is also, visible macroscopically with the quality of the vaginal tissue to show improvement in terms of vascularization, rogation, and secretion **(Fig. 2)**.

STRESS URINARY INCONTINENCE

Stress urinary incontinence (SUI) is a common problem, with an estimated prevalence of 50% in the female population worldwide.[4] The classical treatment for SUI basically, involves strengthening of the pelvic floor. In the past, this was only possible at the muscular level through physiotherapy, Kegels exercise, and, in more severe cases, at a connective tissue level through surgeries in which a mesh or tape was placed parallel to the urethra with the purpose of generating more collagen at this level, thereby improving urethral support and closure. Such surgery proved effective against incontinence but did not address the problem of atrophy. In addition, the presence of tapes or meshes in the tissue ultimately tended to cause pain during sexual intercourse (dyspareunia), thus worsening the sexual health of the patient.

The vaginal carbon dioxide (CO_2) laser combined with platelet-rich plasma and the high-intensity focus electro magnetic (HIFEM) chair **(Fig. 3)** together are very effective in noninvasively treating SUI in women.

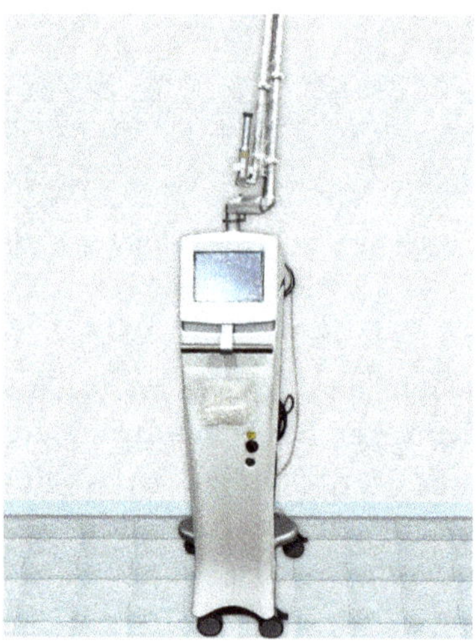

Fig. 2: Carbon dioxide (CO_2) laser.

The laser is a noninvasive, painless, and technically advanced procedure that is able to generate collagen in the connective tissue that affords support and closes the urethra. It is a physical procedure that stimulates the synthesis of new collagen in the connective tissue surrounding the urethra, contributing to its anatomical and functional closure and thus avoiding urine leakage.

All this is done in the clinic on an ambulatory basis, without having to enter the operating room and without leaving any bandages, tapes, or meshes in the body tissues, which over the long term can give rise to more problems.

Furthermore, it is being shown to be effective not only in urinary stress incontinence but also in urinary urgency and in mixed incontinence.

VAGINAL RELAXATION OR HYPERLAXITY

Due to pregnancy and childbirth, the vagina gets loosened and loses its elasticity. Vaginal rejuvenation by energy-based devices leads to restoration of elastin and collagen fibers of vaginal mucosa. This treatment is safe, painless, and does not affect future fertility.

Thermal energy generated from energy-based devices creates microscopic lesions, which promote wound healing, subsequent new collagen, and elastin fiber formation.[5] After the inflammatory phase of wound healing, dermal fibroblasts produce new collagen fibrils at 2 weeks interval and remain high for at least 5 weeks after treatment.[6]

VULVAR LICHEN SCLEROSUS

Lichen sclerosus is a chronic skin inflammatory condition of unknown origin in which the skin clears, hardens, and becomes dry, causing pruritus or intense itching. It is most

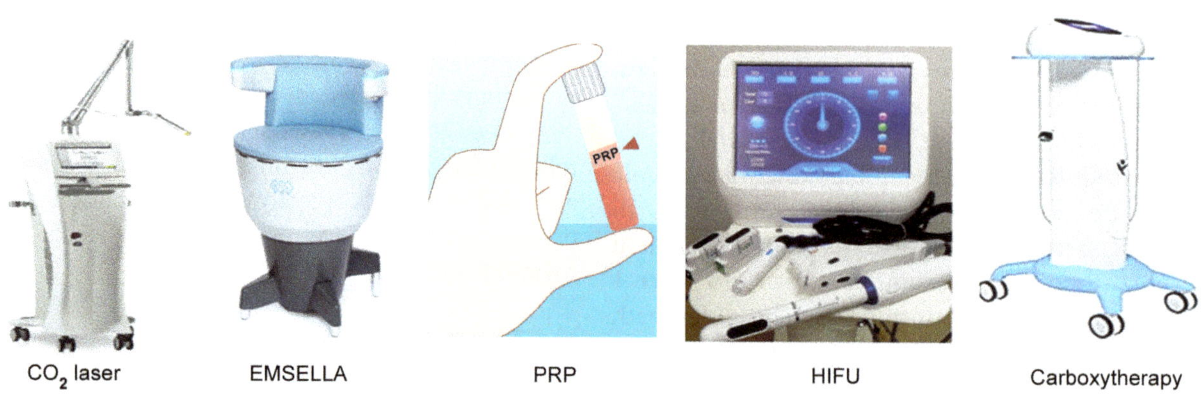

Fig. 3: Nonsurgical options for stress urinary incontinence (SUI). (HIFU: high-intensity focused ultrasound; PRP: platelet-rich plasma)

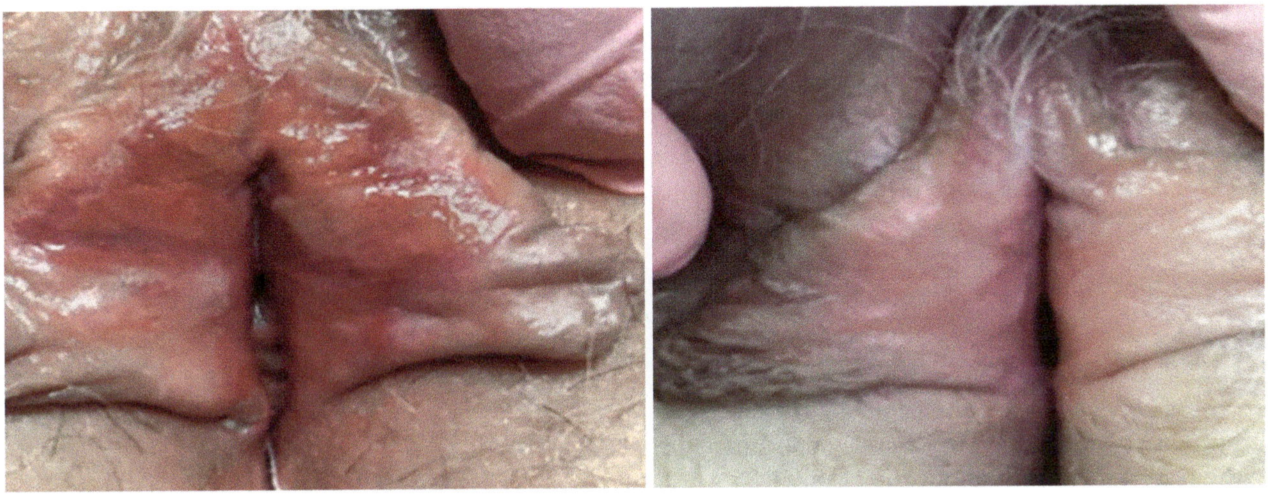

Fig. 4: Lichen sclerosus.

frequent in women in their 50s, though it may appear at any age and even in little girls.

As the disease advances, the skin experiences atrophy and retraction, thereby altering the normal anatomy of the vulva. The labia minora may even disappear, with burying or embedding of the clitoris and urethra. The entry to the vagina narrows and hardens, making penetration impossible.

The disorder must always be distinguished from other vulvar diseases characterized by similar symptoms, such as squamous cell carcinoma of the vulva. A biopsy is therefore required.

Once diagnosed, the reference treatment remains high-potency corticosteroids (clobetasol). However, in many cases, such treatment is not fully effective; some patients are refractory to treatment, or the lichen may evolve despite therapy.

In all these scenarios, the CO_2 laser **(Fig. 4)** is a great treatment alternative for vulvar lichen sclerosus, a common disorder for which conventional medicine has no effective therapy.

The CO_2 laser offers a treatment alternative that is seen to be increasingly effective, since it greatly reduces the symptoms, improves the clinical appearance, and, in most cases, is able to arrest the progression of the disease. Again, three to four sittings, 1 month apart, help. These patients require annual sittings to prevent recurrences.

ELIMINATION OF GENITAL WARTS

In the genital and perianal region, warts (condyloma acuminate) are very common, cosmetically disfiguring, and usually, they are caused by the human papillomavirus (HPV). Vaporization with the CO_2 laser is the treatment of choice for warts in the genital region. It is a painless, quick, and effective method as compared to cold knife excision.

The treatment is carried out in the clinic under local, topical, or infiltrating anesthesia, and depending on the number and extent of the lesions, the procedure is usually brief and simple. Local anesthesia may be used for small isolated vulvar warts. Warts should be vaporized no deeper than the level of the surrounding skin surface using a power level of 40–60 W with a beam diameter of 3 mm. After complete vaporization of the genital warts is accomplished, the 1–2 cm of skin surrounding the individual lesions is brushed lightly with 10 W of power and a 2-mm diameter spot size to destroy subclinical HPV involvement and diminish the recurrence of the disease. For those patients who are immunologically compromised, chronic application of 5-fluorouracil cream is recommended.[7]

VAPORIZATION OF CERVICITIS, ECTOPIA, AND CERVICAL DYSPLASIA

Inflammation of the cervix alters its architecture and results in cervical lesions such as cervicitis, ectopia, and cervical dysplasia, which usually cause intermittent bleeding, especially during and after sexual intercourse. These cellular alterations can only be diagnosed through cytological study for HPV.

Vaporization of the upper layers of the cervix with the CO_2 laser eliminates the inflammatory tissue, resulting in resurfacing of the cervical epithelium, i.e., producing a new and healthy mucosal layer.

This mechanism of action has also led to the idea that cervical vaporization may eliminate HPV, which is often the origin of these lesions and is the cause of cervical cancer and of the dysplasia that precedes cancer. Thus, vaporization with the CO_2 laser is becoming the treatment of choice for cervical lesions, such as low-grade squamous intraepithelial lesion (LSIL), cervicitis, and ectopia **(Fig. 5)**.

CERVIX–CERVICAL INTRAEPITHELIAL NEOPLASIA

Treatment of cervical intraepithelial neoplasia (CIN) can be performed by vaporization or by excisional conization using the laser as a substitute for the scalpel.[6] The CO_2 laser is the laser of choice for this. The major advantages of the CO_2 laser for the treatment of CIN include:

- High degree of clinical efficacy
- Bloodless field
- Microscopic precision
- Sparing of normal tissue
- Rapid healing with minimal scar formation

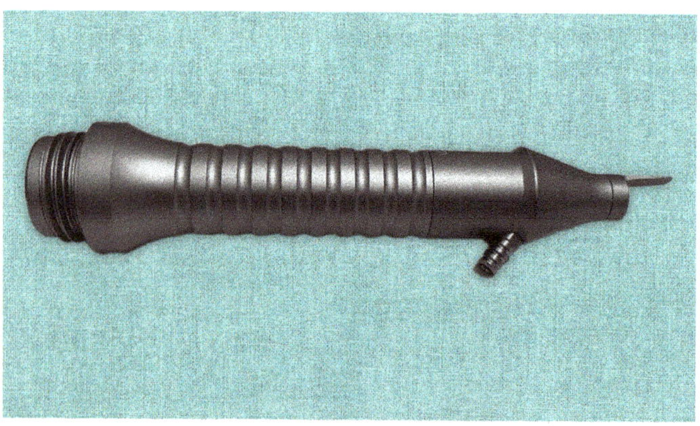

Fig. 5: Laser surgical handpiece.

- Small number of complications
- Outpatient methodology

The main disadvantages of the CO_2 laser include the absence of a histologic sample when vaporization is performed and the expense of the laser machine.

GENITAL PROLAPSE

Pelvic floor defects are visible as a bulge on anterior and posterior vaginal walls with resultant SUI, incomplete defecation/fecal incontinence, chronic pelvic pain, vaginal relaxation, sexual dysfunction, and social isolation.[8] In the case of genital prolapses, it is known that milder prolapse is associated with greater treatment success with the vaginal laser or energy-based devices. The HIFEM chairs are more effective treatments for these problems as they strengthen the pelvic floor muscles.

GENITAL WHITENING

The genital laser eliminates the most superficial layers of the skin that are generally darker and also increases skin permeability, allowing depigmenting chemical agents to penetrate more deeply into the skin. For this reason, the treatment must be continued with topical depigmenting products at home to complete the process and prolong the effect **(Fig. 6)**.

As the skin tone clears, it is up to the patient to decide whether further sessions are needed or not.

TREATMENT OF RECURRENT VAGINAL INFECTIONS

Chronic recurrent vaginal infections can benefit from treatment with the vaginal laser. Vulvovaginal candidiasis (VVC) is considered the second most common genital infection in women after bacterial vaginosis.[6]

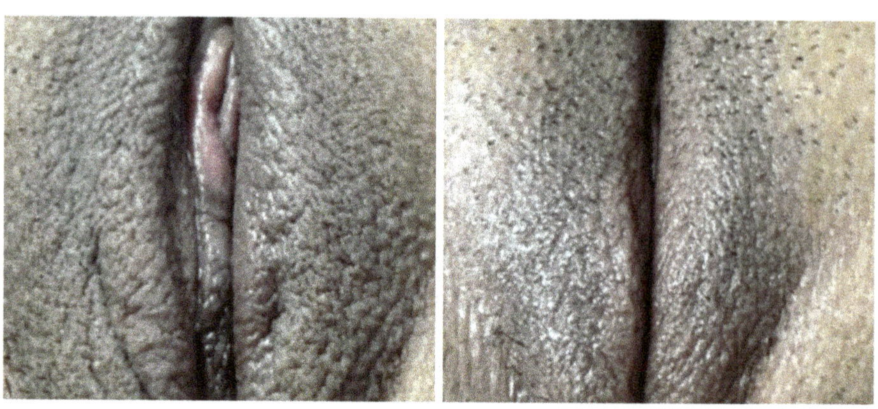

Fig. 6: Genital whitening by carbon dioxide (CO_2) laser.

The authors (Jindal et al.) have observed that after treating vaginal infections, if one sitting of vaginal laser is given, it significantly reduces the incidence of recurrent vaginal infections. The probable explanation is that laser causes rejuvenation of the vaginal mucosa, restoring the microbiota, lubrication, and normal defense mechanisms of the vaginal mucosa.

INTIMATE FEMALE SURGERY

The CO_2 laser is able to cut and coagulate simultaneously and therefore operates in a fine, minimally invasive and very hemostatic manner, making it a great option for gynecological surgeries.

The gynecological surgeries that most often involve the use of the CO_2 laser are:

- Labiaplasty **(Fig. 7)**
- Clitoral hood surgery
- Bartholinitis drainage or
- Removal of Bartholin cysts
- Repair of episiotomies or episiorrhaphies
- Ablation of trigger zones in "vulvodynia"
- Removal of anal tags

HOW THE CARBON DIOXIDE LASER WORKS IN GYNECOLOGICAL TREATMENTS?

The CO_2 laser basically works through three mechanisms of action:

1. *Regeneration:* The essence of its action is that tissue ablation stimulates the formation and regeneration of new healthy tissue.
2. *Vaporization:* It is literally the transformation of tissue into water vapor.
3. *Cutting and coagulation:* It is the basis of surgery.

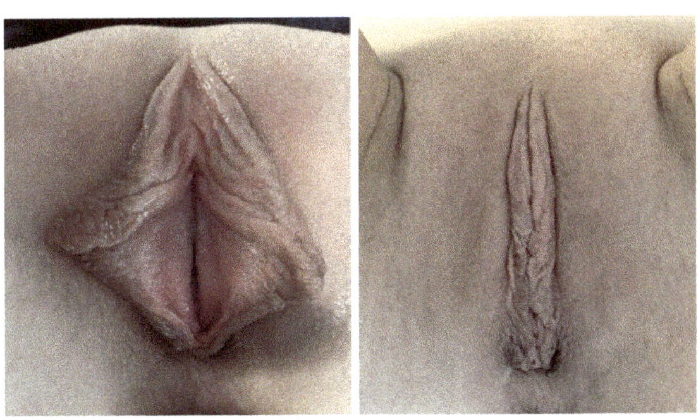

Fig. 7: Labiaplasty (Before and after).
Source: Jindal P et al.[6]

Regeneration

The CO_2 laser emits light at a specific wavelength that can penetrate the vaginal mucosa without damaging the surrounding tissues. This is the mechanism whereby it stimulates the elastin and collagen cells in the lamina propria of the mucosa. The thickness of the vaginal mucosa is 4 mm and the CO_2 laser penetrates up to 400 μm. Hence, there is no way it can damage surrounding structures, provided it is used as per the specifications and following all safety standards **(Fig. 8)**.

Following laser treatment, the number of layers of the vaginal epithelium increases, and this restores the function of the glands in charge of lubrication, as evidenced from the histological sections.

The vaginal mucosa is repaired with fully restored tissue, with the multiple layers it had before atrophy, and with its corresponding glandular elements, thus restoring vaginal mucosal health, lubrication, and function.

In the more internal layers: The energy of the CO_2 laser in turn is transmitted to layers deeper than the mucosa, such as connective tissue, fascias and apparently also to the muscle layer, where it can stimulate regenerative mechanisms and the production of proteins such as collagen and elastin, thereby also restoring vaginal anatomical health, tightening the vagina and restoring prolapses, and also functional health, as for example, urinary retention.

These results have been evidenced from histopathological studies of biopsies obtained after the treatments and have been published in the scientific literature.

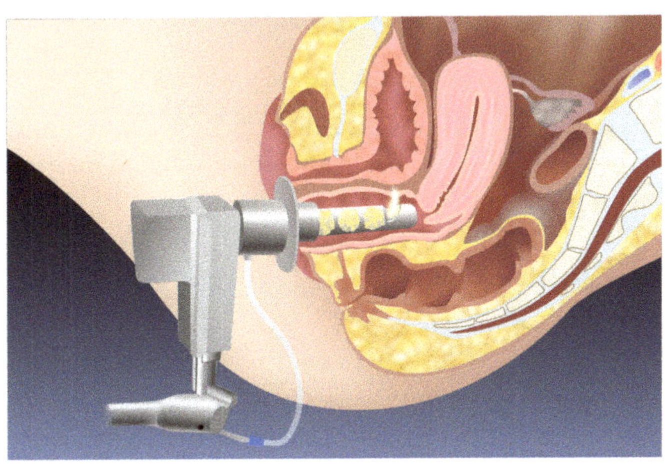

Fig. 8: A nonsurgical fractional laser probe emitting in the vaginal canal.

Vaporization

In the Elimination of Genital Warts, Ectopia, Cervicitis, and Cervical Dysplastic Lesions

The laser ablation effect eliminates tissue layers through vaporization, or their transformation into water vapor. This makes the laser ideal for eliminating raised lesions on the skin, such as genital condylomas, or any other dermatological lesions that may be located in the genital zone or anywhere else on the skin.

Cutting and Coagulation: Surgery

For Intimate Female Surgery, Bartholin Cyst Surgery, Abscesses, etc.

The CO_2 laser is able to cut and coagulate in a precise, fine, minimally invasive, and very hemostatic manner, thus representing a great option for both gynecological surgeries and labiaplasties, or clitoral hood surgeries, or plastic surgeries such as blepharoplasty.

FREQUENTLY ASKED QUESTIONS

How is the Vaginal Laser Used?

It is performed on an ambulatory basis in about 20 minutes. No anesthesia is required. One may use topical local anesthesia in the form of cream in very sensitive patients. The procedure is totally painless, and the patient may just feel little pins and needle sensation or vaginal warmth during the session. The treatment is intravaginal and is applied with a cylindrical autoclavable or disposable headpiece that can access all the vaginal walls with the help of an internal mirror. The patient can return to her normal life after the treatment with minimal or no discomfort.

How Many Sessions are Needed?

The number of sessions needed to obtain the best results varies depending on the disorder involved and on each individual patient, though in most cases, no less than three sessions are advised.

What is the Duration of the Treatment?

The situation should be evaluated again after 1 year or upon request by the patient.

CONCLUSION

Laser if used properly is painless, safe and very effective treatment of the problems like vaginal dryness, atrophy, stress urinary incontinence and warts. Every gynecologist should get trained in using these new modalities.

REFERENCES

1. Hutchinson-Colas J, Segal S. Genitourinary syndrome of menopause and the use of laser therapy. Maturitas. 2015;82:342-5.
2. Mac Bride MB, Rhodes DJ, Shuster LT. Vulvovaginal atrophy. Mayo Clin Proc. 2010;85(1):87-94.
3. Athanasiou S, Pitsouni E, Antonopoulou S, Zacharakis D, Salvatore S, Falagas ME, et al. The effect of microablative fractional CO_2 laser on vaginal fora of postmenopausal women. Climacteric. 2016;19(5):512-8.
4. Markland AD, Richter HE, Fwu C-W, Eggers P, Kuesk JW. Prevalence and trends of urinary incontinence in adults in the United States, 2001 to 2008. J Urol. 2011;186:589-93.
5. Gaspar A, Addamo G, Brandi H. Vaginal fractional CO_2 laser: a minimally-invasive option for vaginal rejuvenation. Am J Cosmet Surg. 2011;28:156-62.
6. Jindal P, Malhotra N, Joshi S (Eds). Aesthetic and Regenerative Gynaecology, 1st edition. USA: Springer; 2022.
7. Krebs HB. Prophylactic topical 5-5-fluorouracil for the treatment of human papilloma virus associated lesions of the vulva and vagina. Obstet Gynecol. 1986;68(6)837-41.
8. Baggish MS. Management of cervical intraepithelial neoplasia by carbon dioxide laser. Obstet Gynecol. 1982; 60(3):378.

Index

Page numbers followed by *b* refer to box, *f* refer to figure, *fc* refer to flowchart, and *t* refer to table.

T

U

V

W

Z

www.ingramcontent.com/pod-product-compliance
Ingram Content Group UK Ltd.
Pitfield, Milton Keynes, MK11 3LW, UK
UKHW051433250425
457755UK00002BA/7

9 781787 791848